Progress in Drug Research
Fortschritte der Arzneimittelforschung
Progrès des recherches pharmaceutiques
Vol. 48

Progress in Drug Research
Fortschritte der Arzneimittelforschung
Progrès des recherches pharmaceutiques
Vol. 48

Edited by / Herausgegeben von / Rédigé par
Ernst Jucker, Basel

Authors / Autoren / Auteurs
Eric J. Lien, Arima Das, Partha Nandy and Shijun Ren · Horst Kleinkauf
and Hans von Döhren · Iradj Hajimohamadreza and J. Mark Treherne ·
Esteban Domingo, Luis Menéndez-Arias, Miguel E. Quiñones-Mateu,
Africa Holguín, Mónica Gutiérrez-Rivas, Miguel A. Martínez, Josep Quer,
Isabel S. Novella and John J. Holland · Vijendra K. Singh · Shijun Ren and
Eric J. Lien · Deborah S. Hartman and Olivier Civelli · Vera M. Kolb

Springer Basel AG

Editor:

Dr. E. Jucker
Steinweg 28
CH-4107 Ettingen
Switzerland

© 1997 Springer Basel AG
Originally published by Birkhäuser Verlag in 1997
Softcover reprint of the hardcover 1st edition 1997

Printed on acid-free paper produced from chlorine-free pulp. TCF ∞
ISBN 978-3-0348-9806-5   ISBN 978-3-0348-8861-5 (eBook)
DOI 10.1007/978-3-0348-8861-5

9 8 7 6 5 4 3 2 1

Contents · Inhalt · Sommaire

Foreword

Volume 48 of „Progress in Drug Research" contains eight reviews and the various indexes which facilitate the use of these monographs and also help to establish PDR as an encyclopaedic source of information in the complex field of drug research.

The articles in volume 48, all written by experts in the respective fields of research, deal with genetic codes, with enzymatic generation of complex peptides, with the important functions of apoptosis, with the increasing problems related to vaccine-escape and drug-resistant mutants, with immunotherapy for brain diseases and mental illnesses, with natural products as cancer chemopreventive agents, and with the dopamine receptor diversity. In the final chapter, Vera Kolb provides a fascinating insight into a selected group of novel and unusual nucleosides as drugs. All these review articles contain extensive bibliographies, thus enabling the interested reader to have easy access to the original literature.

It has always been the aim of the Founder/Editor of PDR to help disseminate information on the vast and fast growing domain of drug research. For the individual scientist it is increasingly difficult to retain an overview of the enormous amount of information available, and PDR enables the reader to keep abreast of the latest developments and trends. This goal has remained unchanged now for 38 years, and I believe that the reviews in PDR are useful to the non-specialist as well as to the specialist readers, who will appreciate the comprehensive bibliographies and, in addition, might even get fresh impulses for their own research.

Since the foundation of the series of monographs, the Editor has enjoyed much appreciated help and advice from the authors, the readers, many colleagues and, last but not least, from the reviewers. To all of them, I would like to express my gratitude.

In addition to the thanks expressed above, I would like to extend my thanks to Birkhäuser Publishers and, in particular, to Mrs. Elizabeth Beckett, Dr. Petra Gerlach, Mrs. L. Koechlin and Mssrs. H.-P. Thür, E. Mazenauer and G. Messmer. Their personal involvement, assistance and advice was of great importance for the successful production of PDR Volume 48.

Basel, May 1997   DR. E. JUCKER

Vorwort

Der vorliegende 48. Band der Reihe «Fortschritte der Arzneimittelfor-schung» enthält acht Beiträge, die wiederum von anerkannten Forschern verfasst wurden. Ausserdem sind auch in diesem Band ein Stichwortver-zeichnis des Bandes sowie ein Autoren- und Titelverzeichnis und ein Titel-verzeichnis aller 48 Bände enthalten. Der Leser hat dadurch die Mög-lichkeit, nicht nur den vorliegenden Band zu konsultieren, sondern auch alle bisher erschienenen Bände quasi als enzyklopädisches Nachschla-gewerk zu benutzen. Da alle Beiträge umfangreiche Literaturnachweise enthalten, ist die Möglichkeit des Zugriffes auf Original-Publikationen gegeben, was dem aktiven Forscher besonders wichtig ist und seinen eige-nen Arbeiten Impulse geben kann.

Die Artikel des 48. Bandes behandeln neue Entwicklungen der Genetik, der enzymatischen Herstellung von komplexen Peptiden und bringen die neuesten Erkenntnisse der Apoptose unserem Verständnis näher. Immun-therapie bei Hirnerkrankungen und psychischen Störungen, der Einsatz von Naturprodukten zur Vorbeugung von Krebserkrankungen, das beun-ruhigende Anwachsen der Arzneimittelresistenz, die Mannigfaltigkeit der Dopamin-Rezeptor-Wirkung und die faszinierende Darstellung einer grösseren Gruppe von neuartigen Nukleosiden als Arzneimittel runden den vorliegenden Band der «Fortschritte der Arzneimittelforschung» ab und bieten dem Leser viel Neuartiges und Interessantes.

Seit der Gründung der Reihe im Jahre 1959 war der Herausgeber stets bemüht, die nicht mehr überschaubare Flut der Informationen über das komplexe Gebiet der Arzneimittelforschung dem interessierten Leser und dem engagierten Forscher näher zu bringen und in Teilgebieten über-schaubar zu machen. Diese Zielsetzung habe ich bis heute beibehalten, obwohl die Themen heute ungleich komplexer sind, als sie vor 38 Jahren noch waren. Wenn es gelungen ist, das angestrebte Ziel wenigstens teilweise zu erreichen, so ist dies in erster Linie den Autoren zu verdanken. Aber auch Leser und Fachkollegen haben mich immer wieder unterstützt, wobei ich ganz besonders an die Rezensenten denke, die mit wohlgemeinter Kri-tik und konkreten Empfehlungen zum Erfolg der «Fortschritte» ganz we-sentlich beigetragen haben. Ihnen allen danke ich auch an dieser Stelle.

Mein Dank geht auch an den Birkhäuser Verlag und insbesondere an die Damen Elizabeth Beckett, Dr. Petra Gerlach und Leslie Koechlin sowie an die Herren H.-P. Thür, E. Mazenauer und G. Messmer. Sie alle haben durch ihren persönlichen Einsatz den 48. Band mitgestaltet und mitgeprägt.

Basel, Mai 1997   DR. E. JUCKER

Progress in Drug Research, Vol. 48 (E. Jucker, Ed.)
© 1997 Birkhäuser Verlag, Basel (Switzerland)

Physicochemical basis of the universal genetic codes – quantitative analysis

By Eric J. Lien[1], Arima Das, Partha Nandy and Shijun Ren

Department of Pharmaceutical Sciences, School of Pharmacy, University of Southern California, 1985 Zonal Avenue, Los Angeles, CA 90033, USA

---

[1]   To whom correspondence should be addressed.

1   Summary

Quantitative mathematic models have been developed to correlate the fragment hydrophobicity contribution constants (f_{aa}) of 20 amino acids with the physicochemical properties (μ, Hb, and $\sqrt{MW}$) of the four bases (U, A, C, G) of the codons, or those of the anticodons. Using the general equation $f_{aa} = a\mu_1 + b\mu_2 + c\mu_3 + d\sqrt{MW_1} + e\sqrt{MW_2} + f\sqrt{MW_3} + g\,Hb_1 + h\,Hb_2 + i\,Hb_3 + j$, where 1, 2, 3 refer to the first, the second and the third base respectively, correlation coefficient of about 0.82 can be obtained for all 20 amino acids coded by 61 different triplet codes.

These correlations are statistically highly significant, even though they do not take into account the involvement of various factors and peptidyl transferases. Furthermore, the reasons for the three stop codons are revealed. The graphic presentation of the codons and the amino acids coded separates the acidic and the basic, the aromatic and the heterocyclic amino acids into different quadrants of an octagon. This is in agreement with the ancient Chinese Ying-Yang theory embedded in the classical I-Ching.

2   Introduction

Recent developments of molecular biology and genetic engineering owe their success to the discovery of the structures of the nucleic acids by Pauling and Corey [1, 2] and Watson and Crick [3, 4]. Without the fundamental knowledge of the molecular structures of these complex biomacromolecules, subsequent decoding of the genetic codes for proteins [5–13] would not be possible.

Over the past five decades the standard universal genetic code has been well established [14–16]. Tables relating the specific amino acids to the triplet bases in DNA or RNA can be found in many textbooks. They are shown in Figures 1 and 2, respectively.

The purpose of this study is to analyze quantitatively how the different physicochemical properties of the nucleic acid bases can affect the selection of a specific amino acid as represented by the hydrophobicity. The physicochemical basis of the termination of the peptide chain by the three stop codons will also be evaluated.

The working hypothesis being tested is that during the translation process, specific molecular recognition exists among codon-anticodon and the amino acid being coded. During the complementary recognition of the specific amino acid, the major molecular attributes involved are the size

($\sqrt{MW}$), the hydrogen bonding ability (Hb) and the dipolar character (μ) of the triplet codon or anticodon. The recognition site may be allosteric to the acylamino acid-acyltranferase binding site, like the remote lock-and-key device next to a driver's seat which controls the locking mechanism of a car trunk. Since codons and anticodons are complementary to each other, either set of triplets should give the same results. Furthermore, the weight carried by each base is different. The third base of the triplet has the least weight, thus giving rise to degeneracy.

3   Structures and physicochemical properties of nucleic acid bases

The discovery of the antiparallel double-helical structure of deoxyribonucleic acid (DNA) paved the road to the development of recombinant DNA technology. In the molecular structures of both DNA and ribonucleic acid (RNA), the backbones (deoxy-ribose-triphosphate, and ribosetriphosphate, respectively) remain constant, only the bases change their permutation and combination. In the case of DNA the base pairs include two purines and two pyrimidines, they are A (adenine) and G (guanine), and T (thymine) and C (cytosine). In the case of RNA, U (uracil) replaces T (thymine), the other base pairs remain the same (see Figures 1 and 2) [15–18].
Among these five different building blocks of nucleic acids, there exist different ranges of physicochemical properties (see Table 1 on page 18). For example, the molecular weight (which reflects both the bulk and the steric effect) ranges from 111.10 to 151.13, the dipole moment (a measure of the separation of charge) ranges from 2.18 D to 6.74 D, the total number of hydrogen bond (Hb) is 7 for all except adenine, which has a value of 10. The hydrophobicity as measured by 1-octanol/water partition coefficient (log P) ranges from –1.73 to –0.09.
By different combination and permutation of the triplet genetic codes, namely codons (mRNA) and anticodons (tRNA), and with the participation of various factors and peptidyl transferase, a specific amino acid gets incorporated into the peptide chain in the ribosome [18]. From the cumulation of the material investigated over the last half century, a standard coding dictionary or universal code has been established (Figures 1 and 2).

**Proteins have unique amino acid sequences
that are specified by genes (DNA)**

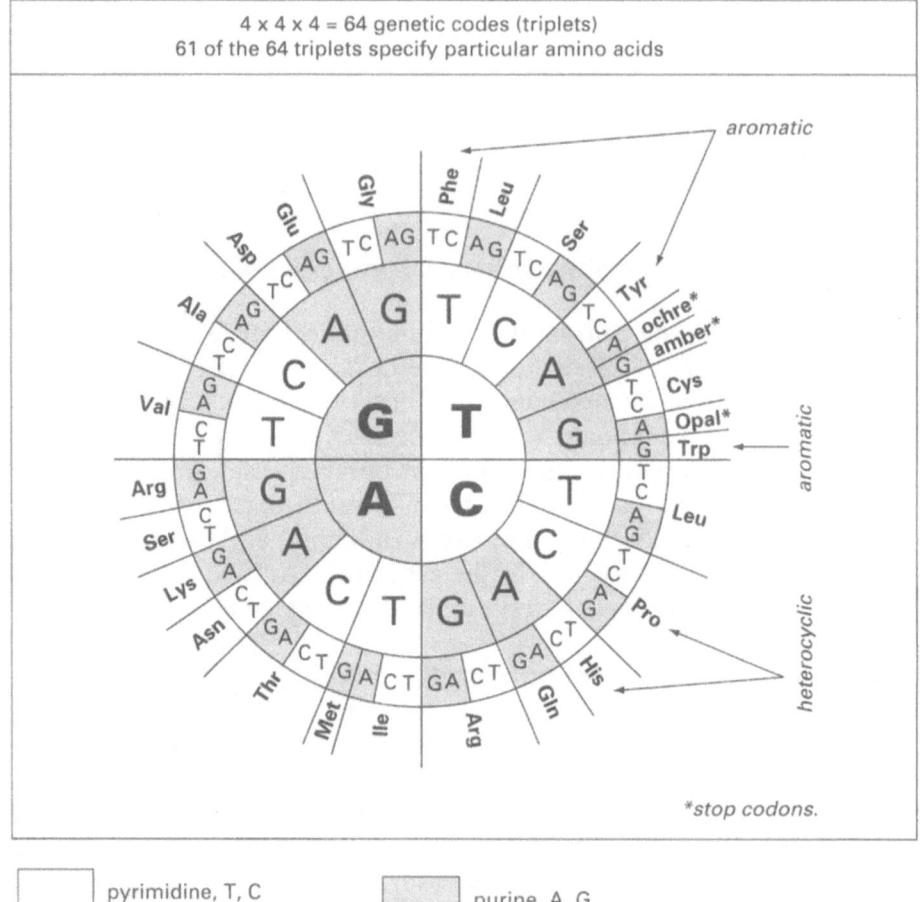

4 x 4 x 4 = 64 genetic codes (triplets)
61 of the 64 triplets specify particular amino acids

*stop codons.

pyrimidine, T, C   purine, A, G

DNA Template	mRNA	tRNA
^{5}T - A^3	→ U ^{5}	A
A - T	→ A	U
C - G	→ C	G
^{3}G - C^5	→ G ^{3}	C

Names of amino acids and chain termination codons are on the periphery of the circle. The first base of the codon is identified in the center ring; the second base of the codon is in the middle ring; and the third base(s) of the codons is in the outer ring of the circle.

NOTE the clustering of aromatic, heterocyclic amino acids in the right hand side.

Fig. 1
The genetic code (DNA).

Proteins have unique amino acid sequences that are specified by genes (mRNA)

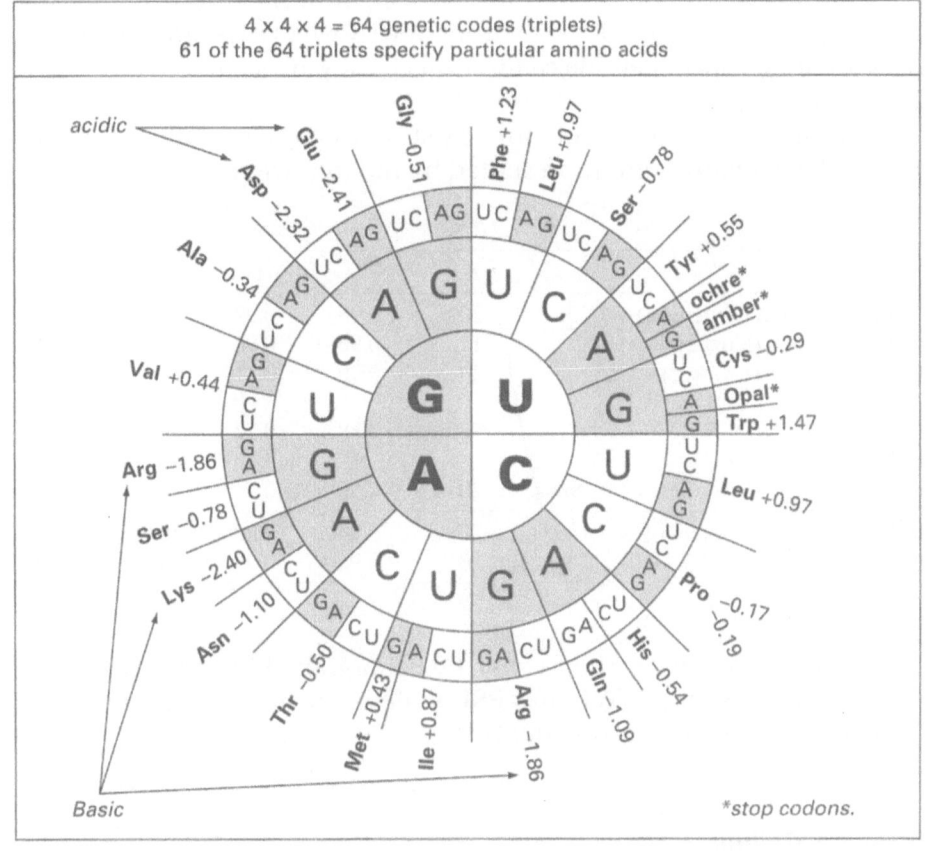

4 x 4 x 4 = 64 genetic codes (triplets)
61 of the 64 triplets specify particular amino acids

| | pyrimidine, U, C | | purine, A, G |

DNA Template	mRNA	tRNA
5'T - A 3' →	U 5'	A
A - T →	A	U
C - G →	C	G
3'G - C 5' →	G 3'	C

Names of amino acids and chain termination codons are on the periphery of the circle. The first base of the codon is identified in the center ring; the second base of the codon is in the middle ring; and the third base(s) of the codons is in the outer ring of the circle. The fragment hydrophobic contribution constants (faa) of the amino acids are indicated right next to them.
NOTE *the acidic and basic amino acids on the left hand side.*

Fig. 2
The genetic code (mRNA).

4   Hydrophobicity scales of amino acids

Over the last quarter century, various investigators have designed various scales for representation of the hydrophobicity when a specific amino acid is incorporated into a peptide chain [19–21]. They are summarized in Table 2 (see page 19).
Statistically significant correlations exist between these different scales. The best correlations are represented by the following equations:

	n	r	r^2	s	$F_{1, n-2}$
GWL = −1.153 (Fauchère) + 1.226	20	0.96	0.92	0.34	217.73
GWL = 0.638 (Nozaki) − 0.603	12	0.96	0.92	0.23	116.18
GWL = −0.170 (Parker) − 0.254	20	0.90	0.81	0.54	75.13
GWL = −0.215 (GES) − 0.126	20	0.88	0.77	0.59	61.63
GWL = 1.607 (Eisenberg) − 0.182	20	0.86	0.74	0.62	52.21
PSL = −1.076 (Fauchère) + 1.123	20	0.94	0.89	0.39	141.98
PSL = 0.915 (GWL) − 0.033	18	0.96	0.93	0.34	196.01

It should be noted that while Nozaki, Eisenberg, and PSL scales have positive correlations with GWL and PSL scales, Fauchère, Parker and GES have negative correlations with GWL and PSL scales.

5   Method

5.1   Quantitative correlation of the hydrophobicity of amino acid with the physicochemical parameters of the genetic code

Long before the process of translation was well understood, it was speculated by Gamow in 1954 [22] that free amino acids from the medium get caught in the 'holes' of DNA molecules. Although this over-simplified model completely missed the important roles of m-RNA, t-RNA and peptidyl transferase in the process, it did invoke the right concept of complementarity between the genetic codes and the amino acids encoded. In our re-examination of the quantitative relationship between the physicochemical properties of the triplet codons and anticodon and the hydrophobicity of the individual amino acids specified, the following general mathematic model was examined:

$$f_{aa} = f_1 \, (\mu_1, \mu_2, \mu_3) + f_2 \, (Hb_1, Hb_2, Hb_3) + f_3 \, (\sqrt{MW}_1, \sqrt{MW}_2, \sqrt{MW}_3)$$
$$+ \text{constant.} \hspace{4cm} \text{Eq. (1)}$$

Where μ, Hb, and MW are the dipole moment, maximum hydrogen bond and MW of the base, respectively, 1,2 and 3 refer to the first, the second and the 3rd base in order.

The parameters used are summarized in Tables 3 and 4.

The f_{aa} values are taken from ref. [20] for all except two amino acids, proline and cysteine. These two f_{aa} values are from ref. [21] (see Table 2 on page 19).

The regression analysis was performed with a nonweighted least squares program using a BMDP Statistical Software [23].

5.2   Results and discussion

The regression analysis based on Eq. 1 resulted in the following statistically significant correlations, insignificant terms have been deleted:

Using the triplet codons:

$$f_{aa} = -0.35 \, \mu_1 - 0.85 \, \mu_2 \quad + 0.86 \, Hb_1 \quad + 2.25 \, Hb_2 \quad + 0.10 \, Hb_3$$
$$\hspace{1.2cm} -1.44 \, \sqrt{MW}_1 \hspace{1.3cm} -3.74 \, \sqrt{MW}_2 \quad -0.30 \, \sqrt{MW}_3 \quad + 42.13 \hspace{1cm} \text{Eq. (2)}$$

$$n = 61 \hspace{2cm} r = 0.82 \hspace{1cm} r^2 = 0.67 \hspace{1.5cm} SEE = 0.66$$
$$\hspace{2cm} F_{8,52} = 13.31 \hspace{0.5cm} \text{significant at } 99.95\%$$

Using the triplet anticodons:

$$f_{aa} = -0.03 \, \mu_1 + 0.29 \, \mu_2 \quad + 0.07 \, \mu_3 \hspace{1.2cm} -0.39 \, Hb_1 \hspace{1cm} -1.45 \, Hb_2$$
$$\hspace{1.2cm} -0.21 \, Hb_3 \hspace{1.8cm} + 0.79 \, \sqrt{MW}_1 \quad + 2.61 \, \sqrt{MW}_2 \quad + 0.45 \, \sqrt{MW}_3$$
$$\hspace{1.2cm} -29.75 \hspace{7.5cm} \text{Eq. (3)}$$
$$\hspace{1.2cm} n = 61 \hspace{2cm} r = 0.82 \hspace{1cm} r^2 = 0.67 \hspace{1.5cm} SEE = 0.67$$
$$\hspace{2cm} F_{9,51} = 11.59 \hspace{0.5cm} \text{significant at } 99.95\%$$

After deleting 3 outliers (#33, 34 tyrosine and #49 tryptophan) slightly different statistics are obtained, only the term with very small coefficient in Eq (3) (i.e. $-0.03 \, \mu$) is dropped in Eq (4).

$$f_{aa} = +0.39 \, \mu_2 \hspace{1.8cm} -0.01 \, \mu_3 \hspace{1.2cm} -0.05 \, Hb_1 \hspace{1cm} -1.70 \, Hb_2$$
$$\hspace{1.2cm} -0.03 \, Hb_3 \hspace{1.8cm} + 0.21 \, \sqrt{MW}_1 \quad + 3.12 \, \sqrt{MW}_2 \quad + 0.23 \, \sqrt{MW}_3$$
$$\hspace{1.2cm} -28.70 \hspace{7.5cm} \text{Eq. (4)}$$
$$\hspace{1.2cm} n = 58 \hspace{2cm} r = 0.89 \hspace{1cm} r^2 = 0.79 \hspace{1.5cm} SEE = 0.52$$
$$\hspace{2cm} F_{8,47} = 23.35 \hspace{0.5cm} \text{significant at } 99.95\%$$

From the results obtained, it is evident that since codons and anticodons are complimentary to each other, similar results can be obtained by using the physicochemical properties of either series. Furthermore, the first two letters of the codons and anticodons play much more significant roles than the third one.

Since only about 67 to 79% (100 r^2) of the variance in the data are accounted for by these equations, the rest of the variance (33 to 21%) is probably due to the participation of peptidyl transferase and other factors (e.g. IF_2, IF_3 and Efs). Nevertheless, it is gratifying to see that the highly complex process of translation in protein synthesis can be rationalized in terms of the structures and the physicochemical properties of the codons and anticodons. The next step of validation would be to use the correlation equation to check what f_{aa} values would be called for by the three stop codons, UAA (ochre), UAG (amber) and UGA (opal). When the appropriate parameters are entered into Eq. (2), the following f_{aa} values are obtained for the three stop codons:

Exceptions

UAA (ochre) predicted $f_{aa} = -0.94$ ⎤ Ciliates code for glutamine
                                      ⎬ $f_{aa} = -1.09$, very close to the pre-
UAG (amber) predicted $f_{aa} = -0.87$ ⎦ dicted f_{aa} values $-0.94, -0.87$

UGA (opal) predicted $f_{aa} = -0.59$

From Figures 1 and 2 one can see that these three stop codons are flanked by two amino acids with aromatic rings, namely tyrosine and tryptophan, both with positive f_{aa} values. Since there are no aromatic amino acids with f_{aa} values of $-0.94, -0.87$ or -0.59, this will stop the process. In contrast to these UGU and UGC call for cysteine with a f_{aa} of -0.29, which may be a compromise for slightly hydrophilic «aromatic amino acid».

6   Conclusion

From the graphic presentations of the genetic codes (Figures 1 and 2), and the correlations obtained (Eqs. 2–4), it is evident that the first two letters of the triplet code have the predominant roles of determining the amino acid to be incorporated into the protein chain. The third letter has a less significant role, this allows the degeneracy to occur, and only 20 amino acids are coded by 61 triplet codes, and three codes result in termination of the chain.

Yan [24] has used a 4 x 4 x 4 cube (the I-gene cube) in a patent to assign the 20 amino acids. This reveals a startling correlation between ancient knowledge of I Ching and modern science. Yan further divided the amino acids into four subgroups, namely, large-polar, large-nonpolar, small-polar and small-nonpolar. There are two amino acids with aromatic rings and positive hydrophobic fragment constants incorrectly classified as large-polar. They are tryptophan (f_{aa} = +1.47) and tyrosine (f_{aa} = +0.55), they should have been classified as large-nonpolar just like phenyalanine (f_{aa} = +1.23). The rest of Yan's classification of amino acids is in agreement with recent work of ours [20,21]. The quantitative correlation in this report appears to be the first attempt in correlating the physicochemical properties of the genetic code with those of the amino acids encoded (i.e. f_{aa} values). This is logical, since the hydrophobicities (log P, π or f) of organic compounds have been shown to be due to the contribution of intermolecular forces measured by electronic (dipole moment μ), hydrogen bond (Hb) and bulk or size ($\sqrt{MW}$ or log MW) parameters [20,21,25–30]. With continuous investigations into the three-dimensional structures of the complexes of protein bio-synthesis involving various elongation factors, GTP and peptidyl transferases [31], some day it may be possible to further improve the correlation coefficient (r) from 0.82 to above 0.95. In order to apply the principles of physical organic chemistry in molecular biology, the rate-limiting step is always in the collection of sufficient numbers of reproducible data points. In this case, it will be the collection of the structural parameters of all the complexes involved in the incorporation of 20 amino acids by 61 codes together with peptidyl transferases and other factors involved [31].

Acknowledgment

This work was supported in part by a grant from the H&L Charitable Foundation. The authors would like to thank Professors Michael M.C. Lai, Curtis Okamoto, Deborah L. Johnson and Michael Bolger for helpful discussions during the course of this study. Skillful typing of the manuscript was performed by Ms. Ruth Ballard, Ms. Jane Radaza, and Ms. Juliet Lai.

Table 1
Structures and properties of nucleic acid bases

			μ^a (D)	Hb[b]	log P[c] (oct/w)
Pyrimidines					
Thymine	$C_5H_6N_2O_2$ M.W.= 126.11		4.13 4.20[d]	7	−0.62
Cytosine	$C_4H_5N_3O$ M.W.= 111.10		4.29	7	−1.73
Uracil	$C_4H_4N_2O_2$ M.W.= 112.09		4.16	7	−1.07
Purines					
Adenine	$C_5H_5N_5$ M.W.= 135.14		2.18[d]	7	−0.09
Guanine	$C_5H_5N_5O$ M.W.= 151.13		6.74[d]	10	−1.07

[a] From A.L. McClellan: Tables of Experimental Dipole Moments. Vol. 3, Rahara Enterprises. pp. 1–1455, 1989.
[b] Maximum number of hydrogen bonds possible, hydrogen donors + acceptors −1.
[c] From C. Hansch, A. Leo and D. Hoekman: Exploring QSAR. Hydrophobic, Electronic and Steric Constants. ACS, Washington, D.C., 1995. pp.1–348.
[d] Calculated with HyperChem[TM] Program, after geometry optimization and energy minimization. Hypercube, Inc., Waterloo, Ontario, Canada, 1994.

Table 2
Hydrophobicity scales[a]

Residue	Source[19]														
	Nozaki	Bull	Wolfenden	Manavalan	Janin	Argos	von Heijne	Kyte-Doolittle	Eisenberg	Fauchère	Parker	Sweet	GES	GWL[20]	PSL[21]
Ala	0.5	-0.2	1.9	13.0	0.3	1.6	-1.0	1.8	0.25	1.52	2.1	-0.40	-1.6	-0.34	0.31
Cys	–	-0.5	-1.2	14.6	0.9	1.2	-1.5	2.5	0.04	1.70	1.4	0.17	-2.0	(-0.29)[21]	-0.29
Asp	–	-0.2	-10.9	10.9	-0.6	0.1	7.4	-3.5	-0.72	2.60	10.0	-1.31	9.2	-2.32	-2.07
Glu	–	-0.3	-10.2	11.9	-0.7	0.2	5.9	-3.5	-0.62	2.47	7.8	-1.22	8.2	-2.41	-1.96
Phe	2.5	-2.3	-0.8	14.0	0.5	2.0	-3.4	2.8	0.61	0.04	-9.2	1.92	-3.7	1.23	1.12
Gly	0.0	0.0	2.4	12.4	0.3	0.6	0.0	-0.4	0.16	1.83	5.7	-0.67	-1.0	-0.51	-0.76
His	0.5	-0.1	-10.2	12.2	-0.1	0.3	3.4	-3.2	-0.40	1.70	2.1	-0.64	3.0	-0.54	0.25
Ile	2.6	-2.3	2.2	15.7	0.7	1.7	-2.5	4.5	0.73	0.03	-8.0	1.25	-3.1	0.87	0.85
Lys	–	-0.4	-9.5	11.4	-1.8	0.2	4.2	-3.9	-1.10	2.82	5.7	-0.67	8.8	-2.43	-2.34
Leu	1.8	-2.5	2.3	14.9	0.5	2.9	-2.4	3.8	0.53	0.13	-9.2	1.22	-2.8	0.97	0.85
Met	1.3	-1.5	-1.5	14.4	0.4	3.0	-2.7	1.9	0.26	0.60	-4.2	1.02	-3.4	0.43	0.17
Asn	–	0.1	-9.7	11.4	-0.5	0.3	2.9	-3.5	-0.64	2.41	7.0	-0.92	4.8	-1.10	-1.44
Pro	–	-1.0	–	11.4	-0.3	0.8	3.3	-1.6	-0.07	1.34	2.1	-0.49	0.2	(-0.17)[21]	-0.17
Gln	–	0.2	-9.4	11.8	-0.7	0.5	2.4	-3.5	-0.69	2.05	6.0	-0.91	4.1	-1.09	-1.27
Arg	–	-0.1	–	11.7	-1.4	0.5	11.3	-4.5	-1.80	2.84	4.2	-0.59	12.3	-1.89	-1.91
Ser	-0.3	-0.4	-5.1	11.2	-0.1	0.8	1.5	-0.8	-0.26	1.87	6.5	-0.55	-0.6	-0.78	-0.94
Thr	0.4	-0.5	-4.9	11.7	-0.2	0.9	0.9	-0.7	-0.18	1.57	5.2	-0.28	-1.2	-0.50	-0.82
Val	1.5	-1.6	2.0	15.7	0.6	1.1	-2.0	4.2	0.54	0.61	-3.7	0.91	-2.6	0.44	0.73
Trp	3.4	-2.0	-5.9	13.9	0.3	1.1	-2.0	-0.9	0.37	-0.42	-10.0	0.50	-1.9	1.47	1.23
Tyr	2.3	-2.2	-6.1	13.4	-0.4	0.7	1.1	-1.3	0.02	0.87	-1.9	1.67	0.7	0.55	0.16

[a] Adapted from ref. [19–21], for details see the references cited therein.
[20] GWL = Gao, Wang and Lien (1993).
[21] PSL = Palekar, Shiue and Lien (1996).

Table 3
Physiochemical parameters of the codons used in correlation with the hydrophobicities of the amino acids.

	123	f	f_{aa} obsd	f_{aa} calcd[a]	μ 1	μ 2	μ 3	MW 1	MW 2	MW 3	Hb 1	Hb 2	Hb 3
1	UUU	Phe	1.23	1.45	4.28	4.28	4.28	112.09	112.09	112.09	7	7	7
2	UUC	Phe	1.23	1.46	4.28	4.28	5.97	112.09	112.09	111.10	7	7	7
3	UUA	Leu	0.97	1.14	4.28	4.28	2.18	112.09	112.09	135.14	7	7	7
4	UUG	Leu	0.97	1.25	4.28	4.28	6.74	112.09	112.09	151.13	7	7	10
5	CUU	Leu	0.97	0.93	5.97	4.28	4.28	111.10	112.09	112.09	7	7	7
6	CUC	Leu	0.97	0.94	5.97	4.28	5.97	111.10	112.09	111.10	7	7	7
7	CUA	Leu	0.97	0.62	5.97	4.28	2.18	111.10	112.09	135.14	7	7	7
8	CUG	Leu	0.97	0.72	5.97	4.28	6.74	111.10	112.09	151.13	7	7	10
9	AUU	Ile	0.87	0.69	2.18	4.28	4.28	135.14	112.09	112.09	7	7	7
10	AUC	Ile	0.87	0.71	2.18	4.28	5.97	135.14	112.09	111.10	7	7	7
11	AUA	Ile	0.87	0.38	2.18	4.28	2.18	135.14	112.09	135.14	7	7	7
12	AUG	Met	0.43	0.49	2.18	4.28	6.74	135.14	112.09	151.13	7	7	10
13	GUU	Val	0.44	0.70	6.74	4.28	4.28	151.13	112.09	112.09	10	7	7
14	GUC	Val	0.44	0.71	6.74	4.28	5.97	151.13	112.09	111.10	10	7	7
15	GUA	Val	0.44	0.39	6.74	4.28	2.18	151.13	112.09	135.14	10	7	7
16	GUG	Val	0.44	0.50	6.74	4.28	6.74	151.13	112.09	151.13	10	7	10
17	UCU	Ser	-0.78	0.19	4.28	5.97	4.28	112.09	111.10	112.09	7	7	7
18	UCC	Ser	-0.78	0.20	4.28	5.97	5.97	112.09	111.10	111.10	7	7	7
19	UCA	Ser	-0.78	-0.12	4.28	5.97	2.18	112.09	111.10	135.14	7	7	7
20	UCG	Ser	-0.78	-0.02	4.28	5.97	6.74	112.09	111.10	151.13	7	7	10
21	CCU	Pro	-0.17	-0.34	5.97	5.97	4.28	111.10	111.10	112.09	7	7	7
22	CCC	Pro	-0.17	-0.33	5.97	5.97	5.97	111.10	111.10	111.10	7	7	7
23	CCA	Pro	-0.17	-0.65	5.97	5.97	2.18	111.10	111.10	135.14	7	7	7
24	CCG	Pro	-0.17	-0.54	5.97	5.97	6.74	111.10	111.10	151.13	7	7	10
25	ACU	Thr	-0.50	-0.57	2.18	5.97	4.28	135.14	111.10	112.09	7	7	7
26	ACC	Thr	-0.50	-0.56	2.18	5.97	5.97	135.14	111.10	111.10	7	7	7
27	ACA	Thr	-0.50	-0.88	2.18	5.97	2.18	135.14	111.10	135.14	7	7	7
28	ACG	Thr	-0.50	-0.78	2.18	5.97	6.74	135.14	111.10	151.13	7	7	10
29	GCU	Ala	-0.34	-0.56	6.74	5.97	4.28	151.13	111.10	112.09	10	7	7
30	GCC	Ala	-0.34	-0.55	6.74	5.97	5.97	151.13	111.10	111.10	10	7	7
31	GCA	Ala	-0.34	-0.87	6.74	5.97	2.18	151.13	111.10	135.14	10	7	7
32	GCG	Ala	-0.34	-0.77	6.74	5.97	6.74	151.13	111.10	151.13	10	7	10

	123	f	f_{aa} obsd	calcd[a]	μ 1	2	3	MW 1	2	3	Hb 1	2	3
33	UAU	Tyr	0.55	-0.64	4.28	2.18	4.28	112.09	135.14	112.09	7	7	7
34	UAC	Tyr	0.55	-0.63	4.28	2.18	5.97	112.09	135.14	111.10	7	7	7
	UAA	Stop			4.28	2.18	2.18	112.09	135.14	135.14	7	7	7
	UAG	Stop			4.28	2.18	6.74	112.09	135.14	151.13	7	7	10
35	CAU	His	-0.54	-1.17	5.97	2.18	4.28	111.10	135.14	112.09	7	7	7
36	CAC	His	-0.54	-1.15	5.97	2.18	5.97	111.10	135.14	111.10	7	7	7
37	CAA	Gln	-1.09	-1.48	5.97	2.18	2.18	111.10	135.14	135.14	7	7	7
38	CAG	Gln	-1.09	-1.37	5.97	2.18	6.74	111.10	135.14	151.13	7	7	10
39	AAU	Asn	-1.10	-1.40	2.18	2.18	4.28	135.14	135.14	112.09	7	7	7
40	AAC	Asn	-1.10	-1.39	2.18	2.18	5.97	135.14	135.14	111.10	7	7	7
41	AAA	Lys	-2.40	-1.71	2.18	2.18	2.18	135.14	135.14	135.14	7	7	7
42	AAG	Lys	-2.40	-1.60	2.18	2.18	6.74	135.14	135.14	151.13	7	7	10
43	GAU	Asp	-2.32	-1.39	6.74	2.18	4.28	151.13	135.14	112.09	10	7	7
44	GAC	Asp	-2.32	-1.38	6.74	2.18	5.97	151.13	135.14	111.10	10	7	7
45	GAA	Glu	-2.41	-1.70	6.74	2.18	2.18	151.13	135.14	135.14	10	7	7
46	GAG	Glu	-2.41	-1.60	6.74	2.18	6.74	151.13	135.14	151.13	10	7	10
47	UGU	Cys	-0.29	-0.27	4.28	6.74	4.28	112.09	151.13	112.09	7	10	7
48	UGC	Cys	-0.29	-0.26	4.28	6.74	5.97	112.09	151.13	111.10	7	10	7
	UGA	Stop			4.28	6.74	2.18	112.09	151.13	135.14	7	10	7
49	UGG	Trp	1.47	-0.47	4.28	6.74	6.74	112.09	151.13	151.13	7	10	10
50	CGU	Arg	-1.86	-0.80	5.97	6.74	4.28	111.10	151.13	112.09	7	10	7
51	CGC	Arg	-1.86	-0.78	5.97	6.74	5.97	111.10	151.13	111.10	7	10	7
52	CGA	Arg	-1.86	-1.11	5.97	6.74	2.18	111.10	151.13	135.14	7	10	7
53	CGG	Arg	-1.86	-1.00	5.97	6.74	6.74	111.10	151.13	151.13	7	10	10
54	AGU	Ser	-0.78	-1.03	2.18	6.74	4.28	135.14	151.13	112.09	7	10	7
55	AGC	Ser	-0.78	-1.02	2.18	6.74	5.97	135.14	151.13	111.10	7	10	7
56	AGA	Arg	-1.86	-1.34	2.18	6.74	2.18	135.14	151.13	135.14	7	10	7
57	AGG	Arg	-1.86	-1.23	2.18	6.74	6.74	135.14	151.13	151.13	7	10	10
58	GGU	Gly	-0.51	-1.02	6.74	6.74	4.28	151.13	151.13	112.09	10	10	7
59	GGC	Gly	-0.51	-1.01	6.74	6.74	5.97	151.13	151.13	111.10	10	10	7
60	GGA	Gly	-0.51	-1.33	6.74	6.74	2.18	151.13	151.13	135.14	10	10	7
61	GGG	Gly	-0.51	-1.22	6.74	6.74	6.74	151.13	151.13	151.13	10	10	10

[a] calculated from eq. 2

Table 4.
Physiochemical parameters of the anticodons used in correlation with the hydrophobicities of the amino acids.

	123	f	f_{aa} obsd	calcd[a]	μ 1	2	3	MW 1	2	3	Hb 1	2	3
1	AAA	Phe	1.23	1.46	2.18	2.18	2.18	135.14	135.14	135.14	7	7	7
2	AAG	Phe	1.23	1.46	2.18	2.18	6.74	135.14	135.14	151.13	7	7	10
3	AAU	Leu	0.97	1.15	2.18	2.18	4.28	135.14	135.14	112.09	7	7	7
4	AAC	Leu	0.97	1.25	2.18	2.18	5.97	135.14	135.14	111.10	7	7	7
5	GAA	Leu	0.97	0.93	6.74	2.18	2.18	151.13	135.14	135.14	10	7	7
6	GAG	Leu	0.97	0.93	6.74	2.18	6.74	151.13	135.14	151.13	10	7	10
7	GAU	Leu	0.97	0.60	6.74	2.18	4.28	151.13	135.14	112.09	10	7	7
8	GAC	Leu	0.97	0.72	6.74	2.18	5.97	151.13	135.14	111.10	10	7	7
9	UAA	Ile	0.87	0.70	4.28	2.18	2.18	112.09	135.14	135.14	7	7	7
10	UAG	Ile	0.87	0.70	4.28	2.18	6.74	112.09	135.14	151.13	7	7	10
11	UAU	Ile	0.87	0.39	4.28	2.18	4.28	112.09	135.14	112.09	7	7	7
12	UAC	Met	0.43	0.49	4.28	2.18	5.97	112.09	135.14	111.10	7	7	7
13	CAA	Val	0.44	0.71	5.97	2.18	2.18	111.10	135.14	135.14	7	7	7
14	CAG	Val	0.44	0.71	5.97	2.18	6.74	111.10	135.14	151.13	7	7	10
15	CAU	Val	0.44	0.40	5.97	2.18	4.28	111.10	135.14	112.09	7	7	7
16	CAC	Val	0.44	0.50	5.97	2.18	5.97	111.10	135.14	111.10	7	7	7
17	AGA	Ser	-0.78	0.19	2.18	6.74	2.18	135.14	151.13	135.14	7	10	7
18	AGG	Ser	-0.78	0.19	2.18	6.74	6.74	135.14	151.13	151.13	7	10	10
19	AGU	Ser	-0.78	-0.12	2.18	6.74	4.28	135.14	151.13	112.09	7	10	7
20	AGC	Ser	-0.78	-0.02	2.18	6.74	5.97	135.14	151.13	111.10	7	10	7
21	GGA	Pro	-0.17	-0.33	6.74	6.74	2.18	151.13	151.13	135.14	10	10	7
22	GGG	Pro	-0.17	-0.33	6.74	6.74	6.74	151.13	151.13	151.13	10	10	10
23	GGU	Pro	-0.17	-0.64	6.74	6.74	4.28	151.13	151.13	112.09	10	10	7
24	GGC	Pro	-0.17	-0.54	6.74	6.74	5.97	151.13	151.13	111.10	10	10	7
25	UGA	Thr	-0.50	-0.57	4.28	6.74	2.18	112.09	151.13	135.14	7	10	7
26	UGG	Thr	-0.50	-0.57	4.28	6.74	6.74	112.09	151.13	151.13	7	10	10
27	UGU	Thr	-0.50	-0.88	4.28	6.74	4.28	112.09	151.13	112.09	7	10	7
28	UGC	Thr	-0.50	-0.78	4.28	6.74	5.97	112.09	151.13	111.10	7	10	7
29	CGA	Ala	-0.34	-0.56	5.97	6.74	2.18	111.10	151.13	135.14	7	10	7
30	CGG	Ala	-0.34	-0.56	5.97	6.74	6.74	111.10	151.13	151.13	7	10	10
31	CGU	Ala	-0.34	-0.87	5.97	6.74	4.28	111.10	151.13	112.09	7	10	7
32	CGC	Ala	-0.34	-0.77	5.97	6.74	5.97	111.10	151.13	111.10	7	10	7

			f_{aa} obsd	f_{aa} calcd[a]	μ 1	μ 2	μ 3	MW 1	MW 2	MW 3	Hb 1	Hb 2	Hb 3
33	AUA	Tyr	0.55	−0.64	2.18	4.28	2.18	135.14	112.09	135.14	7	7	7
34	AUG	Tyr	0.55	−0.64	2.18	4.28	6.74	135.14	112.09	151.13	7	7	10
	AUU	Stop			2.18	4.28	4.28	135.14	112.09	112.09	7	7	7
	AUC	Stop			2.18	4.28	5.97	135.14	112.09	111.10	7	7	7
35	GUA	His	−0.54	−1.16	6.74	4.28	2.18	151.13	112.09	135.14	10	7	7
36	GUG	His	−0.54	−1.16	6.74	4.28	6.74	151.13	112.09	151.13	10	7	10
37	GUU	Gln	−1.09	−1.47	6.74	4.28	4.28	151.13	112.09	112.09	10	7	7
38	GUC	Gln	−1.09	−1.37	6.74	4.28	5.97	151.13	112.09	111.10	10	7	7
39	UUA	Asn	−1.10	−1.40	4.28	4.28	2.18	112.09	112.09	135.14	7	7	7
40	UUG	Asn	−1.10	−1.40	4.28	4.28	6.74	112.09	112.09	151.13	7	7	10
41	UUU	Lys	−2.40	−1.71	4.28	4.28	4.28	112.09	112.09	112.09	7	7	7
42	UUC	Lys	−2.40	−1.61	4.28	4.28	5.97	112.09	112.09	111.10	7	7	7
43	CUA	Asp	−2.32	−1.39	5.97	4.28	2.18	111.10	112.09	135.14	7	7	7
44	CUG	Asp	−2.32	−1.39	5.97	4.28	6.74	111.10	112.09	151.13	7	7	10
45	CUU	Glu	−2.41	−1.70	5.97	4.28	4.28	111.10	112.09	112.09	7	7	7
46	CUC	Glu	−2.41	−1.60	5.97	4.28	5.97	111.10	112.09	111.10	7	7	7
47	ACA	Cys	−0.29	−0.26	2.18	5.97	2.18	135.14	111.10	135.14	7	7	7
48	ACG	Cys	−0.29	−0.26	2.18	5.97	6.74	135.14	111.10	151.13	7	7	10
	ACU	Stop			2.18	5.97	4.28	135.14	111.10	112.09	7	7	7
49	ACC	Trp	1.47	−0.47	2.18	5.97	5.97	135.14	111.10	111.10	7	7	7
50	GCA	Arg	−1.86	−0.79	6.74	5.97	2.18	151.13	111.10	135.14	10	7	7
51	GCG	Arg	−1.86	−0.79	6.74	5.97	6.74	151.13	111.10	151.13	10	7	10
52	GCU	Arg	−1.86	−1.10	6.74	5.97	4.28	151.13	111.10	112.09	10	7	7
53	GCC	Arg	−1.86	−1.00	6.74	5.97	5.97	151.13	111.10	111.10	10	7	7
54	UCA	Ser	−0.78	−1.02	4.28	5.97	2.18	112.09	111.10	135.14	7	7	7
55	UCG	Ser	−0.78	−1.02	4.28	5.97	6.74	112.09	111.10	151.13	7	7	10
56	UCU	Arg	−1.86	−1.34	4.28	5.97	4.28	112.09	111.10	112.09	7	7	7
57	UCC	Arg	−1.86	−1.23	4.28	5.97	5.97	112.09	111.10	111.10	7	7	7
58	CCA	Gly	−0.51	−1.02	5.97	5.97	2.18	111.10	111.10	135.14	7	7	7
59	CCG	Gly	−0.51	−1.01	5.97	5.97	6.74	111.10	111.10	151.13	7	7	10
60	CCU	Gly	−0.51	−1.33	5.97	5.97	4.28	111.10	111.10	112.09	7	7	7
61	CCC	Gly	−0.51	−1.23	5.97	5.97	5.97	111.10	111.10	111.10	7	7	7

[a] calculated from eq. 3

References

1   Pauling, L. and Corey, R.B.: Structure of the nucleic acids. Nature *171*, 346 (1953).
2   Pauling, L. and Corey, R.B.: A proposal structure for the nucleic acid. Proc NAS *39*, 84–97 (1953).
3   Watson, J.D. and Crick, F.H.C.: Molecular structure of nucleic acids. Nature *171*, 737–138 (1953).
4   Watson, J.D. and Crick, F.H.C.: Genetic implications of the structure of deoxyribonucleic acid. Nature *171*, 964–967 (1953).
5   Crick, F.H.C., Barnett, L., Brenner, S. and Watts–Tobin, R.J.: General nature of the genetic code for proteins. Nature *192*, 1227–1232 (1961).
6   Eck, R.V.: Genetic code: emergence of a symmetrical pattern. Science *140*, 477–481 (1963).
7   Söll, D., Ohtsuka, E., Jones, D.S., Lohrmann, R., Hayatsu, H., Nishimura, S. and Khorama, H.G.: Studies on polynucleotides, XLIX stimulation of the binding of aminoacyl–sRNA's to ribosomes by ribotrinucleotides and a survey of codon assignments for 20 amino acids. Proc NAS *54*, 1378–1385 (1965).
8   Nirenberg, M., Leder, P., Bernfield, M., Brimacombe, R., Trupin, J., Rottman, F. and O'Neal, C.: RNA code words and protein synthesis, VII. on the general nature of the RNA code. Proc NAS *53*, 1161–1168 (1965).
9   Crick, F.H.C.: Codon–anticodon pairing. The wobble hypothesis. J. Mol. Biol. *19*, 548–555 (1966).
10   Söll, D., Jones, D.S., Ohtsuka, E., Faulkner, R.D., Lohrmann, R., Hayatsu, H., Khorana, H.G., Cherayil, J.D., Hampel, A. and Beck, R.M.: Specificity of sRNA for recognition of codons as studied by the ribosomal binding technique. J. Mol. Biol. *19*, 556–573 (1966).
11   Crick, F.H.C.: The origin of the genetic code. J. Mol. Biol. *38*, 367–379 (1968).
12   Gorini, L.: Informational suppression. Am. Rev. Genetics *4*, 107–134 (1970).
13   Söll, D., Abelson, J.N. and Schimmel, P.R.: Transfer RNA, Biological Aspects. Cold Spring Harbor Laboratory, 341–362 (1980).
14   Stent, G.S. and Calender, R.: Molecular Genetics, An introductory narrative. San Francisco, W.H. Freeman and Co., 336–566 (1978).
15   Stryer, L.: Biochemistry. 3rd edit. New York, W.H. Freeman and Co., 1089 (1988).
16   Lewin B. Genes IV. New York, Oxford University Press, 1–857 (1990).
17   Sinden, R.R.: DNA Structure and Function. San Diego, Academic Press, 1–279 (1994).
18   Klug, W.S. and Cummings, M.R.: Concepts of Genetics. 4th edit. New York, MacMillan College Publishing Co., 475–476 (1994).
19   Von Heijne, G.: Sequence Analysis in Molecular Biology, Hydrophobicity Scales. New York, Academic Press, 98–100 (1987).
20   Gao, H., Wang, F.Z. and Lien, E.J.: Hydrophobicity of oligopeptides having un–ionizable side chains. J. Drug Targeting *1*, 59–66 (1993).
21   Palekar, D., Shiue, M. and Lien, E.J.: Correlation of physicochemical parameters to the hydrophobic contribution constants of amino acid residues in small peptides. Pharm. Res. *13*, 1191–1195 (1996).
22   Gamow, G.: Possible relation between deoxyribonucleic acid and protein structures. Nature *173*, 318 (1954).
23   Dixon, W.J., Brown, M.B., Engelman, L., Frane, J.W., Hill, M.A., Jennrich, R.I. and Toturk, J.D. (eds.): Regression. In: BMDP Statistical Software, eds. Berkeley, University California Press, 235–283 (1985).

24 Yan, J.F.: DNA and the I Ching: The Tao of Life. Berkeley, North Atlantic Books, 1–1176 (1991).

25 Selassie, C.D., Wang, P.H. and Lien, E.J.: Re–evaluation of bulk parameters, molar fraction, molecular mass, molar volume and parachor. Acta Pharm. Jugosl. *30*, 135–139 (1990).

26 Lien, E.J., Guo, Z.R., Li, R.L. and Su, C.T.: The use of dipole moment as a parameter in drug receptor interaction and QSAR studies. J. Pharm. Sci. *71*, 641–655 (1982).

27 Ou, X.C., Ouyang, Y. and Lien, E.J.: Examination of quantitative relationship of partition coefficient (log P) and molecular weight, dipole moment and hydrogen bond capability of miscellaneous compounds. J. Mol. Sci. (Wuhan, China) *4*, 89–95 (1986).

28 Yang, Q.Z., Lien, E.J. and Quo, Z.R.: Physical factors contributing to hydrophobic constant π. Quantitative Structure–Activity Relationships *5*, 12–18 (1986).

29 Lien, E.J., Gao, H. and Prabhakar, H.: Physical factors contributing to the partition coefficient and retention time of 2',3'–didoexynucleoside analogues. J. Pharm. Sci. *80*, 517–521 (1991).

30 Lien, E.J.: Partition coefficients. In: Swarbick, J. and Boylan, J.C. (eds.): Encyclopedia of Pharmaceutical Technology. New York, Marcel Dekker, 293–307 (1994).

31 Nilssen, P., Kjeldgaard, M., Thirup, S., Polekhina, G., Reshetnikova, L., Clark, B.F.C. and Nyborg, J.: Crystal structure of the termini complex of Phe–tRNA[Phe], EF–Tu, and a GTP analog. Science *270*, 1464–1471 (1995).

Progress in Drug Research, Vol. 48 (E. Jucker, Ed.)
© 1997 Birkhäuser Verlag, Basel (Switzerland)

Enzymatic generation of complex peptides

By Horst Kleinkauf and Hans von Döhren

Technical University of Berlin, D-10587 Berlin, Germany

1   Introduction

Complex peptides have continued to be lead structures in the search of drugs, especially those of microbial sources. In addition, the discovery of active peptides in animal sources including insects and mammals is advancing. As considerable progress has been achieved in the analysis of protein structure, the identification of targets and mechanisms of action is carried out at the molecular levels. For many purposes of structure-function studies the preparation and modification of complex peptides are required, and often chemical strategies are laborious or not available. Efforts have thus been conducted to make use of protein biocatalysts evolved in the producer organisms, exerting their catalytic powers under physiolgical conditions. Such enzymes permit the synthesis of complex metabolites like cyclic peptides in single pot sequential reactions starting from the direct precursor amino acids. In pharmaceutical research recent examples of bioengineering include the *in vitro* synthesis of immunomodulators of the cyclosporin-type and antihelminthics of the ennatin-type, as well as the *in vivo* synthesis of antifungals of the R106-type. The reasons for biocatalyst-assisted production are amongst others (1) the convenient and rapid access to small amounts of analogs, (2) the option to develop a later bioproduction of a certain analog since natural systems are exploited, and (3) the contribution of knowledge on these systems with a view to developing new systems for the generation of compound libraries.

2   Peptide biosynthesis

The generation of peptide bonds follows either ribosomal or nonribosomal mechanisms. The ribosomal path itself is not a subject of this review, although with some justification the ribosome may be referred to as an enzyme system. Likewise, the exploitation of the ribosomal machinery to generate peptides without participation of the mRNA template, or the generation of catalytic RNA molecules for peptide bond formation is in its beginnings and will therefore not be considered here. Enzymes treated here are classical protein catalysts including single-step and multistep systems, which besides their genetic determination are not dependent on nucleic acid structures.

2.1   Overview of biosynthetic mechanisms [1]

The principal difference between enzymatic and chemical synthesis of peptides is the use of unprotected amino and imino acids, hydroxy acids, and
their derivatives. Carboxyl group activation is catalyzed by ATP, while no
protection or deprotection of side chains is required, since these are specifically protected by the catalyst's protein surfaces. We differentiate
systems catalyzing the addition of one amino group donor to an activated
carboxyl acceptor (single-step system) and systems linking three or more
residues in a sequential enzymatic process, thus generating two or more
peptide bonds (multistep systems). Only the latter system is currently of
general interest in the generation of complex peptides, while single-step
systems known from compounds like carnosine, glutathione, or muropep-
tides are easily accessible by conventional chemical processes, but equally
available by the respective enzymes.

Multistep systems consist of single or several interacting multifunctional
proteins and combine activated precursors by directed condensation reactions into the respective linear multimers. An essential feature of the
systems is the covalent attachment of all intermediates on the biocata-
lyst, avoiding the presence of free intermediates. The bound intermediates are then specifically cyclized or modified and thus released from the
enzyme surface. Such processes can be observed in peptide- and poly-
ketide-forming systems, but here we are restricting the discussion to peptide synthetases. Some systems have been characterized as forming mixed
types of compounds, combining both structural features, the formation
of peptide and ester bonds as well as carbon-carbon bonds. Respective
examples are the immunomodulators FK506 (immunomycin) and rapa-
mycin, or the antibiotic pristinamycin M.

Peptides generated by multienzyme systems are known to have sizes of
up to 48 amino acid residues [2]. Their enzymatic origin is inferred from
a composition that includes amino acids not processed by the ribosomal
system. Several unusual residues are known to originate from ribosomally
manufactured peptides, e.g. lanthionine, methyl-lanthionine, D-alanine,
hydroxyproline and hydroxylysine. Some of the respective modifying
enzymes including hydroxylases and an in-chain alanine epimerase have
been characterized.

2.2   Basic features of multienzyme systems

Multienzyme systems are composed of modules, each contributing the
information required for the addition of one carboxyl compound. Repet-

Table 1.
Peptide synthetase domains and their occurrence in related enzyme systems

Domain	Activity	Present in
Adenylate formation	providing acyl-CoA for a variety of biosynthetic reactions	acyl-CoA ligases
	luminescence	insect luciferase
	carboxyl activation	acyl transfer (aromatic acids)
	amino acid activation	peptide synthetases
Carrier protein	covalent transport of acyl intermediates	fatty acid synthases polyketide synthases peptide synthetases pha-synthases
Epimerase	epimerization of acyl intermediates	peptide synthetases
Condensation	peptide bond formation	peptide synthetases
Thioesterase	providing free carboxyls from thioesters	fatty acid synthases free thioesterases
	transferase functions (cyclization?) stereospecific peptide release	peptide synthetases
N-methyl-transferase	methyl transfer to activated amino acids	peptide synthetases

itive operating systems may reuse their modules and thus require less structural space. Examples of such systems are polyhydroxybutyrate synthase and poly-gamma-glutamate synthetase, enniatin synthetase trimerizing a dipeptidol (two modules), or gramicidin S synthetase, dimerizing a pentapeptide (five modules). Modules are composed of functional elements or domains, which have been observed in various biosynthetic systems (Table 1). Sequence analysis of peptide synthetase genes has provided highly similar structures from both pro- and eukaryotic sources. A collection of amino acid sequence motifs has emerged permitting the identification of peptide synthetase genes (Fig. 1). Peptide synthetases contain both adenylate-forming domains, as contained in acyl-CoA synthetases, and condensation domains, which have no close structural relative [2]. These are linked by domains homologous to acyl carrier proteins found in fatty acid and polyketide biosynthetic systems, functioning here in aminoacyl-, hydroxyacyl-, acyl- and peptidyl-transfer reactions.

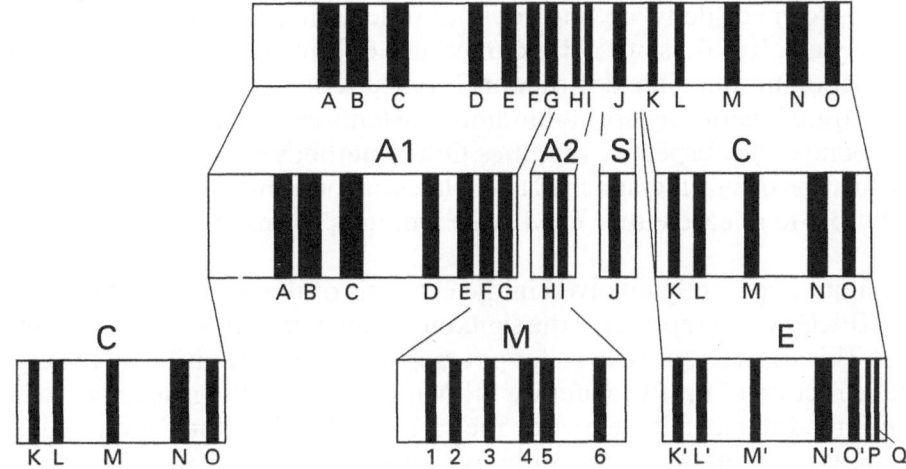

Fig. 1
Domain construction of peptide synthetases. Peptide synthetase sequences can be identified by a spacing of motifs, which have been assigned to adenylate formation, aminoacylation of pantetheine, N-methylation of aminoacyl-residues, and elongation (peptide bond formation). The respective consensus sequences are given in [2, 29].

2.2.1   Peptide synthetase domains

Adenylate domains. Compared to the ribosomal peptide-forming system these domains correspond to aminoacyl-tRNA synthetases and thus represent a major part of the nonribosomal code. Here the respective amino acid or related substrate is selected. Although we are still lacking three-dimensional structures, a major structural determinant resides between motifs C and D (Fig. 1). Sequence alignments may provide tentative information on the respective substrate of unidentified genes or multigene fragments [2, 3]. The recently completed substrate-free crystal structure of the firefly luciferase indicates that the catalytic center is formed by two subdomains connected by a linker region [4]. The binding sites of $MgATP^{2-}$ have been traced on both subdomains by affinity labeling [5, 6]. The substrates form an aminoacyl- or acyladenylate releasing $MgPPi^{2-}$ (1):

(1) $E + RCOOH + MgATP^{2-} \leftrightarrows E \{RCO\text{-}AMP\} + MgPPi^{2-}$

By addition of labeled pyrophosphate the reaction can be reversed and labeled ATP is formed. This reversed activation reaction is widely used to determine the substrate specificity of the respective domain. However, the velocity of ATP formation is a measure of the pyrophosphorylation of the formed adenylate, and does not reflect the rate of formation of the adenylate. It is thus not a direct measure of intermediate formation but rather of intermediate destruction. From kinetic analysis employing two-substrate kinetics substrate-binding constants can be derived, which correspond to the respective affinities. Other methods measuring directly the formation of enzyme-attached adenylates or consumption of ATP by pyro-phosphate release either need large amounts of enzyme or are less sensitive.

A motif apparently involved in the catalysis of the reaction is SGT(S,T) GXPKG, which represents the signature sequence of this type of enzymes [2]. This stretch represents a loop region only partially visible in the crystal structure of firefly luciferase [4]. Mutagenesis of the respective lysine residue dramatically decreases the rate of adenylate formation and enhances the proteolytic susceptibility of the domain in the presence of substrates [7]. Peptide-directed antibodies against this sequence have proved to be highly useful in the detection of this enzyme class in protein extracts [8].

The protected adenylate is then stabilized by formation of a thioester reacting with the cysteamine group of 4'-phosphopantetheine. The cofactor moiety is contained in the carrier protein domain where it is introduced by posttranslational modification [2, 9, 10]. This transfer is thought to introduce an additional selection step in the activation reaction, since Schwecke has shown that an aminoadipate-specific domain does not transfer misactivated valine [11]. Speculatively, a functionally unidentified thioesterase-like gene found in peptide synthetase clusters has been assigned a correcting hydrolytic activity for misactivated thioesters.

Acyl carrier domains. Acyl carrier protein-like domains have been detected in a variety of enzyme systems catalyzing single or sequential condensation reactions. These include fatty acid synthases, polyketide synthases, polyhydroxyalkanoate synthases, and peptide synthetases. For all these regions comprising about 80 to 100 amino acids a three-helix structure is predicted similar to the one found in acyl carrier proteins e.g. from *Escherichia coli* using NMR techniques [9, 12]. Posttranslational modification by a holo-enzyme synthase is required to functionalize this domain. The respective substrate is CoA, and 4'-phosphopantetheine is transferred to a highly conserved serine residue with release of 3',5'-ADP. Holo-enzyme synthases have recently been identified for the acyl carrier protein of *Escherichia coli* [10], the siderophore system of *Escherichia coli*, where EntD modifies EntF [13], peptide synthetase systems of gramicidin S and tyrocidine [14], and various fungal peptide forming systems [15]. The car-

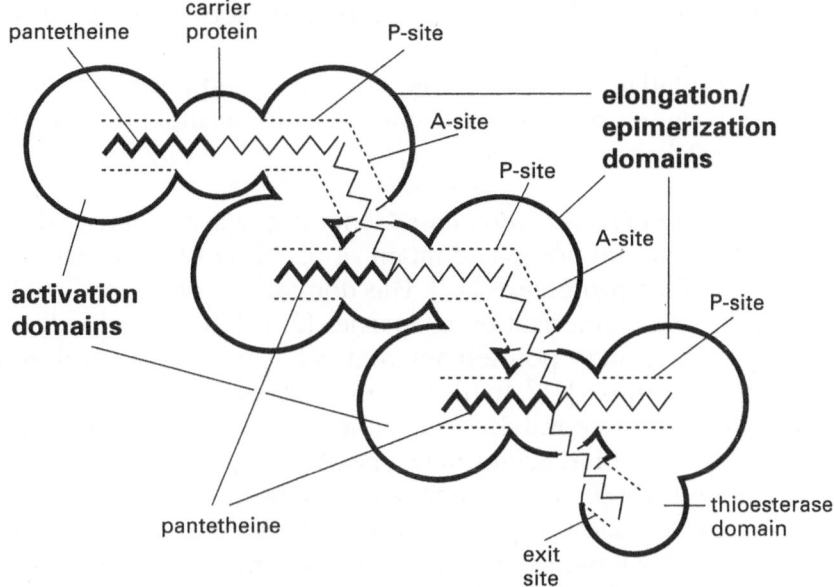

Fig. 2
Scheme of elongation in the nonribosomal system employing the terminology of the ribosomal system. The aminoacyl-residue is attached as thioester to its tRNA-analog cofactor 4'-phos-
phopantetheine. This residue swings to its respective A-site on the elongation domain. The
respective peptidyl-residue, equally thioester-bound to its 4'-phosphopantetheine carrier, swings
to a respective P-site, and condensation is catalyzed by a peptidyl-transferase center, transferring the peptidylresidue onto the aminoacyl residue with peptide bond formation. The free cofactor is now aminoacylated to function in its respective A-site, while the elongated peptide docks
to the following P-site. Contrary to the ribosome, each step has its own peptidyltransferase center on the elongation domain, and A- and P-site may vary in their selection properties.

boxyl moiety of the adenylates is transferred to the acyl carrier domain,
where it presumably is stabilized by protein interactions (2):

(2)   E1 {RCO-AMP} + E2-SH ⇄ E2-S-RCO + AMP + E1

Here E1 and E2 stand for adenylate and acyl carrier domains, respectively. Gene sequence analysis has revealed that contrary to earlier
assumptions each module contains one such domain. The original thio-
template model, as described before in this series [16], has been changed
to a multiple carrier model [9]. Peptide bond formation thus occurs from
adjacent modules by interaction of two neighboring acyl carrier domains
with the respective inserted condensation domain (Fig. 2). The cofactor
is then charged by a respective peptidyl-residue formed in the condensation reaction (3):

(3)   E12-S-AA1 + E22-S-AA2 → E12-SH + E22-S-AA2-AA1

E12 and E22 stand here for the carrier domains of modules 1 and 2, while AA1/2 are the amino acids 1 and 2 condensing to the dipeptidyl intermediate AA1-AA2.

Condensation/epimerization domains. Generally, each acyl carrier domain is followed by an autonomous domain of 55 to 60 kDa, which can be released by limited proteolysis [17]. This domain has been ascribed both condensation and epimerization properties [2, 18]. It seems likely, as de Crécy-Lagard et al. have pointed out, that either reaction is catalyzed by similar catalytic centers [18]. In the case of epimerization of the thioester-bound aminoacyl- or peptidylresidue either a transfer to a second multienzyme is observed, or a specific new type of elongation domain is found, approximately 100 kDa in size, representing a fused epimerization/elongation domain (see below) [2]. As can be seen in the current working model of peptide bond formation, the charged pantetheines are directed towards the active center catalyzing condensation or epimerization by a postulated binding to donor and acceptor site. These sites resemble functionally the A- and P-sites of the ribosomal system in the case of peptide bond formation (Fig. 2). The respective targeting of acyl, aminoacyl- and peptidyl-residues could then account for the direction of peptide bond formation. In the case of acylation of starter amino acids, as e.g. in the case of surfactin or enterobactin, a respective condensation domain is found N-terminal adjacent to the starter activation domain. Transfer is catalyzed either from the acyl-CoA compound requiring an additional transferase protein, or, in the case of aromatic acids, presumably directly from the enzyme-bound acyladenylate.

It has long been thought that epimerization would occur at the thioester stage of the activated amino acid. This had been concluded from the studies on gramicidin S and tyrocidine biosynthesis. Analysis of the configuration of the thioester-bound amino acids yielded L,D-mixtures with the D-configuration dominating [1]. Surprisingly in both actinomycin and ACV synthetases enzyme-bound valine showed L-configuration exclusively (Table 2). Stindl and Keller have shown that the dipeptide intermediate of actinomycin is enzyme-attached as a racemate, indicating that epimerization occurs at the dipeptide stage [19]. In ACV synthesis, the tripeptide is released so fast that no intermediate can be trapped. The modification of the release function is described in the thioesterase domain section. If in the ACV system amino acid analogs Glu or OMe-Ser are used, the dipeptides Cys-D-Val and OMe-Ser-D,L-Val are formed in low

Table 2.
Epimerization in nonribosomal peptide biosynthesis

Enzyme system	Amino acid epimerized	Intermediate	Isolated intermediates	Released products
Gramicidin S	Phe	D-Phe	D,L-Phe (2:1)	–
Tyrocidine	Phe	D-Phe	D,L-Phe (6:4)	–
Actinomycin	Val	R-Thr-D-Val	R-Thr-D,L-Val (1:1)	–
ACV	Val	Aad-Cys-D-Val	L-Val	Aad-Cys-D-Val
ACVS-TE*				Aad-Cys-L,D-Val (9:1)
ACV		Glu(?)Cys-D-Val		Cys-D-Val
ACV		Aad(?)OMe-Ser-D-Val		OMe-Ser-D,L-Val (9:1)

*ACV synthetase with modified thioesterase motif GXSXG

yields [20, 21]. These data seem to indicate that the first peptide bond has not been formed, and the release of the dipeptide is catalyzed by the thioesterase. It has also been suggested that this peptide bond is formed only in the second step. Clarification has to come from the analysis of intermediate thioesters.

Thioesterase domains. In several systems comprising either one or several multienzymes C-terminal domains with structural elements known from thioesterases have been detected [2]. The diversity of peptide structures produced in these systems indicate that this domain should exert a variety of transferase functions including hydrolytic release of thioesters (ACV synthetase), cyclization of peptidylintermediates (surfactin synthetase, gramicidin S synthetase), and cyclic ester formation (enterobactin synthetase). However, other systems that also require such termination reactions lack the respective domain. In addition, some systems have separate thioesterase-like genes. The functions of these domains thus remain to be established. Mutagenesis in the GXSXG-motif of the ACV synthetase thioesterase indicated that this motif is not involved in the hydrolytic release, but rather in the selection of the LLD-epimer to be released. The mutated enzyme released mainly LLL-ACV (Table 2)[22].

N-methyl-transferase domains. Methyl-transferase domains have been found integrated within the adenylate subdomains as a 50-kDa entity [2, 23–26]. N-methylation occurs at the thioester-stage of the aminoacyl groups, as has been demonstrated by the isolation of N-methyl-amino acids

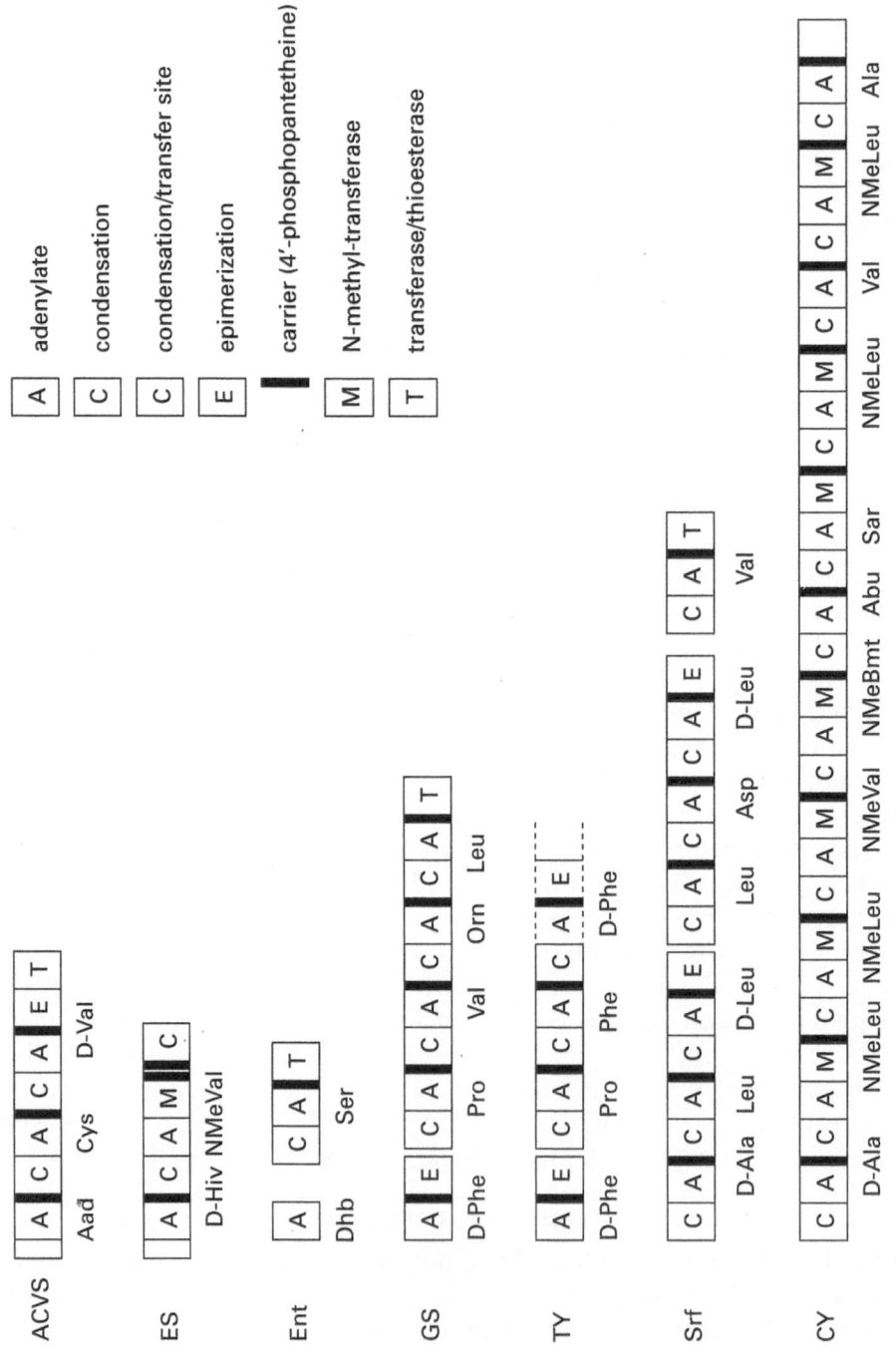

[23]. Inhibition of N-methylation by known methyltransferase inhibitors like sinefungin leads to the formation of unmethylated peptides, which are formed at reduced rates.

2.2.2 Multienzyme systems in peptide biosynthesis

The modular construction of a selection of well-characterized enzyme systems is shown in Figure 3. It is evident that for each constituent amino or hydroxy acid a respective activation domain is present. However, the situation appears to be more complicated when inspecting acyl carrier domains and elongation/epimerization domains. So in enniatin synthetase, two adjacent carrier functions are found in the second module. Since enniatin is a trimer of the dipeptidol-precursor Hiv-NMeVal, the function of this additional cofactor is thought to be a waiting position for the respective intermediates. On the contrary, although formed by the dimerization of two pentapeptides, no such waiting position has been detected in the gramicidin S system. Here the complex formation of multienzymes may be required to facilitate the cyclization. As already indicated above, systems transferring D-amino acids or peptides with terminal D-configuration, elongation and condensation domains are adjacent. The only known example of a residue in D-configuration which is directly transferred is the D-proline starter in HC-toxin formation. Here the respective domain is a fused type of epimerization and elongation domain [27]. A similar domain has recently been detected in the daptomycin biosynthetic cluster of *Streptomyces roseosporus* [28]. Unexpectedly the cyclosporin synthetase has a C-terminal condensation domain, but does not seem to require an acyl transfer for initiation. Although they have a cyclic structure both cyclosporin and HC-toxin synthetases lack the C-terminal thioesterase. We are thus still lacking fundamental insight into these sequential processes.

2.3 *In vivo* generation of peptides

The *in vivo* generation of peptides and analogs includes two fundamentally different approaches: either screening for analog producers or direct-

---

Fig. 3

Modular construction of peptide synthetases. ACVS: ACV synthetase, ES: enniatin synthetase, Ent: enterobactin biosynthetic enzymes, EntE and EntF, GS: gramicidin S synthetases 1 and 2, TY: tyrocidine synthetases 1 and 2, Srf: surfactin synthetases 1,2 and 3, CY: cyclosporin synthetase. Specificity of the domains is indicated. Note that two different types of condensation domains are found, slightly deviating in their consensus sequences, and one very closely related epimerization domain.

Table 3.
Selected cyclosporin producer strains [29]

Strain		Volumetric production*		Remarks
		CycA	CycC	
Tolypocladium inflatum	NRRL8044	100[L]	30[L]	
(*Beauveria niveum*)		500[L]		UV-mutant
Tolypocladium inflatum	ATCC 34291	199[SF]		white strain
(*Beauveria niveum*)		318[S]		epichlorohydrin mutant
Tolypocladium cyclindrosporum	260	79[SF]		
	285	89[SF]		
	286	71[SF]		
	287	113[SF]		
Beauveria bassiana		135[SF]		
Fusarium solanii	ATCC 46829	39[SF]		
Neocosmospora vasinfecta	ATCC 24402	17[S]		
	IFO 8966	–	1.7[S]	
	IFO 31377	0.78[S]		
Neocosmospora boninensis	NHL 2919	19[S]		
Stachybotrys chartarum	No.19392	148[L]		FR 901459

*volumetric production in mg/l; L-liquid culture, SF-shake flask, S-solid culture

ing cells by precursor addition or manipulation. In practice both procedures have been done. Examples for directed biosynthesis include tyro-
cidines (*Bacillus brevis*), actinomycins (*Streptomyces* sp.), viridogriseins
(*Streptomyces viridochromogenes*), ergot peptides (*Claviceps purpurea*),
enniatins (*Fusarium* sp.), cyclosporins (*Beauveria niveum*), and R106
(*Aureobasisium pullulans*). With the exception of the latter ones these have
been reviewed recently [29], and we focus our discussion on the most recent
data.

2.3.1   Cyclosporins and related peptides

Cyclosporins, related cyclopeptides and peptidolactones are immunosup-
pressors with a narrow antifungal spectrum but additional, interesting antiviral and antipsoriasis actions. A number of producing soil fungi have been
identified, some of which are compiled in Table 3 [30]. Productivity of
strains varies considerably depending on the fermentation procedures
applied. Mutagenesis (UV, epichlorohydrin), as well as precursor feeding
(see below), may enhance peptide production several times. The main
products observed are cyclosporin A and C (Fig. 4). Supplying aminobutyrate suppresses cyclosporin C formation and increases the yield of A

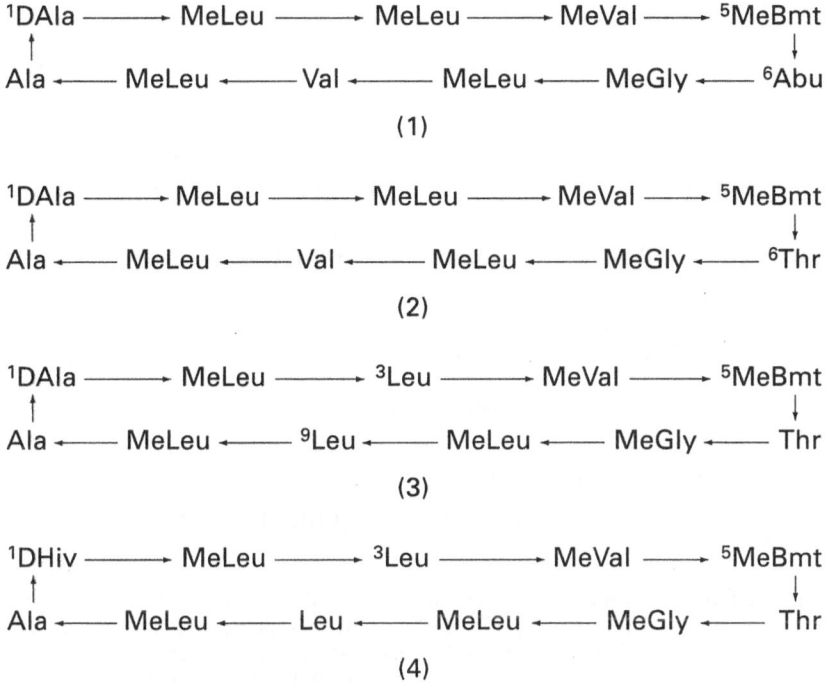

Fig. 4
Structures of cyclosporins A (1) and C (2), the recently-described analog FR 901459 [83] (3), and the peptidolactone analog SDZ 214-103 (4). Note the positional exchange of 9valine by leucine, the loss of N-methylation in position 3, and the replacement of D-alanine by D-hydroxy-isovalerate.

2.5-fold [31]. The feeding of threonine, the apparently limiting substrate of cyclosporin C formation, increases the yield from 30 to 275 mg/l, raising at the same time the cyclosporin A level from 100 to almost 400 mg/l. Strains like *Neocosmospora vasinfecta* IFO 8966 produce only cyclosporin C, half of which is excreted (12.7 mg/l, [32]). In cyclosporin A producers of the same genus, only 15–25% of the peptide produced is excreted.
Screenings have led to analogs with positional exchanges [33] and missing N-methylation in position 10 (Fig. 4). A total number of 32 analogs have been isolated so far from cyclosporin fermentations (Fig. 5). It is evident from the total number of observed changes in these analogs that only a selected set of peptides is formed in fermentation. The 20 alterations shown in Figure 5 permit the prediction of 72,000 structural analogs. However, most of these will not be formed by the system due to unefficient rates of formation leading to the early abortion of intermediates by hydro-

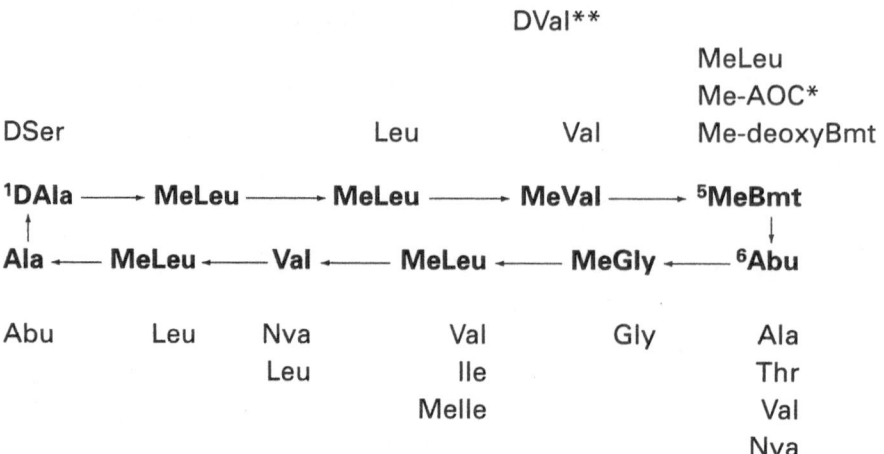

*N-methyl-L-aminooctanoic acid
**artefact during purification due to rearrangement

Fig. 5
Cyclosporins isolated from fermentation broth including feeding studies. All compounds are single-substituted analogs with the exception of cyclosporin F (5deoxy-MeBmt6Abu), cyclosporin K (5deoxy-MeBmt6Val), cyclosporin M (6,9Nva), cyclosporin O (5MeLeu6Nva), 6Nva9Leu-cyclosporin, 5MeLeu6Val-cyclosporin; demethylated cyclosporins are lacking an N-methyl in one position only, with the exception of cyclosporin R (positions 3 and 10).

lysis or side reactions. So e.g. inhibition of the N-methyl-transferase reaction in enniatin biosynthesis by e.g. sinefungin leads to the formation of unmethylated enniatins at a reduced rate of about 10% [34]. Although cyclosporin analogs with unmethylated peptides bonds have been found in six of the seven positions, no analogs have been observed with more than two methylations missing. This indicates that the rate of formation of peptides is then too slow to permit completion of synthesis. Besides the formation of piperazinediones no secondary products have been characterized so far, but can be expected to be present in the investigation of unidentified by-products in enzymatic synthesis [35].

2.3.2   Aureobasidin or R106

Aureobasidins are antifungal nonapeptidolactons produced by the black yeast *Aureobasidium pullulans* R106 [36–40]. So far 29 structural analogs have been isolated from fermentation broth (Fig. 6). Residues in positions 3, 5 and 8 have been exempt from variations, but recently precursor-directed biosynthesis permitted their substitution [41]. Structural varia-

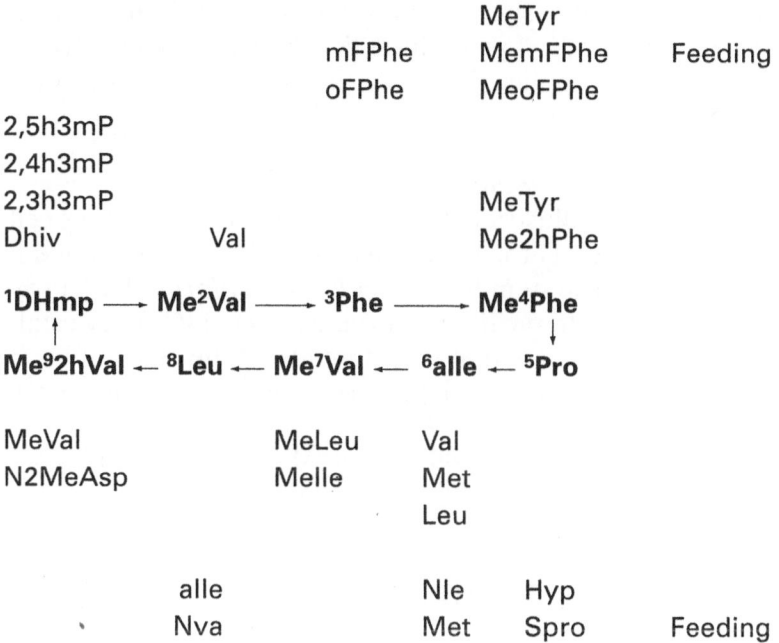

Fig. 6
Structural variations of aureobasidins isolated from fermentation broth with or without feeding of amino acid analogs.

tions direct to some extent the target specificities of these compounds. An interesting chemical approach to their modification is a tandem retro-aldol,aldol reaction replacing the amino acid preceding the lacton bond [42]. This work has demonstrated the importance of the configuration and presence of the tertiary alcohol (2-hydroxy-L-valine) for biological activity. Non-hydroxylated derivatives show no activity against *Cryptococcus*.

2.4   *In vitro* generation of peptides

The current state of the art requires (1) the identification of a growth phase in active production of the metabolite, (2) determination of a suitable time of harvest permitting the isolation of active and stable enzyme(s), and (3) evaluation of conditions for *in vitro* synthesis and stabilization. Generally, fungal systems actively produce peptides for periods of at least days, and are less sensitive for the time of harvest. Bacterial cultures like Bacilli may require harvesting periods of a few hours, only to be met by cooling the broth and using high efficiency flow-through centrifugation. Improvements have come from the design of continuous culture conditions [43, 44]. Once established, standard procedures for the isolation of intracellular enzymes are usually applied; however, they have not been successful in all cases, as illustrated below.

2.4.1   Generation of cell-free enzyme systems

A collection of pitfalls may illustrate the problems met in establishing cell-free systems. In bacitracin (I) formation, Wang et al. have succeeded in preparing a crude enzyme system from *Bacillus licheniformis* [45]. Frøyshov et al. have attempted to purify the enzyme system [46]. They established a period of harvest in a defined medium just at the onset of bacitracin production, permitting the isolation of a soluble multienzyme system.

$$[1](Ile \rightarrow Cys) \rightarrow Leu \rightarrow DGlu \rightarrow Ile \rightarrow Lys \rightarrow DOrn \rightarrow Ile \rightarrow DPhe$$
$$\uparrow \qquad\qquad\qquad\qquad\qquad \downarrow$$
$$Asn \leftarrow DAsp \leftarrow His$$

(I)

Within most of the production phase the enzyme system was membrane-attached and unstable. Although the purification and characterization of the three bacitracin synthetases was successful [47, 48], the purified system failed to produce bacitracin. The linear gramicidin (II) has been synthesized by a combination of enzymatic and chemical synthesis releasing the nascent pentadecapeptide with ethanolamine [49].

$$fVal \rightarrow Gly \rightarrow [3]Ala \rightarrow DLeu \rightarrow Ala \rightarrow DVal \rightarrow Val \rightarrow [8]DVal \rightarrow$$
$$Trp \rightarrow DLeu \rightarrow [11]Trp \rightarrow DLeu \rightarrow Trp \rightarrow DLeu \rightarrow Trp \rightarrow EA$$

(II)

Later it was shown by Kubota that this release is catalyzed from phosphatidylethanolamine in the membrane [50]. In the case of valinomycin (III), cells and protoplasts of *Streptomyces tsushimaensis* could be fed with labeled precursors to produce the labeled depsipeptide; however, all attempts to generate a cell-free system failed [51]. In the case of penicillin biosynthesis, the multienzyme forming the tripeptide precursor ACV (IV) was isolated from *Aspergillus nidulans*, *Acremonium chrysogenum*, and *Streptomyces clavuligerus* [52], but attempts to isolate ACV synthetase from *Penicillium chrysogenum* failed due to proteolysis. Later it was shown that ACV synthetase is at least partially associated with vacuolar membranes, while the enzymes processing ACV to isopenicillin N and penicillin G, isopenicillin N synthase and acyl transferase, respectively, are located in the cytoplasm or microbody-like organelles [53–55].

```
Val→DHiv—DVal→Lac
 |             |
Lac           Val         Aad→Cys→DVal
 ↑             ↓
DVal          DHiv            (IV)
 |             |
DHiv←Val—Lac ← DVal

        (III)
```

A major breakthrough in the development of fungal cell-free systems has been the extraction of freeze-dried mycelia with buffers containing up to 50% glycerol. With this procedure the synthesis of cyclic peptides like cyclosporin, SDZ 214-103 and SDZ 90-215 [56] was achieved. The outstanding sizes of peptide synthetases of about 400 to 1700 kDa could indicate low solubilities of these enzymes and thus permit salting out at relatively low ionic strength. Thus ammonium sulfate cuts (as low as 40% saturation) may be enriched by 10 to 30% in peptide synthetases in the total protein, when high producing strains are available.

Synthetase fractions are incubated with the constituent amino acids and ATP, in the case of N-methylated peptides with the addition of S-adenosyl-methionine [57]. The direct precursors have to be established in advance, since some precursors do have the D-configuration (D-Ala in cyclosporin), or even have to be hydroxylated in advance (D-4-hydroxyproline in neoviridogrisein) [58]. Other modifications, like hydroxylation, O-methylation, and N-hydroxylation remain to be established.

2.4.2   Gramicidin S synthetase

The gramicidin S synthetase system consists of two multienzymes, gramicidin S synthetases 1 and 2, with 125 and 512 kDa. Enzyme systems for the synthesis of the peptide and analogs employed both purified and reconstituted as well as ammonium sulfate preparations. Considerable efforts have been undertaken to stabilize the system and thus to compete with fermentational procedures for peptide production [45, 59]. The use of polymers like dextran and ficoll has been especially promising, achieving an operational stability of several days at room temperature [60, 61]. An overview of analogs produced is shown in Figure 7. Still proof of structural

D-CHA				
D-ThA[1]				
D-Trp				
D-OmTyr				
D-mTyr				
D-oTyr				
D-Tyr				
D-IPhe	Sar	Leu		
D-BrPhe	4S-Pro	Nva		
D-ClPhe	3S-Pro	Nle		
D-oFPhe	hPro	alle		Nle
D-mFPhe	Aze	Nle	Lys	alle
D-pFPhe	3,4ΔPro	Ile	Arg	Ile

$$^1DPhe \longrightarrow {}^2Pro \longrightarrow {}^3Val \longrightarrow {}^4Orn \longrightarrow {}^5Leu$$
$$\uparrow \qquad\qquad\qquad\qquad\qquad\qquad\qquad\qquad \downarrow$$
$$^{5'}Leu \longleftarrow {}^{4'}Orn \longleftarrow {}^{3'}Val \longleftarrow {}^{2'}Pro \longleftarrow {}^{1'}Dphe$$

Fig. 7

Analogs of gramicidin S obtained by *in vitro* enzymatic synthesis. Note that due to the symmetry of the compound in principle both mono- and disubstituted analogs may be found.

identity of most peptides is lacking, and their presence has been concluded from the introduction of labeled precursors and a similar behavior to gramicidin S.

2.4.3   Enniatin and beauvericin synthetases

Enniatin synthetase from *Fusarium oxysporum* was the first depsipeptide synthetase characterized [62], and has been used to produce a number of analogs (V) both in solution and its immobilized form [63, 64].

MeXxx→DHiv—MeXxx   MePhe→DHiv—MePhe
| ↓ | ↓
DHiv←MeXxx—DHiv   DHiv→MePhe—DHiv

(V)   (VI)

Immobilized multienzymes did not differ in stability from soluble enniatin synthetase. Synthetases producing analogs with branched chain amino acids from *Fusarium scirpi* and *Fusarium lateritium* have been purified and shown to differ in substrate selection [65]. The products thus depend primarily on the substrate binding site and less on the precursor availability. Beauvericin (VI), the insecticidal analog with phenylalanine replacing the aliphatic branched chains, is formed by beauvericin synthetase in *Beauveria bassiana*, and various other fungal producers. A respective synthetase has been isolated from a strain infecting larvae from *Lophyrotoma interrupta*, an Australian sawfly [66, 67]. While this enzyme accepted both aromatic and aliphatic substrates, enniatin synthetases did not activate aromatic substrates [66, 67]. Asymmetric enniatins have been prepared with amino acid mixtures [68]. Also the replacement with serine permits chemical modification of the cyclodepsipeptides to obtain more efficient compounds with nematocidal activities [69].

2.4.4 Cyclosporin synthetase

Characterization of the biosynthetic system forming cyclosporin from amino acid precursors was attempted employing procedures developed for fungal peptide synthetases, in particular the extraction of lyophilized mycelia with glycerol-containing buffers. First experiments employed a nitrosoguanidin-mutagenized strain of *Tolypocladium niveum*, and led to a 540-fold purified protein fraction [70]. This high molecular weight fraction catalyzed adenylate formation of the constituent amino acids, including D-alanine and Bmt. In addition, thioester attachment of valine and leucine as well as their N-methylated forms could be demonstrated. The fraction produced cyclo-D-alanyl-N-methyl-leucine, which was later shown to be the initiation point of biosynthesis. This piperazinedione is not usually detected in producer strains, but is found in the mycelium of a nonproducer mutant, *T. niveum* YP 582 [71]. Soon afterwards Billich and Zocher achieved total *in vitro* synthesis of cyclosporins using high glycerol concentrations in the initial extraction step, stabilizing the multienzyme fraction [57].

Characterization of the cyclosporin synthetase as a single polypeptide chain was carried out by Lawen and Zocher with a 72-fold purification to near-homogeneity from the high producer *T. niveum* 7939/45, correlating a very high molecular weight protein with biosynthetic activity [72]. The presence of methyltransferase activity was established by affinity labeling with S-adenosylmethionine. The synthetase also cross-reacted with monoclonal antibodies raised against the related fungal enniatin synthetase, and was shown to contain 4'-phosphopantetheine. The lack of marker proteins delayed correct size estimations considerably. Thus first estimates employing denaturing gel electrophoresis failed. Molecular cloning and sequence determination of ACV synthetases [52] and gramicidin S syn-

MeCys

DLys   MeSer
DPhe   MeaThr
DVal+   Me2a4m4HEA
DCys   MecyclodihydroBmt
DcyclopropylGly+   Me2a3h4buOA
1-Cl-D-vinylGly   MeNva+   Me2a3h4,8m$_2$NA
DtbuAla   MetbuGly   Me2a3h6OEA
2-F-DAla+   MetbuAla   Me2a3h4m$_2$OA+
2-Cl-DAla+   MeallylGly Me2a3h4mOA
β-Ala+   MeCPG+   MeNle
DAbu+   MealIe+   Me3hCHA+
Gly+   MeIle+   MeCHA

                                 Me-dihydroBmt
                                 Meleu
vinylGly   MeAOC*
DSer   Leu   Leu   Val Me-deoxyBmt

¹DAla ⟶ MeLeu ⟶ MeLeu ⟶ Me⁴Val ⟶ ⁵MeBmt
↑   **↓**
Ala ⟵ MeLeu ⟵ ⁹Val ⟵ MeLeu ⟵ MeGly ⟵ ⁶Abu

Abu   Leu   Nva   Val   Gly   Ala
                   Leu   Ile   Thr
                            MeIle   Val
                            Leu   Nva

Gly+   Ile+   allylGly
Nva   alle+   aThr
Nle   CPG   Cys
vinylGly   allylGly   Ile
Val   Abu   PPT
Cys   tbuAla
Phe   tbuGly
βAla

+ molecular mass by FAB-MS

thetase 2 [73, 74] provided reliable sizes for extrapolation, especially when the modular construction of peptide synthetases was employed to predict molecular weights. A size of 1.54 MDa was proposed for cyclosporin synthetase, and 1.46 MDa for SDZ 214-103 synthetase, lacking one methyltransferase function [75]. Cesium chloride density gradient centrifugation gave an estimate of 1.4 MDa, suffering however from variations of the sedimentation coefficients due to denaturation and the unknown shape of the synthetase. The cloning and sequence determination of the cyclodepsipeptide enniatin synthetase, which contains a methyltransferase function [76] permitted excellent estimations of the size, which were verified perfectly by Weber et al. [77] who analyzed the cyclosporin synthetase gene at 1.69 MDa. Thus the cyclosporin synthetase still presents the largest known enzyme polypeptide combining 40 catalytic functions. The multienzyme has been used to synthesize a variety of analogs in the milligram range [35, 78, 79] (Fig. 8).

2.4.5   SDZ 214-103 synthetase

The cyclosporin peptidolactone analog SDZ 214-103 (Fig. 4) differs from cyclosporin in four respects: replacement of the D-alanine in the initiating position by a respective hydroxy acid, omission of the second N-methylation function in position 3, substitution of aminobutyrate for threonine in position 6, and substitution of valine for leucine in position 9. The synthetase can be prepared in analogy to the cyclosporin system [80], and a comparative analysis [35] of substrate specificities has been carried out. With respect to cyclosporin the following observations were made (Fig. 9): substrate binding sites are more restricted, especially the Bmt site (position 5), and the threonine site (position 7). With the same sets of amino acid analogs only about half the number of peptide analogs were formed.

Fig. 8
Cyclosporins synthesized *in vitro*. Changed positions are indicated, and generally single replacements are reported, except for substitutions at positions 5 and 11 showing double replacement, or even triple replacement for 2,5 and 11 in case of e.g. Nva or allyl-glycine. Compounds directly placed at the cyclosporin A-structure were also isolated from fermentations and were available as reference compounds. All other compounds were described by chromatographic evidence or additional mass spectra (+). Abbreviations used are: Abu: aminobutyrate, allylGly: allyl-glycine, 2a3h4buOH: 2-amino-3-hydroxy-4-butyloctanoic acid; 2a3h4,8m2NA: 2-amino-3-hydroxy-4,8-dimethylnonanoic acid; 2a3h6OEA: 2-amino-3-hydroxyoct-6-enoic acid; 2a3h4m 2OA: 2-amino-3-hydroxy-4,4-dimethylocanoic acid; 2a4m4HEA: 2-amino-4-methylhex-4-enoic acid; AOC: aminooctanoic acid; CHA: cyclohexyl-alanine; 2-Cl-DAla: 2-chloro-D-alanine; CPG: cyclopropyl-glycine; cyclopropylGly: cyclopropyl-glycine; D: D-configuration; 2-F-DAla: 2-fluoro-D-alanine; 3hCHA: 3-hydroxy-cyclohexyl-alanine; Me: N-methyl-; Nle: norleucine; PPT: phosphinothricine; tbuAla: t-butyl-alanine; tbuGly: t-butyl-glycine (for details see [35]).

2hiCap+

D2h3mVa+	MetbuAla	
D2hVa+	MeallylGly	Me-dihydroBmt
D2hBu+	MeCPG	Me2a3h4mOA
vinylGly	MeaIle+	MeLeu*
DLac	MeAbu+	MeCHA

^{1}DHiv $\longrightarrow$ MeLeu $\longrightarrow$ Leu $\longrightarrow$ Me^{4}Val $\longrightarrow$ Me^{5}Bmt

Ala $\longleftarrow$ MeLeu $\longleftarrow$ ^{9}Leu $\longleftarrow$ MeLeu $\longleftarrow$ MeGly $\longleftarrow$ ^{6}Thr

Abu+	Leu	3hNva
vinylGly		Abu
Nva		Nva
Cys		Nle

+molecular mass by FAB-MS

Fig. 9
Analogs of SDZ 214-103 synthesized *in vitro* [35]. For abbreviations compare Fig. 8.

Perhaps the cyclization of a lactone is more restricted than the cyclization of a peptide.

2.4.6   *SDZ 90-215 synthetase*

Similar to cyclosporin and SDZ 214-103 this synthetase was prepared from freeze-dried mycelia of *Septoria* sp. as a 1.2 MDa polypeptide [81]. An ammonium sulfate fraction was partially purified by gel chromatography and found to produce the peptolide SDZ 90-215 (VII) from the set of precursors using both tyrosine and O-methyl-tyrosine. Efficiency, however, was reduced by about 90% in the incorporation of tyrosine, which implies that the modified compound is the actual substrate used *in vivo*. Thus it may be concluded that the respective O-methyl-transferase is still present in this enzyme fraction.

^{1}DLac→Pip→MeVal→Val→MeAsp

OMeTyr←MeVal←Gly←MeIle←MeIle

(VII)

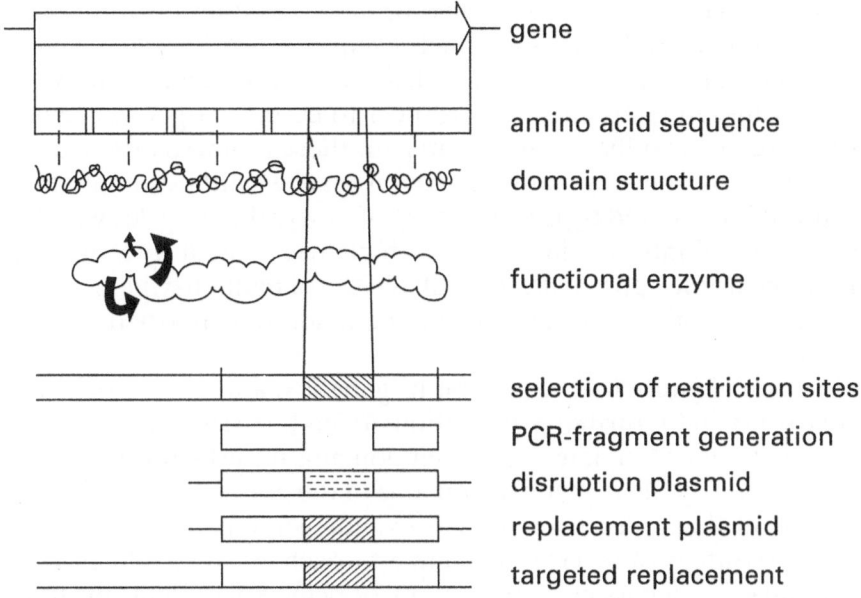

gene

amino acid sequence

domain structure

functional enzyme

selection of restriction sites

PCR-fragment generation

disruption plasmid

replacement plasmid

targeted replacement

Fig. 10
Domain replacement strategy in the construction of new peptide synthetases. This approach assumes that exchanged protein domains function properly within the given synthetase framework. After identification of the respective gene sequence, the amino acid sequence is deduced and permits the localization of modules and domains. The synthesis of peptides is accomplished by the interaction of domains in transferring activated intermediates. A respective enzyme site to be replaced by e.g. a domain of altered amino acid activating properties is selected, and suitable restriction sites next to its boundaries are determined or introduced. The respective homologous sequences for recombination are prepared by PCR A disruption segment, e.g. conferring a resistance marker is introduced and a suitable vector plasmid is constructed. By recombination this plasmid will knock out biosynthetic activity and express the introduced trait instead. The altered sequence is then introduced by a similar replacement plasmid, and has to be counterselected for loss of property, thus restoring the biosynthetic activity [82].

3 Perspectives

It is now well established that many peptides originate from a nonribosomal enzymatic system with common features throughout all available sources. The organization of this system represents sequential condensation processes met also in polyketide biosynthesis, and is directed at the gene level by the modular arrangement of encoded functional units. Although apparently of less restricted specificity than the ribosomal mechanism with its proofreading functions, the process is nevertheless highly restrictive in some respects. Certain positions are strictly conserved, and no alterations have been found *in vivo* or *in vitro*. Other positions may be readily exchanged by analogs. Such exchanges are directed by the respective enzyme sites selecting the substrates. These findings imply the selection of these metabolites with respect to certain target molecules, and the conserved residues seem essential for those required interactions. Thus the multienzyme templates are useful for the synthesis of analogs, but their use is restricted by the efficiency of biosynthetic cycles with the respective altered intermediates. These efficiencies obviously limit their use in combinatorial approaches, but still the use of multienzymes for peptide synthesis has proved an elegant and simple solution in structure function analysis.

The alteration of multienzyme systems by genetic manipulation offers an attractive solution for further exploitations. It has been shown by Stachelhaus et al. [82] that adenylate and carrier domains in surfactin synthetase may be replaced by the respective domains of the gramicidin S system or the fungal penicillin precursor synthetase, yielding new peptide structures. The general strategy of this replacement approach is shown in Figure 10. Current studies are focussing on the general principles underlying the functioning of these systems so as to permit the construction of enzyme systems for any desired structure.

References

1   Kleinkauf, H., and von Döhren, H.: Eur. J. Biochem. *192*, 1 (1990).
2   Kleinkauf, H., and von Döhren, H.: Eur. J. Biochem. *236*, 335 (1996).
3   Cosmina, P., Rodriguez, F., de Ferra, F., Grandi, G., Perego, M., Venema, G., and van Sinderen, D.: Mol. Microbiol. *8*, 821 (1993).
4   Conti, E., Franks, N., and Brick, P.: Structure *4*, 287 (1996).
5   Pavela-Vrancic, M., Pfeifer, E., van Liempt, H., Schäfer, H.-J., von Döhren, H., and Kleinkauf, H.: Biochem. *33*, 6276 (1994).
6   Pavela-Vrancic, M., Pfeifer, E., Schröder, W., von Döhren, H. and Kleinkauf, H.: J. Biol. Chem. *269*, 14962 (1994).
7   Dieckmann, R., Pavela-Vrancic, M., von Döhren, H., and Kleinkauf, H. (submitted 1996).
8   Etchegaray, A.: Thesis, University of Sheffield 1995.
9   Stein, T., and Vater, J.: Amino Acids *10*, 201 (1996).
10   Lambalot, R., and Walsh, C.: J. Biol. Chem. *270*, 24658 (1995).
11   Schwecke, T.: Thesis Technical University Berlin 1993.
12   Holak, T.A., Kearsley, S.K., Kim, Y., and Prestegard, J.H.: Biochem. *27*, 6135 (1988).
13   Lambalot et al., manuscript submitted.
14   Marahiel et al., manuscript in press.
15   Pfeifer et al., unpublished data.
16   Kleinkauf, H., and von Doehren, H.: Progr. Drug Res. *41*, 287 (1990).

17 Dieckmann et al., manuscript in preparation.
18 de Crécy-Lagard, V., Marliere, P., and Saurin, W.: C.R. Acad. Sci. Paris, Life Sci. *318*, 927 (1995).
19 Stindl, A., and Keller, U.: Biochem. *33*, 9358 (1994).
20 Shiau, C.-Y., Baldwin, J.E., Byford, M.F., Sobey, W.J., and Schofield, C.J.: FEBS Lett. *358*, 97 (1995).
21 Shiau, C.-Y., Baldwin, J.E., Byford, M.F., and Schofield, C.J.: FEBS Lett *375*, 303 (1995).
22 Kallow et al., manuscript in preparation.
23 Billich, A., and Zocher, R.: Biochem. *26*, 8417 (1987).
24 Haese, A., Schubert, M., Herrmann, M., and Zocher, R.: Mol. Microbiol. *7*, 905 (1993).
25 Weber, G., Schoergendorfer, K., Schneider-Scherzer, E., and Leitner, E.: Curr. Genet. *26*, 125 (1994).
26 Burmester, J., Haese, A., and Zocher, R.: Biochem. Mol. Biol. Int. *37*, 201 (1995).
27 Scott-Craig, J.S., Panaccione, D.G., Pocard, J.-A., and Walton, J.D.: J. Biol. Chem. *267*, 26044 (1992).
28 Baltz, R.H.: 6th Conf. Genetics Mol. Biol. Industr. Microorg., Bloomington, Indiana 1996.
29 Thiericke, R. and Rohr, J.: Natural Prod. Rep. *12*, 265 (1993).
30 Kleinkauf, H., and von Döhren, in: Fungal Biotechnology (T. Anke, ed.) Chapman & Hall, Weinheim, in press (1996).
31 Kobel, H., and Traber, R.: Eur. J. Appl. Microbiol. Biotechnol. *14*, 237 (1986).
32 Nakajima, H., Hamasaki, T., Tanaka, K., et al.: Agr. Biol. Chem. *53*, 2291 (1989).
33 Sakamoto, K., Tsuji, E., Miyauchi, M., Nakanishi, T., Yamashita, M., Shigematsu, N., Tada, T., Izumi, S., and Okuhara, M.: J. Antibiot. *46*, 1788 (1993).
34 Billich, A., and Zocher, R.: in Biochemistry of Peptide Antibiotics (Kleinkauf, H., von Döhren, H., eds.) pp. 57–80, de Gruyter, Berlin 1990.
35 Lawen, A., and Traber, R.: J. Biol. Chem. *268*, 20452 (1993).
36 Yoshikawa, Y., Ikai, K., Umdea, Y., Ogawa, A., Takesako, K., Kato, I., and Naganawa, H.: J. Antibiot. *46*, 1347 (1993).
37 Takesako, K., Kuroda, H., Inoue, T., Haruna, F., Yohikawa, Y., Kato, I., Uchida, K., Hiratani, T., and Yamaguchi, H.: J. Antibiot. *46*, 1414 (1993).
38 Ikai, K., Takesako, K., Shiomi, K., Moriguchi, M., Umeda, Y., Yamamoto, J., Kato, I., and Naganawa, H.: J. Antibiot. *44*, 925 (1991).
39 Ikai, K., Shiomi, K., Takesako, K., Mizutani, S., Yamamoto, J., Ogawa, Y., Ueno, M., and Kato, I.: J. Antibiot. *44*, 1187 (1991).
40 Awazu, N., Ikai, K., Yumamoto, J., Nishimura, K., Mizutani, S., Takesako, K., and Kato, I.: J. Antibiot. *48*, 525 (1995).
41 Takesako, K., Mizutani, S., Sakakibara, H., Endo, M., Yoshikawa, Y., Msuda, T., Sono-Koyama, E., and Kato, I.: J. Antibiot. *49*, 676 (1996).
42 Rodriguez, M.J., Zweifel, M.J., Farmer, J.D., Gordee, R.S., and Loncharich, R.J.: J. Antibiot. *49*, 386 (1996).
43 Tzeng, C.H., Thrasher, K.D., Montgomery, J.P., Hamilton, B.K., and Wang, D.I.C.: Biotechnol. Bioeng. *17*, 143 (1975).
44 Chiu, C.W., Bernhard, T., and Dellweg, G., in: Peptide Antibiotics – Biosynthesis and Functions (H. Kleinkauf, H. von Döhren, eds.), p. 149, De Gruyter, Berlin 1982.
45 Wang, D.I.C., Stramondo, J., and Fleischaker, R., in : Biotechnological Applications of Proteins and Enzymes (Z. Bohak, N. Sharon, eds.) p.183, Academic Press, New York 1977.

52   Horst Kleinkauf and Hans von Döhren

46   Frøyshov, Ø.: FEBS Lett. *81*, 315 (1977).
47   Frøyshov, Ø.: Eur. J. Biochem. *59*, 201 (1975).
48   Roland, I., Frøyshov, Ø., and Laland, S.G.: FEBS Lett. *84*, 22 (1977).
49   Bauer, K., Roskoski, R., Jr., Kleinkauf, H., and Lipmann, F.: Biochem. *11*, 3266 (1972).
50   Kubota, K.: Biochem. Biophys. Res. Comm. *144*, 203 (1987).
51   Mamutoglu, I.: Thesis TU Berlin 1978.
52   Aharonowitz, Y., Bergmeyer, H., Cantoral, J.M., Cohen, G., Demain, A.L., Fink, U., Kinghorn, J., Kleinkauf, H., MacCabe, A., Palissa, H., Pfeifer, E., Schwecke, T., van Liempt, H., von Döhren, H., Wolfe, S., and Zhang, J.: Bio/technol. *11*, 807 (1993).
53   Müller, W.H.. van der Krift, T.P., Krouwer, A.J.J., Wösten, H.A.B., van der Voort, L.H.M., Smaal, E.B., and Verklej, A.J.: EMBO J. *10*, 489 (1991).
54   Müller, W.H., Bovenberg, R.A.L., Groothuis, M.H., Kattevilder, A., Smaal, E.B., van der Voort, L.H.M., and Verklej, A.J.: Biochim. Biophys. Acta *1116*, 210 (1992).
55   Lendenfeld, T., Ghali, D., Wolschek, M., Kubicek-Pranz, E.M., and Kubicek, C.P.: J. Biol. Chem. *268*, 665 (1993).
56   Lee, C., and Lawen, A.: Biochem. Mol. Biol. Int. *31*, 797 (1993).
57   Billich, A., and Zocher, R.: Biochem. *26*, 8417 (1987).
58   Okumura, Y., in : Biochemistry and Genetic Regulation of Commercially Important Antibiotics (L.C. Vining, ed.) p. 147, Addison-Wesley, Reading, MA 1983.
59   Kleinkauf, H., and von Döhren, H., in: Advances in Biotechnology, Vol. 3 (Vezina C., and Singh, K., eds.) pp.83, Pergamon Press, Oxford 1981.
60   Kirchner, A.: Thesis TU Berlin 1989.
61   Kirchner, A., Simonis, M., and von Döhren, H.: J. Chromatogr. *396*, 199 (1987).
62   Zocher, R., Keller, U., and Kleinkauf, H.: Biochem. *21*, 43 (1982).
63   Madry, N., Zocher, R., Grodzki, K., and Kleinkauf, H.: Appl. Microbiol. Biotechnol. *20*, 83 (1984).
64   Siegbahn, N., Mosbach, K., Grodzki, K., Zocher, R., Madry, N., and Kleinkauf, H.: Biotechnol. Lett. *7*, 297 (1985).
65   Pieper, R., Kleinkauf, H., and Zocher, R.: J. Antibiot. *45*, 1273 (1992).
66   Peeters, H.: Thesis TU Berlin 1988.
67   Peeters, H., Zocher, R., Madry, N., Oelrichs, P.B., Kleinkauf, H., and Kraepelin, G.: J. Antibiot. *36*, 1762 (1983).
68   Krause, M., Miyamoto, K., Stindl, A., Zocher, R., Jeschke, P., Thielking, G., and Bonse, G.: Proc. Symp. Enzymology of biosynthesis of natural products, Technical University Berlin, abstract 67 (1996).
69   Jeschke, P., Kleinkauf, H., Zocher, R., Harder, A., Bonse, G., Etzel, W., Schindler, M., Göhrt, A., Gau, W., and Thielking, G.: Proc. Symp. Enzymology of biosynthesis of natural products, Technical University Berlin, abstract 68 (1996).
70   Zocher, R., Nihira, T., Paul, E., Madry, N., Peeters, H., Kleinkauf, H., and Keller, U.: Biochem. *25*, 550 (1986).
71   Dittmann, J., Lawen, A., Zocher, R., and Kleinkauf, H.: Biol. Chem. Hoppe-Seyler *371*, 829 (1990).
72   Lawen, R., and Zocher, R.: J. Biol.Chem. *265*, 11355 (1990).
73   Turgay, K., Krause, M., and Marahiel, M.A.: Mol. Microbiol. *6*, 529 (1992).
74   Saito, F., Hori, K., Kanda, M., Kurotsu, T., and Saito, Y.: J. Biochem. *116*, 357 (1994).
75   Schmidt, B., Riesner, D., Lawen, A., and Kleinkauf, H.: FEBS Lett. *307*, 355 (1992).
76   Haese, A., Schubert, M., Herrmann ,M., and Zocher, R.: Mol. Microbiol. *7*, 905 (1993).
77   Weber, G., Schmorgendörfer, K., Schneider-Scherzer, E., and Leitner, E.: Curr. Genet. *26*, 120 (1994).

78   Lawen, A., Traber, R., Geyl, D., Zocher, R., and Kleinkauf, H.: J. Antibiot. *42*, 1283 (1989).
79   Lawen, A., Traber, R., Reuille, R., and Ponelle, M.: Biochem. J. *300*, 395 (1994).
80   Lawen, A., Traber, R., and Geyl, D.: J. Biol. Chem. *266*, 15567 (1991).
81   Lee, C., and Lawen, A.: Biochem. Mol. Biol. Int. *31*, 797 (1993).
82   Stachelhaus, T., Schneider, A., and Marahiel, M.A.: Science *269*, 69 (1995).
83   Sakamoto, K., Tsuji, E., Miyauchi, M., Nakanishi, T., Yamashita, M., Shigematsu, N., Tada, T., Izumi, S., and Okuhara, M.: J. Antibiot. *46*, 1788–98 (1993).

Progress in Drug Research, Vol. 48 (E. Jucker, Ed.)
© 1997 Birkhäuser Verlag, Basel (Switzerland)

The role of apoptosis in neurodegenerative diseases

By Iradj Hajimohamadreza and J. Mark Treherne

Department of Discovery Biology, Pfizer Central Research, Sandwich, Kent
CT13 9NJ, UK

1   Introduction

Apoptosis is a single word that describes the complex contortions of the membrane and organelles of a cell as it goes through the process of programmed cell death. During this process, the cell activates an intrinsic suicide programme and systematically destroys itself. Apoptosis occurs rapidly, usually taking between a few minutes and a couple of hours, and can be fascinating to watch in real time down a microscope. The following series of events can be observed: the cell surface begins to bleb and express pro-phagocytic signals, and the cell then separates from its neighbours. The nucleus also goes through a characteristic pattern of morphological changes as it commits genetic suicide: the chromatin condenses and is specifically cleaved to fragments of DNA (Fig. 1). The whole apoptotic cell then fragments into membrane-bound vesicles that are rapidly and cleanly disposed of by phagocytosis, so that there is minimal damage to the surrounding tissue.

Although the word "apoptosis" was first used in this context almost a quarter of a century ago (see section 2 below), it is only in the last five years that research into this phenomenon has really taken off in terms of understanding the underlying molecular mechanisms. Consequently, publications have continued to increase exponentially with time with the realisation that apoptosis research has moved from mostly descriptive cell biology to detailed studies on the mechanisms driving the machinery of cell death. Nevertheless, there is still much that is unknown about what must be a very tightly controlled process, if the number of cells that make up an organism are to remain constant. The recent flurry of research has produced a prodigious number of important mediators and inhibitors of cell death but the precise mechanisms by which they all interact to regulate the process is still far from clear. For example, oncoproteins, tumour suppresser proteins, growth factors and intracellular signalling pathways all seem able to induce apoptosis and yet the same group of factors can also suppress it. However, all these diverse factors that can modulate the apoptotic process do, eventually, trigger a relatively simple downstream suicide programme that appears to have remained well conserved throughout evolution [1].

The intense rate at which publications on apoptosis are appearing in the literature has resulted in a number of good reviews [e.g. 2–11] on the subject but comparatively few have focused on neuronal and glial apoptosis [12–14] and comprehensively tackled the vexing questions relating to the role of apoptosis in neurodegenerative diseases. Consequently, we decided to write this review, with particular reference to the therapeutic potential that will come from a better understanding of the cellular mechanisms underlying the neuropathology. There is certainly no shortage of poten-

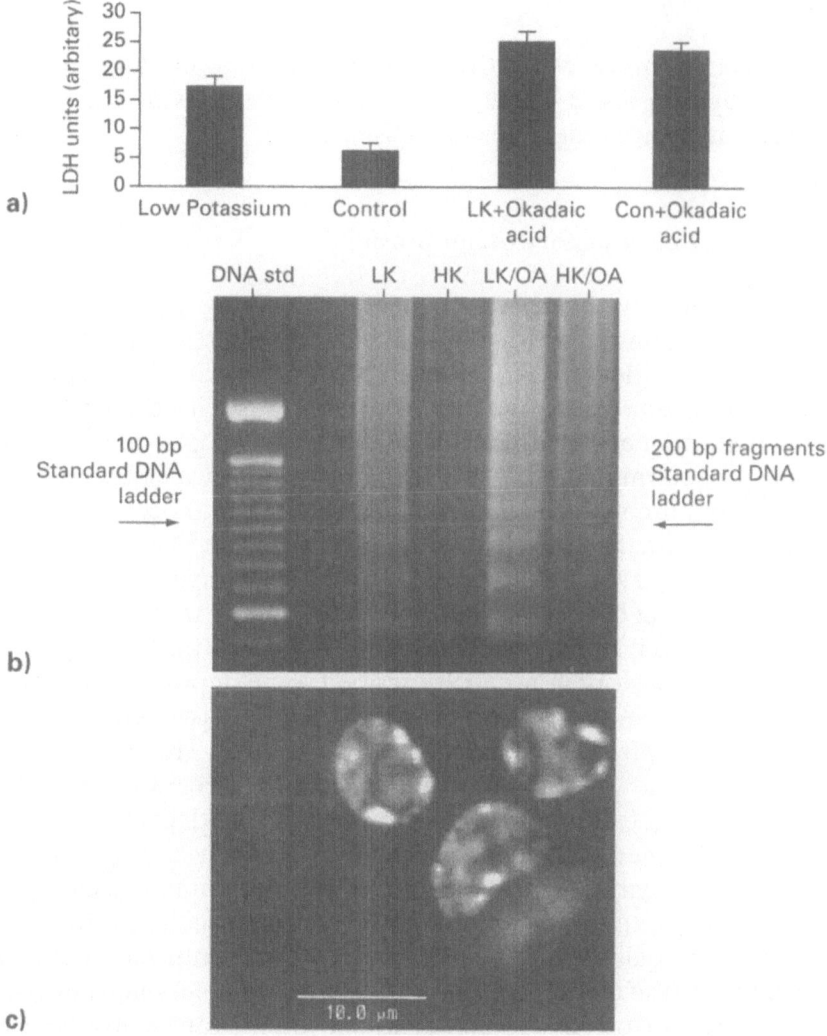

Fig. 1
Apoptosis is induced in cerebellar granule neurones by either a lack of depolarising stimulus (i.e. low-potassium, 5 mM) or 100 nM okadaic acid (a potent protein phosphatase 1 and 2A inhibitor) for 2 hours. Apoptosis is readily evident in these primary neuronal cultures 24 hours after the challenges mentioned above. (a) lactate dehydrogenase measurement in culture media and (b) corresponding DNA laddering following exposure to low-potassium and okadaic acid challenges. Control cultures are maintained in media containing depolarising concentration of potassium (i.e. 30 mM KCl). (c) Apoptotic nuclei in SH-SY5Y cells. Chromatin condensation is another hallmark of apoptosis which can be visualised by various dyes (e.g. bis-benzimide/-Hoechst 33258 and SYTO11). Human neuroblastoma cells (SH-SY5Y) undergo apoptosis with an oxidative challenge (i.e. H_2O_2). Nuclear condensation is visualised by SYTO11 staining in SH-SY5Y cells 4 hours after 200 µM H_2O_2 addition. Three cells with condensed nuclei can be seen (centre of field). Normal nuclei, which are larger and less intensely stained, appear in the same field. We would like to acknowledge Dr Paul Hayter (Pfizer Central Research) for his contribution in obtaining these results.

tial mechanisms by which drugs could be used to modulate the cell biology of apoptosis but which ones are the most relevant for the potential treatment of neurodegenerative diseases?

2   A brief history of apoptosis

Researchers have been describing and classifying the morphology of cell death during ontogeny for almost half a century [e.g. 15] but the term programmed cell death was first used to describe larval metamorphosis in insects [16]. As with many other invertebrate species, the strikingly organised pattern of cell death during silk-moth development appeared to follow a predetermined sequence. Protein synthesis was subsequently shown to be a requirement for programmed cell death to occur [17], which was consistent with the cell actively committing suicide. The term apoptosis was first coined in 1972 [18], from the Greek *apo* (away from) and *ptosis* (falling), which can be used to describe leaves falling from a tree but it is still not clear how it should be pronounced [19, 20]: is the second "p" silent or not? This new word, however, described some important new discoveries in cell biology: Kerr, Wyllie and Currie identified two separate patterns of cell death when studying hepatic ischaemia [17]. The first was described as necrosis and was characterised by a rapid increase in cell volume and the early loss of membrane integrity once the death process started. Mitochondria swelled, the nucleus became pyknotic, lysosomal contents were lost and the dying cell was associated with inflammatory changes, resulting in damage to the surrounding tissue. Apoptosis, by contrast, was characterised by maintenance of membrane integrity until very late in the death process and the membrane showed pronounced blebbing and cell volume decreased (up to a 30% reduction in cell volume can be observed). Shrinkage of cells during apoptosis was thought to be due to the net movement of fluid out of the cell (a possible mechanism to account for this displacement of fluid is inhibition of the Na^+-K^+-Cl^- co-transporter system). The structure of organelles was preserved but the chromatin condensed in the nucleus, which went on to fragment. As cellular fragments continued to bud off and form apoptotic bodies, their lysosomal contents remained intact. *In vivo*, these fragments are consumed by phagocytosis but in most *in vitro* systems, this cannot occur and consequently swelling and lysis is observed (which is also referred to as "secondary necrosis").
This fundamental process of cell biology appeared to occur during normal turnover of adult tissues as well as during pathological conditions [18] but perhaps the most obvious physiological role of apoptosis was found to be

during development. For example, apoptosis of the interdigital webs is required for normal development of hands and paws of mammals but an even more dramatic example is found in invertebrate species: when larvae completely remodel to take on the adult form, such as when the tadpole loses its tail to become a frog [17]. Apoptosis was also found to play an important role in the turnover of rapidly dividing tissue, such as intestinal villi [18] and lymphocytes [21]. These observations led to the idea that a decrease in the rate of apoptosis could have severe pathological consequences and lead to the growth of tumours, such as in B-cell lymphoma [21].

Immunologists have also developed a strong interest in the apoptotic process, as it can play an important role in the development of the appropriate immune response and host's response to viral infection. For example, when the initial antibody response to infection with relatively low-affinity antibodies is replaced by the production of high-affinity antibodies (affinity maturation), it was found that the selection of the B-cells depended on apoptosis. The cells that only produce low-affinity antibodies against the antigen died by apoptosis [22]. This process selects against the manufacture of low-affinity antibodies, so that higher affinity antibodies are produced to more effectively combat the infection. A further example of the relevance of apoptotic cell death to immunology is that cells infected by viruses often die by apoptosis. Infection with HIV (human immunodeficiency virus) was found to kill CD4 cells by priming them for antigen-mediated apoptosis [23, 24]. When an infected cell dies through apoptosis, this can stop or slow down the replication of the virus, so a number of viruses have developed mechanisms to slow apoptosis of the host cell. Thus, when baculovirus infects insect cells, apoptosis is inhibited by the *p35* gene [25] and if *p35* was expressed early enough following baculovirus infection, cells that would have died within hours were found to survive for several days. This allowed viral production to increase by up to 15,000-fold [26]. Subsequently, a further series of viral anti-apoptotic genes have been discovered: cowpox virus *crmA*, adenovirus *e1b*, Epstein-Barr virus *bhrf1* and *lmp-1*, and from the SV40 virus, the large T antigen gene. These genes will be discussed later on, as they have proved to be useful tools to dissect the molecular mechanisms that drive the machinery of apoptosis (see section 7.1).

3   Apoptosis versus necrosis

As mentioned above, Kerr, Wyllie and Currie were the first to draw a clear distinction between the morphology of apoptosis and necrosis in 1972 [18].

Today, however, patterns of cell death are often observed which do not exactly fit the two stereotyped extremes described by Kerr and colleagues. This is not entirely surprising, as the word apoptosis, now as then, essentially describes what a cell looks like as it commits to die and does not identify the precise molecular mechanisms involved. As multiple "death mechanisms" can be activated within a dying cell in different orders and at different rates, not all dying cells look the same. Consequently, features of apoptosis and necrosis can both be observed in a single cell as it undergoes the process of dying. To a lesser or greater extent, the patterns of cell death observed and mechanisms employed vary with the type of cell and the initial triggers of the death process. This means that, although there are many common features of apoptosis between all cell types, lesson learned about the cell biology of, say, a dying fibroblast cannot be simply transferred to a neurone dying during a neurodegenerative disease. This is an important point because it is consistent with the existence of specific neuronal drug targets for the treatment of chronic neurodegeneration, inhibition of which would not inhibit apoptosis throughout the body. Chronic administration of a drug that inhibited or slowed all apoptosis throughout the body, could have potentially serious consequences for tumour growth, the immune response and the turnover of the intestinal lining, for example.

Although there has been some blurring of the differences between apoptosis and necrosis, there are distinct themes that remain true. Apoptosis is more likely to occur during more physiological events such as ontogeny or cell turnover in adult tissues, where there are clear advantages in minimising damage to surrounding cells. In these circumstances, apoptosis can be seen, from the perspective of neighbouring cells, as a more "friendly" form of death. In pathology, cells that are challenged by virtually any insult below the threshold for inducing classical necrosis, may well undergo apoptosis. A simple example of this is when cultured cells are heated at 43°C for an hour and are often observed to undergo apoptosis, whereas heating the same cells to 45°C for an hour results in necrosis [27]. Similar responses have been observed when using hydrogen peroxide as a challenge: low concentrations produce apoptosis whereas higher concentrations produce necrosis. Calcium ionophores and toxic agents can also be used to demonstrate a similar phenomenon [28].

The criteria for rigorously defining apoptosis still depends heavily on the morphological characteristics described in the previous section [18], particularly as genetic and biochemical markers can vary from one cell type to another [29]. However, a distinctive feature of apoptosis at the biochemical level is DNA fragmentation [30, 31]. Initially, DNA is cleaved into

100 to 300 kilobases [32] and then further cleaved by endonucleases into internucleosomal fragments. Chromatin is made up of stands of DNA which are surrounded by histone octomers at regular intervals. During apoptosis, cleavage between histone octomers results in single nucleosome lengths of DNA, approximately 180 base-pairs long. Although internucleosomal DNA fragmentation is an early event in apoptosis, it does not appear to be essential, as some cells can undergo apoptosis without any internucleosomal cleavage [29]. However, when endonucleases are inhibited by non-specific agents such as zinc or aurintricarboxylic acid (ATA), apoptosis can be blocked in most cells [33, 34]. The apoptotic process in cells is energy dependent and can often depend on the synthesis of new proteins. This is a key difference from necrosis, where the cells' energy supply fails and protein synthesis is halted.

4   Apoptosis during neuronal development

Neuronal cell death is a striking feature of ontogeny and plays an important role in ensuring that the nervous system develops normally [35, 36]. It appears that the death of developing neurones depends on the size of the target that they innervate: cells with fewer synaptic partners are more likely to die than those that have formed multiple synapses [37]. This may reflect a process which balances the relative number of pre- to postsynaptic neurones in the developing nervous system. Although neuronal cell death was assumed to be apoptotic by most developmental biologists, it was only comparatively recently that neurones in developing rodent brain were conclusively shown to undergo apoptosis, as classified by morphology and DNA fragmentation [38, 39]. As cell death during development is clearly not a pathological process, it makes sense that cells die by apoptosis rather than by necrosis and, therefore, limit damage to neighbouring cells. Apoptosis during ontogeny is a fascinating subject but is not directly relevant to this review and, consequently, it has only been described very briefly here.

5   Methods for detecting neural apoptosis

Before examining the evidence for the role for apoptosis during neurodegenerative diseases, it is worth discussing the relative merits of the different techniques used to detect apoptosis in neurones and glia. A variety of methods have been widely used to detect apoptosis, since there is no single experiment that can definitively classify the phenomenon. There are three broad groupings of these techniques: 1) changes in nuclear morphology and DNA labelling; 2) morphological changes, such as perturbations in the plasma membrane and expression of cell surface markers used in cellular recognition by phagocytes; 3) pharmacological experiments, where protection from or delaying death can be demonstrated by nuclease inhibition, manipulation of anti-oxidant enzymes, transcriptional or translational inhibitors, and suicide enzyme inhibitors or modulation of other protein components (e.g. *bcl-2*, see section 7.5.2) of the apoptotic pathways. None of these techniques on their own can be thought of as a definitive test for apoptosis for two reasons: 1) the complexity of the cell death process means that multiple biochemical pathways direct cell fate and so inhibitors of, or markers for, a particular pathway may not always work; 2) the detection methods themselves also have certain limitations. A good example to illustrate this is the problems that have been encountered with commonly used DNA labelling assays (e.g. TdT mediated dUTP-biotin nick end labelling or TUNEL). Some cells can be observed with swollen intracellular organelles, a hallmark of necrosis, but they can also show positive TUNEL staining, since the terminal deoxynucleotidyl transferase can sometimes gain access to the fragmented DNA. Consequently, cells that are dying by necrosis could be counted as apoptotic false positives. This can be particularly confusing *in vivo*, where it is more difficult to follow the time course or ultimate fate of cells undergoing apoptosis. Furthermore, the number of apoptotic cells may be relatively few and far between in brain sections derived from *in vivo* experiments, making it difficult and time consuming to generate accurate data.

In vitro experiments can also be fraught with difficulties. Quantification of apoptosis in cell lines can be complicated by the phenomenon of "secondary necrosis". In cultures containing no phagocytic cells, previously apoptotic cells are not engulfed by phagocytes and live on to become necrotic: these cells are then miscounted as necrotic instead of apoptotic. By contrast, apoptotic cells can usually be cleared by phagocytosis in primary cultures or *in vivo*, so counting apoptotic bodies at a single time point may considerably underestimate the proportion of cells that die by apoptosis. As mentioned above, a lack of evidence for DNA laddering should not always be taken as definitively exposing of a lack of apoptosis and this is particularly true where multiple signalling pathways are involved. A further complication is that both apoptotic and necrotic cell death may play a parallel role in the pathology of a particular neurodegenerative disease.

There is often disagreement between different laboratories when the relative importance of necrosis and apoptosis to various neurodegenerative diseases are discussed. Even when similar methods of inducing and detecting neuronal cell death are used, there are often conflicting results reported from different laboratories, particularly when whole animal and primary cell culture models are used. The severity and the duration of the "pathological challenge" can have a major effect on the pattern of death observed. When cortical neurones are maintained in primary culture and exposed to peroxynitrite, they have been shown to die by necrosis or apoptosis, depending on the intensity of the insult [40]. A major source of variation between different laboratories probably results from slight differences in the culture methods used: such as differences in serum, growth factors, the age of cultures and plating densities, which can all affect the propensity of cells to die. When using primary cultures, it is equally important to standardise the developmental age of neural tissue used, since developmental differences may well affect their intrinsic survival: younger tissues are generally more resistant to injury. As many of these variables as possible should be standardised, if valid comparisons are to be made between different experimental protocols. Consequently, all these factors must be considered when comparing experiments described in the literature and we have applied these criteria as rigorously as we can to our analysis of the data described in the following sections.

6   Apoptosis during neurodegenerative diseases

Neurones of the central and peripheral nervous system are relatively unique in the body, since they are post-mitotic and, therefore, largely irreplaceable. Although there are many commonalties which can be observed in the apoptotic process between different neurodegenerative diseases, we have chosen to discuss each disease separately to allow analysis of the evidence for the role of apoptosis in the course of pathology on a case by case basis. A more detailed analysis of the cellular mechanisms involved follows in section 7.

6.1   Parkinson's disease

Parkinson's disease is characterised by a progressive degeneration of dopaminergic neurones in the substantia nigra and these neurones in postmortem sections from Parkinson's patients have demonstrated some of the characteristics of apoptosis: cell shrinkage and chromatin condensation.

Furthermore, the expression of factors involved in mediating apoptosis, such as *bcl-2* (see section 7.5) and TNF-α (tumour necrosis factor-α) were detected in the substantia nigra of these patients [41]. *In vivo* models of Parkinson's disease have also been used to suggest a role for apoptosis in the human pathology. For example, degeneration of striatal dopamine neurones was induced in the rat by systemic reserpine treatment and the dying neurones showed morphological characteristics of apoptosis and DNA fragmentation was observed [42]. Since this striatal apoptosis was also blocked by glutamate antagonists, it is possible that removal of dopaminergic inhibition in the striatum may lead to higher levels of endogenous glutamate, which would induce apoptosis in striatal projections. In mice, MPTP (1-methyl-4-phenyl-1,2,3,6-tetrahydropyridine) is used to kill dopaminergic neurones and produce a model of Parkinson's disease. MPTP produces selective degeneration of dopaminergic neurones and apoptosis has been observed following this challenge by measuring DNA fragmentation [43]. However, another report found no evidence for apoptosis in MPTP-induced death in dopaminergic neurones [44].

In addition to the *in vivo* work described above, much work has focused on the use of dopaminergic cells in culture to model this degenerative process in man. When cultures of dopaminergic neurones are deprived of specific growth factors, they are observed to undergo apoptosis [45, 46]. Consequently, when the levels of growth factors available to neurones are limiting, this mode of death may predominate and amelioration by exogenous growth factor administration may eventually prove useful in the clinic [47, 48]. Further evidence is consistent with the hypothesis that neuronal loss may also be initiated in the disease by as yet unidentified endogenous neurotoxins. Neurotoxic death can be induced by the selective dopaminergic neurotoxin 6-hydroxydopamine (which is also used to create animal models of the disease). 6-Hydroxydopamine causes apoptosis in catecholaminergic PC-12 cells and this can be inhibited by endonuclease inhibitors as well as by actinomycin D [49].

The precursor to dopamine, L-DOPA, is commonly used in the treatment of Parkinson's disease but recent evidence suggests that it may also contribute to neuronal apoptosis. Treatment of PC-12 cells with L-DOPA produced chromatin condensation, DNA laddering and membrane blebbing, which was not inhibited by treatment with similar concentrations of carbidopa. The concentration range of carbidopa used (25 to 100 μM) inhibits the conversion of L-DOPA to dopamine, suggesting the pro-apoptotic effect is mediated directly by L-DOPA. This pattern of toxicity may, apparently, be specific for catecholaminergic cells since other cell types were not affected [50]. If similar toxicity were to occur in man, L-DOPA administration could have serious consequences for disease progression and treatment to prevent the exacerbation of pre-existing neuronal damage should be seriously considered. The mechanism of L-DOPA toxicity may depend on increased free radical production, and in this respect, elevated levels of iron found in the substantia nigra of Parkinson's patients may contribute to enhanced oxidative stress [51]. This possibility has been pursued in dopaminergic PC-12 neurones using rotenone and MPP+ [52]. Apoptotic death predominated at lower concentrations of both these inhibitors, where their effects may elevate reactive oxygen species, but increasing concentrations caused necrosis. This is a similar effect to that induced by glutamate and may reflect the importance of mitochondrial metabolism and ATP levels in dictating cell fate. Primary cultures of rat cerebellar granule cells are commonly used for apoptosis research and MPP+ has also been shown to cause apoptosis in these neurones [53].

6.2   Alzheimer's disease

Samples of human postmortem brain have proved to be a valuable source of information in determining the role of apoptosis in Alzheimer's disease. The entorhinal cortex and hippocampus from Alzheimer's brain have been found to contain neurones with the distinct morphology of apoptotic cells, and DNA fragmentation was also observed [54]. Some of the apoptotic neurones contained tangles whereas others did not. When the morphology of Alzheimer's hippocampus was analysed in more detail, DNA nick end labelling revealed that most apoptotic nuclei were located within neurones in grey matter and most tau-positive neurones were reported to be associated with apoptosis [55]. In contradiction with this observation, it has also been reported [56] that no correlation could be found between TUNEL-positive and tau-positive cells in Alzheimer's hippocampus. The use of double-labelling techniques found that *c-jun* is associated with DNA strand breaks in Alzheimer's disease tissue [57] but there were no clear differences between Alzheimer's and control tissue following electrophoretic analysis of genomic DNA. Further reports suggest a potential role for early inducible genes in the pathology of Alzheimer's disease [reviewed in 13]. Detailed histochemistry of Alzheimer's brain has also shown that DNA fragmentation can be detected in oligodendrocytes and microglia as well as neurones [58]. The observation that microglial apoptosis might play a role in the demise of these cells, suggests that some thought should be given to the consequences of an inhibitor of apoptosis prolonging the life of activated microglia. A further report has indicated that while DNA damage was observed in several

Alzheimer brain regions, localisation did not necessarily correlate with areas of β-amyloid plaques, tangles or neuronal loss [59]. The apparent lack of agreement in these studies could be influenced by variations in postmortem delay, since this has been shown to affect DNA nick end labelling [57].

The use of immunohistochemistry has allowed the detection of proteins associated with apoptosis to be located in Alzheimer's brain and can be used to help elucidate the role of the protein components that drive the mechanisms by which cells die. For example, it has been reported that *bcl-2* expression increases in pathological tissue relative to controls [60–62] but the interpretation of these studies is complicated by some of the limitations of using post-mortem brain samples [for reviews, see 13 and 63]. As already discussed in this section, factors such as the relative sparcity of apoptotic cells in a particular brain section and variations in postmortem delay can complicate the interpretation of these studies.

In addition to the post-mortem studies described above, *in vivo* models can help elucidate pathological mechanisms that could trigger apoptosis in the human disease. Transgenic mice have been used to express β-amyloid in neurones and to correlate this with neurodegeneration in brain regions affected by Alzheimer's disease [64]. The involvement of neuronal apoptosis was implicated in this model by detecting internucleosomal cleavage of DNA and nuclear chromatin condensation in the affected areas. The role of two interesting Alzheimer's-related genes, *ALG-2* and *ALG-3*, has been investigated in a mouse T-cells [65]: *ALG-3* is the mouse homologue of the familial Alzheimer's disease gene *STM2* found on chromosome 1 and *ALG-2* is a Ca^{2+}-binding protein. The *ALG-3* gene was transiently transfected into *3DO* T-cell hybridoma cells, which have been used to evaluate genes involved in apoptosis. When a truncated *ALG-3* transcript was expressed in these cells, they were found to be more resistant to T-cell receptor and Fas-induced apoptosis. The human *STM2* gene may, therefore, play a role in mediating apoptosis during Alzheimer's disease but the mechanism by which this could occur remains to be elucidated.

As already discussed with research into Parkinson's disease, cell culture models have been used extensively to study pathological features associated with Alzheimer's disease. Often this type of research into the potential role of neuronal apoptosis has followed the pattern of cell death observed after exposure to β-amyloid or manipulation of the processing of its precursor protein. Conclusions from these studies can sometimes be difficult to compare with each other, due to the following factors: 1) lack of agreement on the exact structure of the active "pathological agent" in the human disease; 2) differences in the concentration of the pro-apoptotic agent or the vehicle used; and 3) inconsistencies in cell culture protocols. For example, one study found that multiple exposures to a synthetic β-peptide (25–100 μM) was required to induce laddering and chromatin condensation in E17 rat hippocampal and cortical neurones [66] whereas another study demonstrated membrane blebbing, typical chromatin condensation and internucleosomal fragmentation of E14-15 mouse cortical and E18-19 rat hippocampal cells between 1 and 14 days *in vitro*, following exposure to a synthetic β-amyloid peptide at 25 μM [67]. Cell degeneration was detectable at 6 hours and was maximal at 24 hours. The two studies clearly agree that synthetic β-peptides induce apoptosis and that neurones were exposed to some aggregated peptide but the degree of toxicity of the peptides does vary. One important difference is the approximately three-fold lower cell plating density in the latter study which may correlate with an increased susceptibility to the toxic challenge. Apparently in direct contradiction with these two studies, another group found that exposure to 20 μM β-peptide induced an entirely necrotic death in primary cultures of rat cortex and PC-12 cells [68]. Necrosis was assessed by electrophoretic DNA analysis and electron microscopy and compared with apoptosis induced by NGF deprivation in the PC-12 cells. It was concluded in this paper [68] that differences between culture methodologies in different laboratories were not responsible for the lack of observable apoptosis. Furthermore, it was proposed that inflammatory events produced by mature amyloid deposits resulted in neuronal necrosis, rather than apoptosis, being observed. Differences do exist, however, between cell types in both their susceptibility and their mode of death following exposure to β-amyloid. Apoptosis has been demonstrated in PC-12, B104 and $NB_2\alpha$ cells by DNA laddering and morphology but IMR32 cells died by necrosis when exposed to β-peptide under similar conditions [69]. Since these are all neuroblastoma cell lines, they are relatively poor models of "real" neurones. It remains to be clarified, however, whether more consistent results can be obtained under standardised conditions. Mutations in the amyloid precursor protein (APP) gene (which produces increased carboxy terminal fragments within cells) have shown to induce apoptosis, when expressed in PC-12 cells [70]. Whether this effect is mediated by extracellular or intracellular mechanisms is unclear at present. Currently, limitations in culture technologies and insufficient understanding of β-amyloid biochemistry preclude an unqualified affirmation of the role of apoptosis in β-amyloid toxicity but the balance of evidence is currently in favour of apoptotic involvement. It should be remembered, however, that cells may die both by necrosis and apoptosis in this disease. In the future, identification of

robust differences in cellular response to the β-peptide, including neuronal and glial differences, may ultimately elucidate additional therapeutic targets for this disease.

6.3   Cerebral ischaemia

The proposed cascade of pathological events initiated by brain ischaemia
is now well documented [e.g. 71]. The consensus hypothesis is that ischaemia induces excitotoxicity and compromises cellular metabolism, which
results in high concentrations of extracellular glutamate, which in turn
leads to high intracellular concentrations of calcium. Abnormally high fluctuations in cytosolic calcium are thought to play a major role in promoting cell death. Extracellular glutamate released from dying neurones,
causes excitotoxic stimulation of neighbouring neurones and inhibition
of cysteine uptake leading to depletion of intracellular glutathione [72].
Consequently, oxidative stress can also contribute to ischaemic cell death.
It should be emphasised, however, that the complexity of these cascades
and their modulation by excitotoxicity and, particularly, by inflammatory
events significantly complicates the interpretation of the pattern of cell
death observed [73]. Studying the role of apoptosis in ischaemic brain
injury has, therefore, provided a new impetus to stroke research.

When excitotoxic injury is induced *in vivo*, morphological changes are
observed that are mostly consistent with necrosis but apoptosis has also
been detected in several animal models of ischaemia [74–76]. These stroke
models have been used to estimate the possible contributions of apoptosis to ischaemia-induced cell death by using a combination of biochemical, morphological, and pharmacological techniques to quantify the relative proportion of apoptotic versus necrotic cells [reviewed in 77]. Many
of these *in vivo* studies have not yet definitively assessed the relative contribution of apoptosis but there is now good evidence that apoptosis can
be observed in ischaemic brain tissue.

In vitro cultures are commonly used to mimic *in vivo* ischaemia: cell death
usually being induced following direct exposure to glutamate or oxygen-
glucose deprivation (which leads to "indirect" extracellular glutamate elevation). In primary cultures of embryonic rat cortex, sustained exposure
to mM concentrations of glutamate has been demonstrated to induce DNA
laddering with approximately 50% of cells dying within two days [78]. Furthermore, cell death was inhibited by exposing cells to endonuclease and
RNA synthesis inhibitors. In cultures of cerebellar granule neurones, on
the other hand, actinomycin D, cyclohexamide or endonuclease inhibitors did not block cell death following exposure to 100 μM glutamate for

15 minutes [79]. In addition, there was no evidence for internucleosomal cleavage in this study. In further support of these findings, the relative contribution of necrotic versus apoptotic death was assessed following exposure of rat cortical neurones to graded levels of N-methyl-D-aspartate (NMDA), AMPA or kainate: the data were consistent with a mostly necrotic mode of death [80]. Despite obvious variations between the above studies (e.g cortical versus cerebellar cultures and chronic versus acute glutamate exposure), apoptosis and necrosis have been detected in relatively pure neuronal cultures of cerebellar granule cells after similar glutamate insults [81]. When these neurones were exposed to low micromolar glutamate for half an hour, a substantial proportion of cells died by necrosis following glutamate removal. Necrosis was assessed by swollen intracellular organelles, loss of membrane integrity and loss of cytoplasmic contents. Neurones which survived this initial wave of necrosis were found to die by apoptosis 6 hours after removal of the glutamate challenge. Apoptosis was characterised by DNA laddering and morphology. A reduction in mitochondrial membrane potential was found to identify a sub-population of neurones which were destined to die by apoptosis. When mitochondrial potential was restored, this protected a population of neurones from necrosis but did not spare them from their ultimate death by apoptosis. Neuronal cells lines (PC-12, R2 and GT1-7) can be almost completely protected by up regulation of *bcl-2* (see section 7.5), following exposure to 10 μM glutamate. Oxygen-glucose deprivation is another challenge used to mimic *in vivo* ischaemia: necrotic and apoptotic modes of death have been demonstrated in primary cultures of mouse cortical cells and apoptosis predominated following protection by addition of several glutamate antagonists [82]. In contrast to the effects of NMDA receptor stimulation, activation of metabotropic glutamate receptors blocks apoptosis in depolarised rat cerebellar neurones [83]. A similar protection is observed in mouse cortical neurones [84].

In conclusion, therapies that only protect neurones from acute death by necrosis may only be delaying subsequent death by apoptosis and so it is important to further understand the role of apoptosis in stroke. Furthermore, there is only a narrow temporal window of opportunity to inhibit necrosis following ischaemia, so that therapies to inhibit apoptosis may turn out to be a more practical therapeutic intervention in man.

6.4   Traumatic head injury

In comparison with research into the mechanisms of cell death in stroke, the possibility that apoptosis may also play a role in traumatic head injury is only beginning to be realised. However, the evolution of the pathology of head trauma has many commonalties with stroke, since excitotoxic neuronal cell death is also an important feature of both pathologies [reviewed in 85]. In animal models of head trauma, such as the fluid percussion model, both acute and delayed neuronal death have been observed [86], with apoptotic cell death being detected in different brain regions when defined by DNA fragmentation [87]. On further analysis, cellular morphologies consistent with both apoptotic and necrotic cell death were observed and DNA fragmentation confirmed by TUNEL staining [88]. NGF was found to reverse the apoptosis observed in similar trauma models, when assessed by TUNEL staining and detailed morphology [89].

6.5   Multiple sclerosis

For the normal propagation of action potentials along myelinated axons to occur, oligodendrocytes must ensheath the paranodal regions of axons in the mature CNS. In multiple sclerosis (MS), oligodendrocytes die and subsequent demyelination contributes to the axonal conduction block observed in the disease [e.g. 90]. Remyelination of the demyelinated lesions by the surviving oligodendrocytes often takes place during the course of the disease but stable remyelination is unlikely to be maintained indefinitely [91]. Since the extent of myelination is in a state of flux during the progression of the disease, the ability to inhibit the death of oligodendrocytes might not only reduce the rate of demyelination but also promote remyelination.

There is good evidence that oligodendrocytes die by apoptosis during normal development in rats [92] and in myelin-deficient jimpy mice [93]. Apoptotic cells have also been detected in different animal models of MS (e.g. experimental allergic encephalomyelitis), which are probably oligodendrocytes [94] but there are, as yet, no reports of apoptotic oligodendrocytes in sections from multiple sclerosis postmortem samples.

In vitro, both apoptosis and necrosis have been detected in cultured oligodendrocytes when exposed to factors implicated in the pathology of MS. Tumour necrosis factor-α (TNF-α) is elevated in serum from MS patients and induces nuclear fragmentation in human, rat and bovine oligodendrocytes [95, 96]. Exposure to TNF-α in MS could well initiate oligodendrocyte death by apoptosis and contribute to demyelination. Fibroblast growth factor (bFGF) also triggers nuclear fragmentation in mature rat oligodendrocytes. As bFGF stimulates division of oligodendrocyte precursor cells, it is possible that, in mature cells, this signalling pathway also induces entry into the cell cycle [97] but, in adult cells, mitosis is likely to be inappropriate and so the cycle is aborted by apoptosis. Human oligo-dendrocyte precursor cells also abort entry into the cell cycle following serum deprivation or TNF-α exposure and so die by apoptosis [96]. Apo-ptosis as the result of an abortive cell cycle may significantly contribute to the death of mature oligodendrocytes during MS. Oligodendrocytes can also die by necrosis, particularly after lethal exposure to homologous complement in rats [98–100] but a similar mechanism has not been clearly demonstrated in human cells. It is possible, therefore, that inhibiting apo-ptosis in oligodendrocytes after a pathological stimulus or abortion of the cell cycle could have a major impact on the dynamics of myelination and tilt the balance towards demyelination. Nevertheless, the importance of the role of complement attack in multiple sclerosis, coupled with the obser-vations that complement-induced death is uniquely necrotic, suggests that the role of necrosis should not be ignored. Potential therapies should, there-fore, consider intervening in both apoptotic and necrotic pathways.

The pathology of MS is characterised by an inappropriate immune res-ponse, in particular, the role of T-lymphocytes in infiltrating the blood brain barrier and their subsequent interaction with myelin and oligodendro-cytes. The role of apoptosis in terminating T-cell function can therefore play an important role. For example, apoptosis is responsible for the spe-cific elimination of autoreactive V-beta-8.2-encephalitogenic T-cells from the total cell population in Lewis rats, following inoculation with a CD4+V-beta 8.2+ T-cell clone. This clone is specific for a 72-89 amino acid pep-tide fragment of pig myelin basic protein [101]. Furthermore, T-lympho-cytes specific for myelin basic protein have been taken from MS patients and found to undergo antigen-specific apoptosis [102]. These studies are consistent with specific populations of autoreactive T cells being removed from the circulating pool by apoptosis. Enhancing antigen-induced apo-ptosis could, therefore, inhibit T-cell-mediated damage to myelinated nerves and may be of some therapeutic value.

6.6   Motoneurone disease

Motoneurone disease (MND or amyotrophic lateral sclerosis) is a pro-gressive fatal disease characterised by degeneration of upper and lower motoneurones. There are some interesting data derived from postmor-tem samples that link apoptosis with MND, such as *in situ* hybridisation studies with *bcl-2* and *bax* (see section 7.5). It was found that expression of *bcl-2* was increased in neurones, glia and vascular cells in brain and spi-nal cord sections from MND patients [60]. In a similar study, *bcl-2* mRNA levels were lower in MND motoneurones, compared with controls, whereas levels of *bax* expression were higher [103]. Axotomy has also been used to model MND and using a facial nerve preparation, it was found that axotomy-induced degeneration was prevented in transgenic animals over-expressing *bcl-2* [104]. This is yet another example of the neuroprotective effects of *bcl-2* and the use of transgenic models in characterising apoptosis in various disease models.

About 5–10% of MND cases are familial with autosomal dominant inheritance. Mutations in the gene for Cu/Zn superoxide dismutase (SOD1) have been found in approximately 20% of families with the autosomal dominant form of familial MND. This discovery has led to a number of investigations into a role for a degenerative mechanism based on elevation of reactive oxygen species (ROS) or mitochondrial dysfunction in various culture systems. For example, apoptosis in NGF-treated as well as untreated PC-12 cultures is increased by antisense inhibition of SOD1 [105] or decreased in NGF-deprived cells by microinjection of SOD1 protein, SOD1 cDNA or a *bcl-2* expression vector [106]. Furthermore, antisense oligonucleotides have been used to inhibit natural SOD1 activity and metal-chelating agents to potentiate oxygen radical mediated toxicity in organotypic cultures of rat spinal cord [107]. Chronic inhibition of SOD1 activity by antisense oligonucleotides reduced levels of SOD1 to 50% of controls and resulted in apoptotic death of spinal cord motoneurones. Immortalised rat nigral neurones have been transfected with mutations in SOD1 that are associated with familial MND and this manipulation was found to stimulate apoptosis [108]. Although these experiments support the role of ROS in apoptosis, concluding that familial MND mutations in SOD1 lead to apoptosis in vivo is not entirely straightforward [e.g. 108]. In summary, however, these mutations appear to convert the wild-type dismutase into a pro-apoptotic form in neurones and suggest a role for apoptosis in mediating the pathology of MND.

6.7   Other neurodegenerative diseases

There are other neurodegenerative diseases in which comparatively little is known about the role of apoptosis but there are sufficient data for a brief mention in this review. For example, an apoptotic mode of death has also been found in human foetal Down's syndrome cortical neurones. These cells appear to have a defect in the way they handle ROS, which apparently accelerates the demise of the Down's syndrome cells and provides further evidence for the role of ROS in this disease [109]. Further potential roles for apoptosis are in the pathologies of scrapie [110, 111] and Huntington's disease [112].

7 Cellular mechanisms of apoptosis

There have been numerous hypotheses to implicate a specific mediator or pathway responsible for neuronal apoptosis. These include proteases, kinases (stress-activated kinases (SAPKs)), and cyclin-dependent kinases (CDKs), proto-oncogenes (Bcl$_2$ and family members), calcium signalling and free radicals. Details of these pathways are outlined below:

7.1 Multiple protease activation in neuronal apoptosis

Apoptosis is an event that requires disassembly of the cellular scaffolding, thus the involvement of proteolysis is clearly necessary for this to occur. In addition, a number of proteins including poly(ADP-ribose) polymerase (PARP) [113], the 70 kDa protein component of the U1 small nuclear ribonucleoprotein [114], lamin B1, α-fodrin (spectrin) [115], and β-actin, have been reported to become proteolysed in association with the onset of apoptosis. Cytotoxic T-cells produce a series of serine proteases (granzymes) which are necessary for target cell killing by the induction of apoptosis [116]. Protease inhibitors of different specificities including serine and cysteine protease inhibitors, have been shown to inhibit apoptosis which shows that apoptosis may require the participation of several classes of proteases [117].

Genetic studies on the nematode worm, *Caenorhabditis elegans* (*C. elegans*), have been fundamentally important in identifying molecules that play a key role in apoptotic cell death. Homology between the *C. elegans* *ced-3* gene product, which is required for developmental cell death in worms and the human cysteine protease, interleukin-1β converting enzyme (ICE-1), suggested a role for cysteine proteases in apoptosis [118]. Involvement of ICE/*ced3*-like proteases in apoptosis of sympathetic neurones results from studies that have shown protection by *crmA* [119] and *p35* [120], two viral inhibitors of these proteases, and tetrapeptide inhibitors (e.g. Ac-YVAD-CMK, Z-DEVD-FMK). ICE-1 was the first member of a family of cysteine proteases with the distinguishing feature of a near-absolute specificity for aspartate in the S$_1$ subsite. Subsequently, further proteases of the ICE-1 family were identified as *ced-3* homologues: (ICH-1/NEDD2), TX (ICH-2, ICErel-II), Mch2, Mch3 (also known as ICE-LAP-3 and CMH-1), Mch4, Mch5, ICErel-III, and CPP-32/Yama/apopain and been implicated as mediators of all apoptotic deaths [for review see 121, 122]. A complex interaction may exist for all members of ICE-like proteases in mediating apoptotic death (see Fig. 2). CPP-32 is the ICE-like protease for which most literature evidence exists for a role in apoptosis and this protease (along with the Mch family) also has the greatest difference in sequence homology to ICE-1. It seems very likely, therefore, that CPP-32 is the key executioner protease in apoptosis.

Among other proteases, calpains and proteasomes have been shown to play a role in neuronal apoptosis. Calcium-activated neutral proteinase (calpain) has been implicated in the death of neurones in stroke. This enzyme is inactive under normal Ca^{2+} conditions but is activated by the high levels of calcium observed during an ischaemic insult, and targets key structural and regulatory proteins for proteolysis (e.g. spectrin). Calpain I activation has been implicated in lymphocytic apoptosis induced by dexamethasone, low level irradiation and macromolecular synthesis inhibition [123]. While calpain inhibitors reduce the apoptotic death in these models, calpain may not be a critical enzyme in all types of neuronal apoptosis. The neuroprotective potential of calpain inhibitors in ischaemic brain damage (i.e. excitotoxicity, hypoxia, global ischaemia, focal ischaemia) has been shown by various laboratories [for review see 124] and implicates calpain as a key mediator in necrotic rather than apoptotic neuronal death. It is also tempting to speculate that calpain may interact directly or indirectly with other pathways, such as ICE-like proteases or kinases involved in neuronal death. For example calpstatin (endogenous calpain inhibitor) may be a substrate for proteolytic cleavage (and inactivation) by one of the ICE-like proteases, resulting in sustained calpain activation (Figs 2 and 3).

Multicatalytic protease (proteasome) is a ATP-ubiquitin-dependent proteolytic pathway found in both the cytosol and nucleus of eukaryotic cells [125]. The proteasome is a large (20S) hollow cylindrical complex, which degrades ubiquitin-conjugated proteins in an ATP-dependent fashion [126]. In this pathway, proteins are first modified by covalent conjugation to ubiquitin, which marks them for rapid hydrolysis by the proteasome. A ubiquitin-proteasome-dependent system degrades abnormal or incorrectly synthesised proteins as well as damaged proteins and short-lived polypeptides [127]. Sadoul et al. have shown that specific inhibitors of the proteasome (lactacystin) provide neuroprotection against apoptotic death of sympathetic neurones induced by NGF-deprivation and prevent cleavage of PARP. Sadoul et al. also demonstrated that proteasome inhibition by lactacystin blocks activation of ICE-1 (and release of IL-1β) in macrophages stimulated by lipopolysaccharide (LPS) and ATP. Thus, another major pathway leading to apoptosis in sympathetic neurones involves proteasome enzyme activity. It has been suggested that the proteasome acts prior to the activation of ICE-like proteases. The proteasome has also been implicated in UV or dexamethasone-induced apoptosis of thymocytes. The

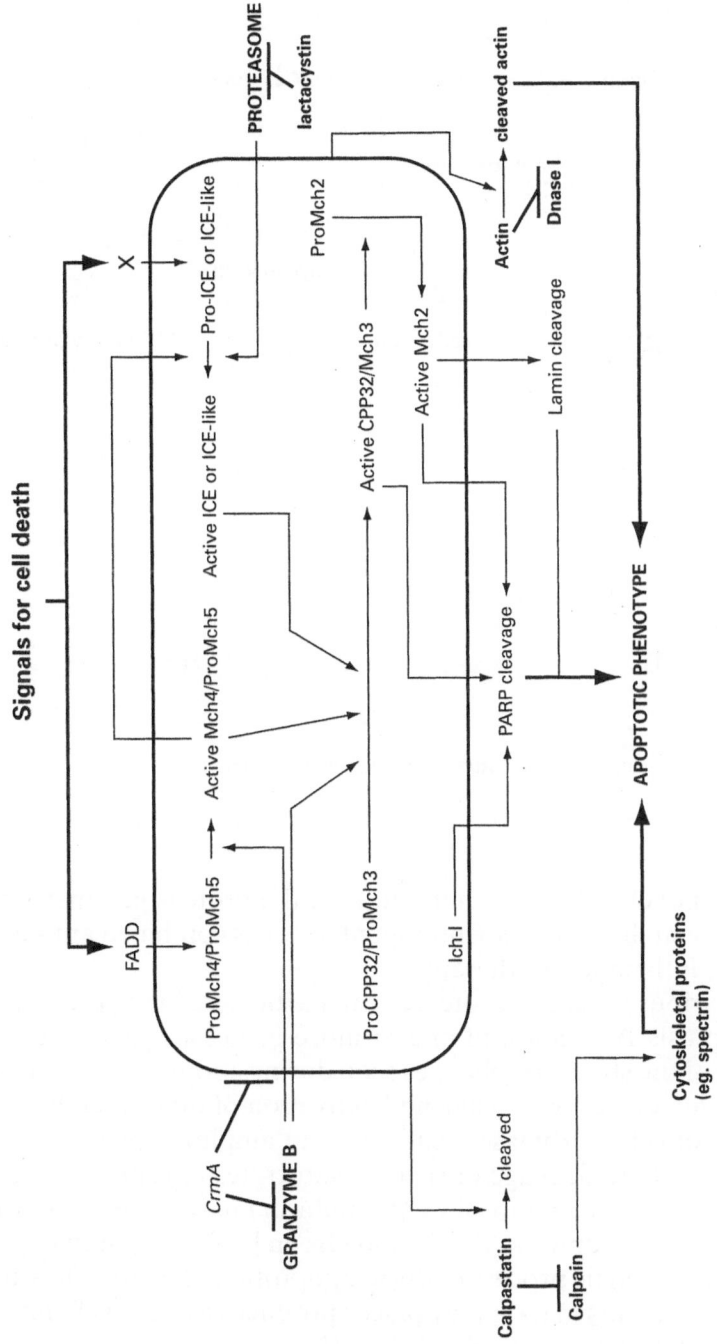

Fig. 2
Complex interaction between different ICE-like protease family members and other types of proteases may exist in cells undergoing apoptosis. Multiple ICE-like proteases may coexist in cells which could generate an amplifiable protease cascade and provide proper elimination of cells during development or pathological apoptosis.

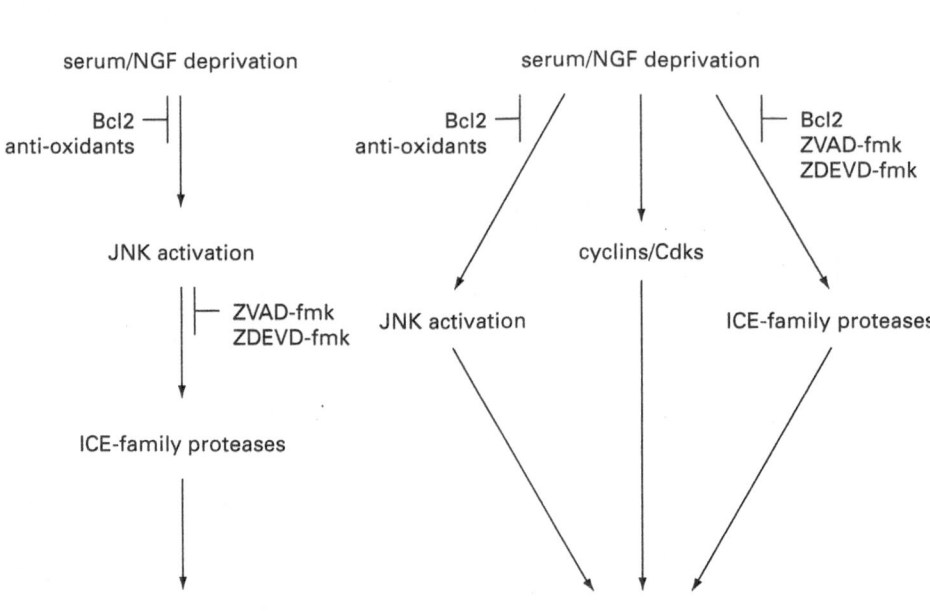

Fig. 3
Two possible models for cell death pathways activated during apoptosis.

formulation of novel and specific inhibitors of the proteasome may provide a useful research and therapeutic agent to act as combined anti-apoptotic and anti-inflammatory therapy.

In summary, various groups of proteases can participate in the process of neuronal apoptosis. Activation of one or more proteases could directly produce some of the structural changes seen during apoptosis. Activation of a protease can lead to processing and activation of other members of the same class or other proteases, leading to an amplified protease cascade [128]. Proteolytic cleavage of specific substrates (e.g. processing of pro-forms of a protein or removal of an inhibitor) may further contribute to the process of apoptosis. Martin and Green [128] suggest that such an amplifying proteolytic process exists in apoptotic cell death. Thus, too many proteolytic events in too many places produces a critical change in the cell which ends in apoptotic death (see Figs 2 and 3).

7.2   Non-neuronal cells and neuronal apoptosis

The pathophysiology of neurodegenerative and neurological disorders is quite complex and components of ion channel modulation, excitotoxicity and inflammation play major roles in cell death. Although most of the research into apoptotic cell death is focused on neurones, non-neuronal cells such as, microglia and astrocytes, are also involved. The central nervous system (CNS) has long been regarded as an immunologically privileged site. Accumulating evidence suggests, however, that the privilege is certainly not total, and that immune functions involving systemic immune cells and resident glial cells can operate in the CNS. The nervous and immune systems interact during normal development, but in the mature brain their interaction is restricted mainly to cases of pathogenic infections and traumatic lesions. Elevated concentrations of cytokines (e.g. IL-1β and TNF-α) have been found in brain after both trauma and cerebral ischaemia. It is likely that these cytokines may participate in subsequent neurodegeneration. It is becoming ever more apparent that there is a major inflammatory component to stroke and that IL-1β greatly exacerbates the cell death observed in ischaemia. Microglia are thought to be the major source of ICE-1 and IL-1β production in ischaemia.

It is possible that activated microglia participate in selective neuronal cell death, and a number of studies have shown that these cells appear before neuronal death [129–131]. Microglia can release a number of cytotoxins including glutamate, hydrogen peroxide, nitric oxide, TNF-α and a novel class of compounds as yet not fully characterised [132]. Inhibition of microglial activity by chloroquine and colchicine leads to a reduction of ischaemic neuronal loss in the rabbit spinal cord [133]. Additionally, macrophages (microglia) may also be involved in tissue remodelling, which involves apoptosis in the eye *in vivo* [134]. It is possible that neurones undergoing apoptosis, but not necrosis, express unique antigens which may serve as a signal for their phagocytosis by microglia. Alternatively, dying neurones may release substances that initiate the cytotoxic activities of microglia. Thus, microglia may function to clear debris and regulate gliosis and tissue repair in severe cortical ischaemia, and participate in selective neuronal apoptotic death in a mild ischaemic insult [135].

The development of an infarct also involves the death of glia cells, which are more resistant to oxygen deprivation than neurones. Damage to glial cells might be indirect and perhaps due to the loss of trophic support. Oligodendrocytes have been shown to be dependent on axon-derived growth factors for survival, and can be rescued by insulin growth factor-1 (IGF-1) or ciliary neurotrophic factor (CNTF) after axotomy [136]. This hypothesis is supported by data showing that exogenous IGF-1, when added 2 hours post-hypoxia, reduces the rate of infarction in a dose-dependent manner following head injury in the adult rat [137].

Therefore microglia and astrocytes are essential elements of the immune surveillance of the nervous system, which can also influence neuronal survival and death in brain injury. Understanding the exact inter-relationship between neurones and glia in health and disease, immunologically or otherwise, should aid us to devise successful interventions for a wide spectrum of nervous system diseases.

7.3   Cell cycle components and apoptosis

It has been postulated by a number of groups that apoptosis can result from conflicting growth regulatory signals. This hypothesis is supported by several pieces of data, which implicate genes normally thought to be involved in cell-cycle control and proliferation in apoptosis. The wild-type transcription factor, and tumour suppresser gene, *p53*, is thought to be involved in regulation of progression through the cell cycle and, in particular, may serve as a detector for damaged DNA [138]. There is some indication that *p53* may be involved in the death of neurones after excitotoxic injury by kainic acid [139]. However, it appears that either *p53* is redundant or is not an important determinant for developmental or NGF-induced apoptosis in neurones [140]. Altered expression of the retinoblastoma gene product (*Rb*), which is another cell cycle related gene, has been associated with neuronal death. Hypo-phosphorylated (i.e. active) *Rb* is associated with cell cycle arrest, however, overexpression of *cyclin D1* can reverse this phenotype. This is not surprising as *cyclin D1* is a subunit of the active *cdk* involved in the phosphorylation and thus inactivation of the *Rb* protein [141].

7.3.1   *Cyclins and cyclin-dependent kinases in apoptosis*
Cyclin D1, a cyclin-dependent kinase regulatory subunit, has been shown to be important for progression through the G1 phase in the cell cycle [142]. In addition, its expression appears to be selectively induced in dying neurones during apoptosis induced by NGF withdrawal [143, 144]. *Cyclin D1* mRNA levels peak 15–20 hours after nerve growth factor withdrawal, concurrent with the time that neurones become committed to die by apoptosis (in contrast the mRNA levels for *cyclin D3* and *cyclin E* remain the same or fall as the neurones undergo apoptosis). Although the mRNA of the associated *cyclin D1*-dependent kinase remains constant the activ-

ity increases in apoptotic neurones as a direct result of the increase in *cyclin D1* levels. This activity could be inhibited by 21 kDa E1B and *bcl-2* (which are known to protect from apoptotic cell death) and the endogenous *cyclin D*-dependent kinase inhibitor, p16INK4 [143].

D-type *cyclins* have also been implicated during programmed cell death in non-neuronal cell types. The IL-2 dependent murine cytotoxic T cell line, CTLL-2, undergoes programmed cell death when deprived of its specific cytokine with the levels of *cyclin D2, cyclin D3, cyclin B1, c-myc* all declining at 1.5–3 hours, rising again at 10–14 hours. This pattern closely followed the time of the first detection of apoptotic DNA degradation following IL-2 deprivation, at 8 hours, but preceded actual loss of viability, at 14 h. Measurement of protein synthesis at a late stage of the apoptotic programme revealed that the mRNA re-induced at these later points was not translated and that accumulation was merely triggered by relaxation of the chromatin in the dying cells [145]. In the hematopoietic cell line 32Dcl, cell death resulting from withdrawal of IL-3 has been demonstrated to be delayed by overexpression of *cyclins D2, D3* and also *cdk-4* and *bcl-2* [146].

The cyclin-dependent kinase *cdc2* has also been implicated in the apoptotic process. Shimizu et al. [147], demonstrated that DNA damage promotes the transient and unscheduled stimulation of *cyclin B1/Cdc2* kinase activity in HL60 cells prior to apoptosis. Apoptosis induced by granzyme B and perforin has also been shown to be inhibited by expression of the *cdc-2* inhibitor Wee1. The apoptosis-resistant cells exhibited markedly increased *cdc2* tyrosine phosphorylation as expected due to the direct action of Wee1 kinase on the *cdc-2* [148]. In addition, in AGF cells it was observed that *cdc-2, cyclin A*, and PCNA proteins were associated mostly with the plasma membrane and the cytoplasm during the log phase. However, in cells undergoing apoptosis, these proteins were found exclusively in the nuclei of apoptotic cells [149].

There are a number of *cdc-2*-like kinases, including a neuronal equivalent known as *cdk5*. This neuronal *cdc2*-like kinase can associate with *D*- and *E*-type *cyclins* and a novel protein p35 which is found exclusively in postmitotic cells [150]. Although *cdk5* can be found in a number of different tissues it has only been demonstrated to have activity in brain. Recent evidence suggests that association of the kinase with the novel cyclin *p35* may be responsible for this selective activity. *cdk5* activity has also been observed as a complex with a *p25* protein which is derived from *p35* via proteolysis. Association of *p35* with *cdk5* appears to prevent its inhibition by the endogenous inhibitor *p27*, but not Wee1 [151]. As the crystal structure of *p27* in complex with *cyclin A-cdk-2* has been resolved at 2.3 Å, it would be interesting to attempt to discover how selectivity could be achieved.

7.4   Mitogen-activated protein kinases (MAPKs)

MAPKs (mitogen-activated protein kinases) are serine/threonine kinases that are activated by dual phosphorylation on threonine and tyrosine residues. In mammalian cells, there are at least three separate but parallel pathways that convey information generated by extracellular stimuli to the MAPKs. These three pathways consist of kinase cascades leading to activation of the ERKs (extracellular regulated kinases), the JNK's (c-Jun N-terminal kinases) and the p38/CSBP kinases. While both the JNK and p38 pathways are involved in relaying stress-type extracellular signals, the ERK pathway is primarily responsible for transducing mitogenic/differentiation signals to the cell nucleus.

SAPK cascades represent a sub-family of the mitogen-activating protein kinase family, that are activated by different external stimuli including DNA damage following UV irradiation, TNF-α, IL-1β, ceramide, cellular stress, and reactive oxygen species and have distinct substrate specificities. Signal transduction via MKK4/JNK or MKK3/p38 results in phosphorylation of inducible transcription factors, c-Jun and ATF2 which then act as either homodimers or heterodimers to initiate transcription of downstream effectors.

c-Jun is a protein that forms homodimers and heterodimers (with e.g. c-Fos) to produce the transactivating complex AP-1 required for the activation of many genes (e.g. matrix metalloproteinases) involved in the inflammatory response. The JNKs were discovered when it was found that several different stimuli such as UV light and TNF alpha stimulated phosphorylation of c-Jun on specific serine residues in the N-terminus of the protein.

A number of recent publications have suggested that activation of stress-activated signal transduction pathways are required for neuronal apoptosis induced by NGF withdrawal in rat PC-12 and superior cervical ganglia (SCG) sympathetic neuronal cells. Inhibition of specific kinases, namely MAP kinase kinase 3 (MKK3) and MAP kinase kinase 4 (MKK4), or c-Jun (part of the MKK-4 cascade) may be sufficient to block apoptosis. Within a few hours of NGF deprivation in SCG neurones, c-Jun becomes highly phosphorylated and protein levels increase. Similarly in rat PC-12 cells deprived of NGF, JNK (c-Jun NH$_2$-terminal kinase) and p38 undergo sustained activation while ERKs are inhibited. In these studies, dominant negative mutants of c-Jun (in SCG), p38 and JNK (PC-12)

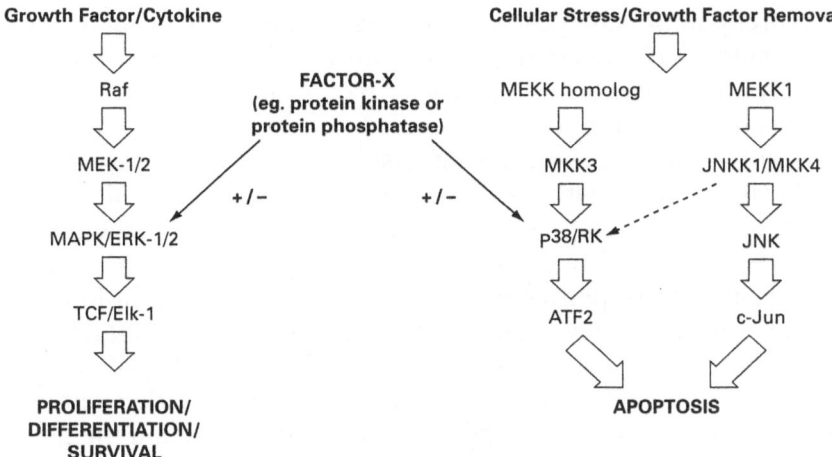

Fig. 4
Mitogen-activated protein kinase signalling pathways in apoptosis and cell proliferation.

protected cells against apoptosis [152, 153]. A summary of the pathways involved in this complex field is shown in Figure 4.

7.5   Proto-oncogene *bcl-2* and family members

Members of the gene family that includes *bcl-2* are involved in the control of apoptosis in a range of different cell types [154, 155]. *Bcl-2* was initially described as the oncogene present in the immunoglobulin locus as a result of a translocation seen in human B-cell leukaemias and lymphomas. Upon cloning, the normal and oncogenic genes were found to be the same; therefore, inappropriate expression of the normal protein was causing tumour formation. The *bcl-2* gene product is a 26 kDa protein that localises to the mitochondrial, ER and perinuclear membranes. It has been shown that most growth factor-dependent cell lines transfected with *bcl-2* can remain in a quiescent state following growth factor withdrawal, but can be induced to proliferate by reintroduction of growth factor. The ability of *bcl-2* to block this form of apoptosis sets it apart from other oncogenes in that its expression can affect normal homeostasis by allowing cells, that are destined to die, to survive, instead of affecting the proliferation rate of the cell. The fact that *bcl-2* can block apoptosis induced by a variety of signals (hypoxia/anoxia, glutamate, lipid peroxidation, elevated calcium, and trauma) suggests that it plays a central role in the regulation of cell death from diverse signalling mechanisms.

Overexpression of *bcl-2* potently inhibits apoptosis in a broad range of model systems. *Bcl-2* overexpressing neurones can survive without NGF for >7 days. Knockout of *bcl-X$_L$* (a *bcl-2*-like protein) is lethal due to massive neurodegeneration. Transgenic mice which overexpress *bcl-2* under the control of a neurone-specific enolase promoter were observed to develop fairly normally with no excessive tumourgenesis but developed a larger brain (50% larger in some areas, including the cerebellum and the optic nerve), presumably due to reduced apoptosis during development. Ischaemia induced by permanent middle cerebral artery occlusion (MCA-O) in these animals shows a 50% reduction in penumbral infarct volume compared to wild-type controls, but some cells still die. Facial nerve axotomy in these animals produces no neuronal death in marked contrast to wild type, but the cell bodies appear slightly atrophied and the glial cell response still occurs. Work has also been done to show that animals overexpressing *bcl-2* were protected from β-amyloid toxicity. Crossing these animals with disease model animals gave variable results: Lurcher mice/*bcl-2* progeny showed no rescue to the Purkinje cells, but inferior olive cells were rescued; progeny from crosses between *bcl-2*/PMN (progressive motor neuropathy) mice showed a total rescue of all motoneurones, but with no effect on axonal degeneration.

Overexpression of *bax*, *bak* or *bik* induces apoptosis in a wide variety of cell systems, and marked *bax* overexpression is observed following NGF withdrawal from neuronal cell cultures. Low *bax* levels are also observed in many tumours. *Bax* knockout mice develop normally, but display lymphoid hyperplasia consistent with a role for *bax* in the promotion of apoptosis [156]. This work suggests that up-regulation of *bcl-2* and *bcl-2*-like activity (or down regulation of *bax* and *bax*-like activity) may be an attractive target for neurodegenerative disease therapy which may also have implications for Alzheimer's therapies.

7.5.1   Bcl-2-like gene family

Currently, about a dozen human genes have been isolated which are related to *bcl-2*, as well as several viral homologues. These gene products can be separated into cytotoxic or cytoprotective proteins (see Fig. 5). Many proteins of the *bcl-2* gene family are capable of homodimerisation and heterodimerisation. This proposed model suggests that the presence of equal or greater amounts of the cytoprotective protein pushes the balance towards cell survival, whereas an excess of the cytotoxic forms leads to cell death.

For all the known sequences of *bcl-2*-like proteins, three conserved regions exist – BH1, BH2, and BH3. In addition, all (except *bad*) contain a C-ter-

Cytoprotective human homologues	Interacts with
Bcl-2 kinase	Bcl-2, Bcl-X_L, Bcl-X_s, Bax, A1, R-Ras, Raf
Bcl-XL	Bcl-X_s, Bax, Bad, Bik
Mcl-1	Bax
BAG-1	Bcl-2, Raf kinase
Bcl-Y ?	?
Bcl-W ?	?
Bfl-1 ?	?
Cytotoxic human homologues	
Bax	Bcl-2, Bcl-X_L, Bcl-X_s, Bax, A1, Mcl-1, Bad
Bcl-XS	Bcl-2, Bcl-X_L
Bak	Bcl-2
Bik	Bcl-2, Bcl-X_L
Bad	Bcl-X_L, Bcl-2 (weaker interaction)
A1	Bcl-2, Bax
Nip 1 (homology to Ca/CaM PDE's)	Bcl-2
Nip 2 (homology to RhoGAP)	Bcl-2
Nip 3 (homology to calbindin D)	Bcl-2

Fig. 5
Bcl-2 and family members.

minal putative membrane anchor sequence. The homology between the BH1-3 regions is conserved throughout most of the family, but is greatest within cytotoxic or cytoprotective forms. Work has recently been done on deletion and site-directed mutagenesis of some of these proteins [157]. In summary, all *bcl-2* and *bcl-X_L* mutations which showed lack of death repression, were also unable to bind *bax*. The BH3 domain of the *bax/bak/bik* proteins appears to mediate cytotoxic activity, and the most conserved domains, BH1 and BH2, are not required for cytotoxicity or *bcl-X_L* binding.

Deletions in BH3 domain ablate cytotoxicity and small peptides corresponding to this region are cytotoxic in their own right. The cytotoxicity of these small peptides corresponds with their ability to bind to *bax* and not their ability to bind to *bcl-X_L*. The BH3 domain appears to be the most important for cell death activation and/or homodimerisation of these proteins.

7.5.2   *Bcl-2 family members involved in neuronal death*
Although there have been several *bcl-2*-like proteins found, only a limited number have been found in neurones: *bcl-X_L*, *bax* and *bad* (smaller

quantities of *bcl-2* and *bcl-X$_S$* have been seen also, but these may be attributable to glial contamination in the samples studied). *Bcl-X$_L$* expression is higher in the CNS than in any other area of the body.

There appears to be differential expression of some of these proteins during development. Developing rat embryonic neurones show high levels of *bcl-2* and *bcl-X$_L$*; after birth, levels of *bcl-2* drop off, but *bcl-X$_L$* levels increase dramatically [158]. This implies that the *bcl-2* is involved mainly in developmental regulation, whereas the *bcl-X$_L$* is required for neuronal survival. This is supported by work using *bcl-X$_L$* knockout mice, which proved lethal due to massive cell death in post-mitotic immature neurones of the brain, spinal cord and dorsal root ganglion [159], whereas *bcl-2* knockout mice survive with apparently normal neuronal development [160].

As for the cytotoxic proteins expressed in neurones, *bax* appears to be the pre-dominant "death activator". However, *bad* displaces *bax* from *bcl-X$_L$*, the suggestion being that this leads to a surplus of *bax*, restoring apoptosis. When 50% or more of the *bax* was heterodimerised with *bcl-X$_L$*, cell death is again inhibited [161]. High levels of *bax* are seen in some cell populations that are highly sensitive to transient global ischaemia, such as the CA1 sector of the hippocampus and Purkinje cells of the cerebellum [162]. *Bax* levels increased significantly from 0.5–3 hours after an ischaemic episode in neurones showing morphological features of degeneration in hippocampus, cortex and cerebellum, and from 3 hours onwards, all degenerating neurones showed increased levels of *bax* and decreased levels of *bcl-2* and *bcl-X* immunostaining; these elevated levels of *bax* remain for several days after the episode. These elevated levels of *bax* have also been seen in the frontoparietal cortex in rats following cardiac arrest [163].

7.6   Calcium and free radicals as mediators of neuronal apoptosis and necrosis

A high level of intracellular calcium ($[Ca^{2+}]_i$) is thought to be the primary causative event in mediating necrotic neuronal death [164, 165]. There is substantial evidence that excess entry of Ca^{2+}, and consequent neuronal cell Ca^{2+} overload, is a key early step in the injury induced by excess exposure to glutamate in the hypoxic/ischaemic brain. Disruption of $[Ca^{2+}]_i$ homeostasis effects various signalling pathways including protein kinases/phosphatases and proteases which in turn activate other biochemical cascades.

Many processes that control $[Ca^{2+}]_i$ homeostasis are interrelated and make it unlikely that blockade of a single mechanism can prevent all cellular necrosis. Neuronal cell cultures subjected to prolonged ischaemia (hypoxia and hypoglycaemia) ultimately die even in the presence of combination of drugs that inhibit many of the pathways associated with Ca^{2+} overload [166].

Substantial amounts of Ca^{2+} ions can be stored and released from mitochondria. Mitochondrial stores for Ca^{2+} are thought to participate in Ca^{2+} homeostasis in conditions of calcium overload (i.e. when Ca^{2+} exceeds the "set point" of 0.5–1.0 mM). The accumulated Ca^{2+} is then released when $[Ca^{2+}]_i$ is reduced by extrusion from the cell [164]. Under normal conditions the increase in $[Ca^{2+}]_i$ is moderate and transient and homeostasis is carried out by calcium binding proteins (e.g. calbindin), Na^+-Ca^+ exchanger and sequestration by endoplasmic reticulum and/or mitochondria. Apart from the buffering of Ca^{2+} by calcium-binding proteins, the mechanisms mentioned are directly or indirectly energy-dependent. Following $[Ca^{2+}]_i$ overload, intramitochondial calcium accumulation triggers a MPT (mitochondrial permeability transition pore) which leads to a cascade of terminal events, resulting in either apoptosis or necrosis.

Under normal conditions the mitochondrial respiratory chain produces reactive oxygen species (ROS), which includes superoxide radicals. Superoxide is then dismutated by superoxide dismutase which results in the production of hydrogen peroxide in the mitochondria. Reduction of hydrogen peroxide via transition metal-catalysed Fenton-type reaction generates the strong and toxic hydroxyl radical [167]. The overload of mitochondria by Ca^{2+} leads to increased production of ROS and, since Ca^{2+} mobilises intramitochondial Fe^{2+}, hydroxyl radicals are formed [168]. A consequence of these events is the activation of MPT, accompanied by increased Ca^{2+} cycling across the mitochondrial membranes in a process which is autocatalysed. Essentially, mitochondria stop producing ATP and become a source of free radicals. Furthermore, the opening of large conductance pores in the inner mitochondrial membrane leads to loss of small molecules from the matrix and induces swelling. Depletion of intramitochondrial glutathione pools due to the MPT contributes to making the mitochondria more vulnerable to free radical attack [169]. Recently the link between calcium overload of cells and mitochondria, enhanced free radical production, and cell death was reported in *in vitro* models of excitotoxicity [169, 170]. Neuronal mitochondria exposed to NMDA and glutamate markedly increase superoxide radical formation. Interestingly, neurones *in vitro* exposed to different glutamate concentrations showed necrotic or apoptotic cell death, dependent on the severity of the insult. Thus, necrotic neuronal death is the result of excessive Ca^{2+} overload, while delayed apoptotic neuronal death is triggered by a milder calcium overload [165].

8   Strategies for therapeutic intervention and conclusions

As we discussed in the Introduction, there is certainly no shortage of potential mechanisms by which drugs could be used to modulate neuronal apoptosis, but which targets are the most relevant for the potential treatment of neurodegenerative diseases? As far as we are aware, there are no compounds in clinical development that directly inhibit apoptosis at the time of writing this review. So the only data we have to rely on were obtained in *in vitro* and animal studies. Based on this information, inhibitors of the ICE-like protease family of enzymes (in particular CPP-32) could well present a possible way forward for the treatment of stroke, since inhibition of apoptosis in non-neuronal cells for a period of acute intervention (say 5 days) would potentially have a more favourable side-effect profile than might be expected from chronic administration. Chronic administration of a drug that inhibited or slowed all apoptosis throughout the body, could have potentially serious consequences for tumour growth, the immune response, the turnover of the intestinal lining and other physiological processes dependent on apoptosis. Furthermore, a number of chemical starting points for medicinal chemistry programmes based around the ICE family exist [e.g. 171]. By inhibiting ICE-1 as well as CPP-32 (therefore inhibiting IL-1β production as well as apoptosis) a combined anti-inflammatory/anti-apoptotic agent could well have increased efficacy for the treatment of cerebral ischaemia. Nevertheless, selectivity for CPP-32 over ICE-1 could be achieved, if required (Fig. 6).

However, there are potentially many additional drug targets by which neuronal apoptosis could be selectively modulated in the clinic (for some possible chemical starting points see Fig. 7). In a very controversial area, one statement will probably remain true: research into the mechanisms and pharmacology of neuronal apoptosis will continue to be an area of intense scientific interest and of considerable importance to the pharmaceutical industry.

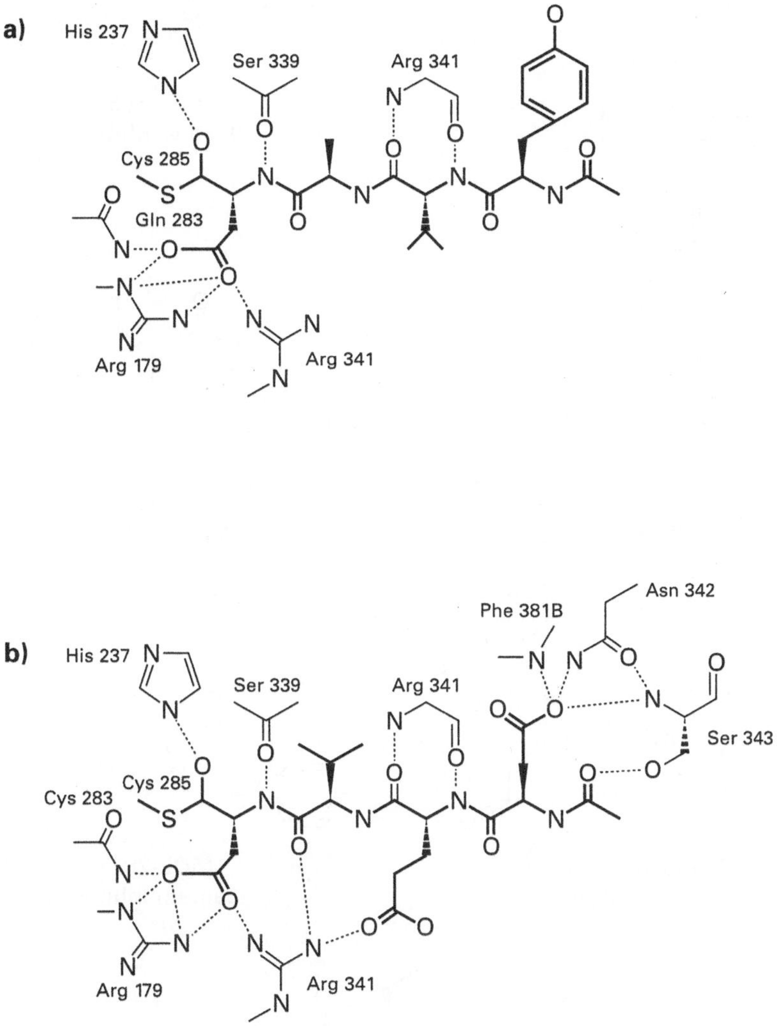

Fig. 6
A diagram of binding of two ICE-like protease inhibitors (drawn in bold) to the active sites of ICE-1 and CPP-32 (amino acids not in bold). a) The binding of YVAD-CHO to the active site of ICE-1. b) The binding of DEVD-CHO to the active site of CPP-32, note that the hydrophilic P4 pocket (Phe 381B, Asn 342 and Ser 343) would allow the binding of selective CPP-32 inhibitors to the active site [adapted from 172].

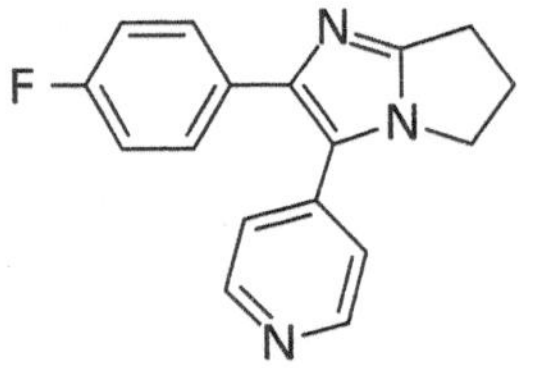

SK&F-104351
(SAPK inhibitor)

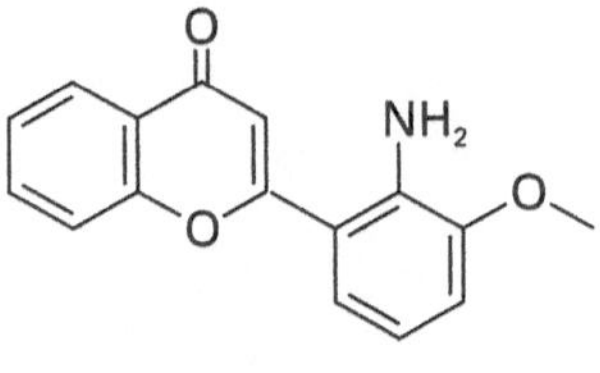

PD-98059
(MAPK inhibitor)

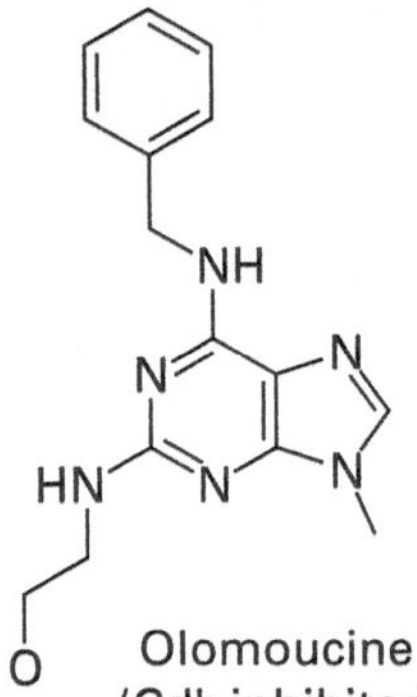

Olomoucine
(Cdk inhibitor)

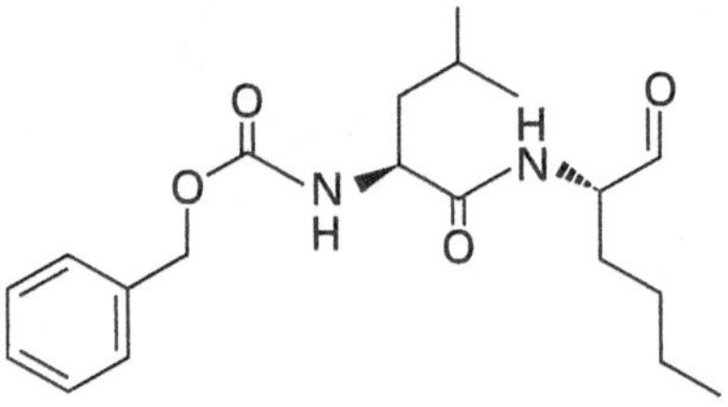

Calpeptin
(calpain inhibitor)

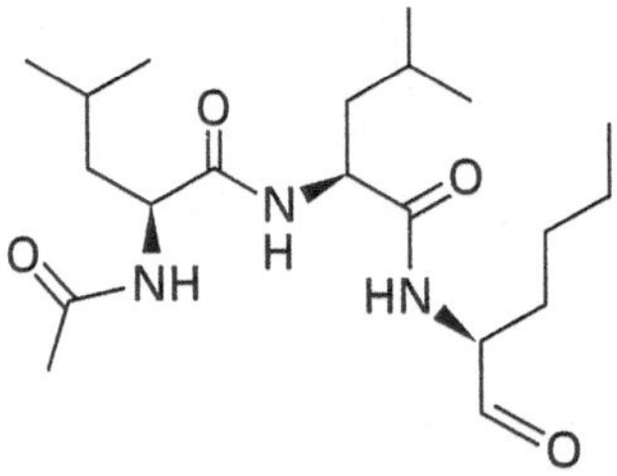

Calbiochem calpain-
inhibitor-I

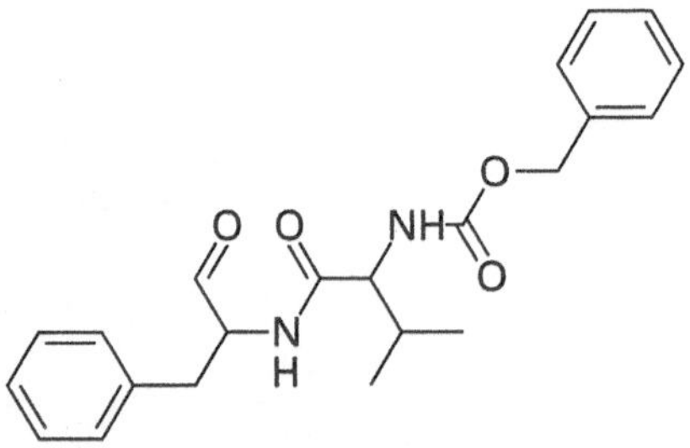

MDL-28170
(calpain inhibitor)

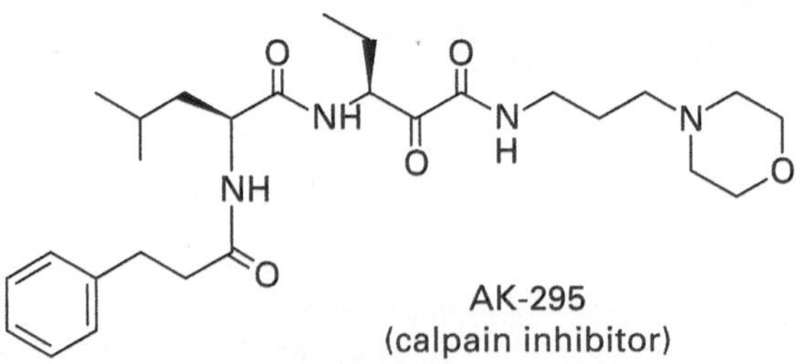

AK-295
(calpain inhibitor)

Fig. 7
The structures of some inhibitors of cell death.

References

1   A. Fraser and G.Evan: A license to kill. Cell *85*, 781–784 (1996).
2   R.E. Ellis, J. Yuan, H.R. Horvitz: Mechanisms and functions of cell death. Ann. Rev. Cell Biol., 663–698 (1991).
3   A.H. Wyllie, M.J. Arends, R.G. Morris, S.W. Walker and G. Evan: The apoptosis endonuclease and its regulation. Semin. Immunol. *4*(6), 389–379 (1992).
4   D.L. Vaux: Toward an understanding of the molecular mechanisms of physiological cell death. Proc. Natl. Acad. Sci., USA *90*(3), 786–789 (1993).
5   A.H. Wyllie: The genetic regulation of apoptosis. Curr. Opin Genet. Dev. *5*(1), 97–104 (1995).
6   D. Hockenbery: Defining apoptosis. Am. J. Pathol. *146*(1), 16–19 (1995).
7   S. Kumar: ICE-like proteases in apoptosis. Trends Biochem. Sci. *20*(5), 198–202 (1995).
8   D.R. Dowd: Calcium regulation of apoptosis. Adv. Second Messenger Phosphoprotein Res. *30*, 255–280 (1995).
9   S. Orrenius: Apoptosis: molecular mechanisms and implications for human disease. J. Intern. Med. *237*(6), 529–536 (1995).
10 C.B. Thompson: Apoptosis in the pathogenesis and treatment of disease. Science *267*, 1456–1462 (1995).
11 A.C. Lo, L.J. Houenou and R.W. Oppenheim: Apoptosis in the nervous system: morphological features, methods, pathology and prevention. Arch. Histol. Cytol. *58*(2), 139–149 (1995).
12 D.E. Bredesen: Neural apoptosis. Ann. Neurol. *38*(6), 839–851 (1995).
13 C.W. Cotman and J.A. Anderson: A potential role for apoptosis in neurodegeneration and Alzheimer's disease. Mol. Neurobiol. *10*, 19–45 (1995).
14 P. Spence, R. Franco, A. Wood and J.A. Moyer: Mechanisms of apoptosis as drug targets in the central nervous system. Exp. Opin. Ther. Patents *6*(4), 345–366 (1996).
15 A. Glüksmann: Cell death in normal vertebrate ontogeny. Biol. Rev. *26*, 59–86 (1951).
16 R.A. Lockshin and C.M. Williams: Programmed cell death. II. Endocrine potentiation of the braekdown of the intersegmental muscles of silkmoths. J. Insect Physiol. *10*, 643–649 (1964).
17 J.R. Tata: Requirement for RNA and protein synthesis for induced regression of tadpole tail in organ culture. Dev. Biol. *13*, 77–94 (1966).
18 J.F.R. Kerr, A.H. Wyllie, A.R. Currie: Apotosis: a basic biological phenomenon with wide ranging implications in tissue kinetics. Br. J. Cancer *26*, 239 (1972).
19 J. Funder: Apoptosis: two p or not two p. Nature *371*, 98 (1994); S. Norby: Opting for Silence. Nature *372*, 132 (1994).
20   J. Funder: Apoptosis forever. Nature *373*, 379 (1994).
21 D. Hockenbery, G. Nunez, C. Milliman et al.: Bcl-2 is an inner mitochondrial membrane protein that blocks programmed cell death. Nature *348*, 334–336 (1990).
22 Y.J. Liu, D.E. Joshua, G.T. Williams et al.: Mechanisms of antigen driven selection in germinal centres. Nature *342*, 21–28 (1989).
23 J.C. Ameisen and A. Capron: Cell dysfunction and depletion in AIDS: the program cell death hypothesis. Immunol. Today *12*, 102–105 (1991).
24 M.L. Gougeon, R. Oliver, S. Garcia et al.: Demonstration of an engagement process towards cell death by apoptosis in lymphocytes of HIV-infected patients. C. R. Acad. Sci. *312*, 529–537 (1991).
25   R.J. Clem, M. Fechheimer and L.K. Miller: Prevention of apoptosis by a baculovirus gene during infection of insect cells. Science *254*, 1388–1390 (1991).

26   P.A. Hershberger, J.A. Dickson and P.D. Friesen: Site-specific mutagenesis of the 35-kilodalton protein gene encoded by *Autographa californica* nuclear polyhedrosis virus: cell line-specific effects on virus replication. J.Virol. 66, 5525–5533 (1992).

27   J.F.R. Kerr and B.V. Harmon: Definition and incidence of apotosis an historical perspective. In L.D. Tomei and F.O. Cope, eds. Apoptosis: the molecular basis of cell death. Cold Spring Harbor Laboratory Press, Plainview, NY 1991, 5–29.

28   S.V. Lennon, S.J. Martin and T.G. Cotter: Dose-dependent induction of apoptosis in human tumor cell lines by widely diverging stimuli. Cell Prolif. *24*, 203–214 (1991).

29   L.D. Tomei, J.P. Shapiro and F.O. Cope: Apoptosis in C3H/10T 1/2 mouse embryonic cells: evidence for internucleosomal DNA modification in the absence of double-strand cleavage. Proc. Natl. Acad. Sci. USA. *90*, 853–857 (1992).

30   A.H. Wyllie: Glucocorticoid-induced thymocyte apoptosis is associated with endogenous endonuclease activation. Nature *284*, 555–556 (1980).

31   D.J. McConkey and S. Orrenius: Cellular signaling in thymocyte apoptosis. In L.D. Tomei and F.O. Cope, eds. Apoptosis: the molecular basis of cell death. Cold Spring Harbor Laboratory Press, Plainview, NY 1991, 227–246.

32   L.D. Tomei: Apoptosis: a program for death or survival? In L.D. Tomei and F.O. Cope, eds. Apoptosis: the molecular basis of cell death. Cold Spring Harbor Laboratory Press, Plainview, NY 1991, 279–316.

33   A. Batistatou and L.A. Greene: Aurintricarboxlyic acid recuses PC-12 cells and sympathetic neurones from cell death caused by nerve growthfactor deprivation: correlation with suppresion of endonuclease activity. J. Cell Biol. *115*, 461–471 (1991).

34   M.L. Gaido and J.A. Cidowski. Indentification, purification and characterisation of a calcium-dependent endonuclease (NUC18) from apoptotic rat thymocytes. NUC18 is not histone H2B. J. Biol. Chem. *266*, 18580–18585 (1991).

35   R.W. Oppenheim: Cell death during the development of the nervous system. Ann. Rev. Neurosci. *14*, 453–501 (1991).

36   E. Janec and R.E. Burke: Naturally occuring cell death during postnatal development of the substantia nigra pars compacts of the rat. Molec. Cell Neurosci. 4, 30–35 (1993).

37   A. Macaya, F. Munell, R.M. Gubits. and R.E. Burke: Apoptosis in substantia nigra following developmental striatal excitotoxic injury. Proc. Natl. Acad. Sci, USA *91*(17), 8117–21 (1994).

38   K.A. Wood, B. Dipasquale and R.J. Youle. In situ labeling of granule cells for apoptosis-associated DNA fragmentation reveals different mechanisms of cell loss in developing cerebellum. Neuron *11*(4): 621–632 (1993).

39   C.M. Waters, W. Moser, G. Walkinshaw and I.J. Mitchell. Death of neurons in the neonatal rodent and primate globus pallidus occurs by a mechanism of apoptosis. Neurosci. *63*(3): 881–894 (1994).

40   A.G. Estevez, R. Radi, L. Barbeito, J.T. Shin, J.A. Thompson and J.S. Beckman: -Peroxynitrite-induced cytotoxcity in PC-12 cells: evidence for an apototic mechanism differentially modulated by neurotrophic factors J. Neurochem. *65*, 1543–1550 (1995).

41   Y. Agid: Aging, disease and nerve cell death. Bull. Acad. Natl. Med. 179(6), 1193–203 (1995).

42   I.J. Mitchell, S. Lawson, B. Mose, S.M. Laidlaw, A.J. Cooper, G. Walkinshaw and C.M. Waters: Glutamate-induced apoptosis results in a loss of striatal neurons in the Pakinsonian rat. Neurosci. *63*(1), 1–5 (1994).

43   A.M. Janson: Apoptosis-like neuronal death in vivo in the MPTP mouse model of Parkinson's disease. 25th Soc. Neurosci. San Diego, USA *21*, 1273 (1995).

44 V. Jackson-Lewis, M.W. Jakowec, R.E. Burke and S. Przedborski: Time course and morphology of MTPT-induced neuronal death. 25th Soc. Neurosci. San Diego, USA *21*, 2002 (1995).

45 Y.A. Barde: Trophic factors and neuronal survival. Neuron *2*, 1525–1534 (1989).

46 H. Thoenen, F.A. Barde, A.M. Davies and J.E. Johnson: Neurotrophic factors and neuronal death. In: Selective neuronal death. Ciba Found. Symp. *126*, 82–95 (1987).

47 R.M. Lindsay: Neuron saving schemes. Nature *373*, 289–290 (1995).

48 M. Baringa: Neurotrophic factors enter the clinic. Science *264*, 272–274 (1994).

49 G. Walkinshaw and C.M. Waters: Neurotoxin-induced cell death in neuronal PC-12 cells is mediated by induction of apoptosis. Neurosci. *63*(4), 975–987 (1994).

50 G. Walkinshaw and C.M. Waters: Induction of apoptosis in catecholeaminergic PC-12 cells by L-DOPA: implications for the treatment of Parkinson's Disease. J. Clin. Invest. *95*, 2458–2464 (1995).

51 D.T. Dexter, A, Carayon, M. Vidailhet, M. Rugerb, F. Agid, A.J. Lees, F.R. Wells, P. Jenner and D. Marsden: Decreased ferritin levels in the brain in Parkinson's Disease. J. Neurochem *55*, 16–20 (1990).

52 A. Hartley. J.M. Stone, C. Heron, J.M. Cooper, A.H.V. Schapira: Complex inhibitors induce dose-dependent apoptosis in PC-12 cells: relevance to parkinson's disease. J. Neurochem. *63*, 1987–1990 (1994).

53 B. Dipasquale, A.M. Marini and R.J. Youle: Apoptosis and DNA degradation induced by MTPT in neurons. Biochem. Biophys. Res. Commun. *181*, 1442–1448 (1991).

54 J.H. Su, A.J. Anderson, B.J. Cummings and C.W. Cotman: Immunohistochemical evidence for apoptosis in Alzheimer's disease. NeuroReport *5*, 2529–2533 (1994).

55 J.H. Su, A.J. Anderson and C.W. Cotman: Quantitative assessment of apoptotic-like nuclei in hippocampal formation of Alzheimer brain. 25th Soc. Neurosci. San Diego, USA *21*, 1727 (1995).

56 M. Dragunow: DNA fragmentation in Alzheimer's disease hippocampus correlation with tau and β-amyloid immunoreactivity. 25th Soc. Neurosci. San Diego, USA *21*, 1724 (1995).

57 A.J. Anderson, J.H. Su and C.W. Cotman: DNA damage and apoptosis in Alzheimer's disease: colocalisation with c-JUn immunoreactivity, relationship to brain area and effects of postmortem delay. J. Neurosci. *16*(5), 1710–1719 (1996).

58 H. Lassman, C. Bancher, H. Breitschopf, J. Wegiel, M. Bobinski, K. Jellinger and H.M. Wisniewski: Cell death in Alzheimer's disease evaluated by DNA fragmentation in situ. Acta Neuropathol. *89*, 35–41 (1995).

59 L.S. Perlmutter, A.F. Bushnell, Y.-P. Li, S. Webster and S. Wong: Evidence for DNA damage, but not apoptosis, in Alzheimer's diseased brain. 25th Soc. Neurosci. San Diego, USA *21*, 1721 (1995).

60 A. Mighelia, P. Cavalla, R Piva, M.T. Giordana and D. Schiffer: Bcl-2 protein expression in aged brain and neurodegenerative diseases. NeuroReport *5*, 1906–1908 (1994).

61 T. Satou, B.J. Cummings and C.W. Cotman: Bcl-2 protein immunoreactivity increases in Alzheimer's disease brain with disease severity. 25th Soc. Neurosci. San Diego, USA *21*, 1726 (1995).

62 S. O'Barr, J. Schultz, M. McKinley and J. Rogers: Expression of Bcl-2 oncoprotein in Alzheimers disease. 25th Soc. Neurosci. San Diego, USA *21*, 740 (1995).

63 E.M. Johnson: Possible role of neuronal apotosis in Alzheimer's disease. Neurobiol. Aging 15(2), S187–S189 (1994).

64 F.M. Laferla, B.T. Tinkle, C.J. Bieberich, C.C. Haudenschild and G. Jay: The

Alzheimer's Aβ-peptide-induced neurodegeneration and apoptotic cell death in transgenic mice Nat. Genet. 9, 21–30 (1995).

65   P. Vito, E. Lacana and L. D'Adamio: Interfering with apoptosis: Ca²⁺-binding protein ALG-2 and Alzheimer's disease gene ALG-3. Science 271, 521–525 (1996).

66   G. Forloni, R. Chiesa, S. Smiroldo, L. Verga, M. Salmona, F. Tagliavini and N. Angeretti: Apoptosis mediated neurotoxicity induced by chronic application of β-amyloid fragment 25–35. NeuroReport 4, 523–526 (1993).

67   D.T. Loo, A. Copani, C.J. Pike, R.R. Whittemore, A.J. Walencewicz and C.W. Cotman: Apoptosis is induced by β-amyloid in cultures central nervous system neurons. Proc. Natl. Acad. Sci. USA 4, 523–526 (1993).

68   C. Behl, J.B. Davis, F.G. Klier and D. Schubert: Amyloid β-peptide induces necrosis rather than apoptosis. Brain Res. 645, 253–264 (1994).

69   M. Gschwind and G. Huber: Apoptotic cell death induced by β-amyloid peptide is cell type dependent. J. Neurochem. 65(1), 292–300 (1995).

70   J.W. Kuisak, S.S. Sisodia and B. Zhao: Apoptosis is induced by expression of mutant amyloid precursor protein in neuronal cells. In: neurodegenerative disorders: common molecular mechanisms, the decade of the brain. Rios, Jamaica 1995; IX: Apoptosis and neurodegenerative disorders.

71   D.W. Choi: Cerebral hypoxia: some new approaches and unanswered questions. J. Neurosci. 10, 2493–2501 (1990).

72   J.T. Coyle and P. Puttfarcken: Oxidative stress, glutamate and neurodegenerative disorders. Science 262, 689–695 (1993).

73   N.R. Sims and E. Zaidan: Biochemical changes associated with selective neuronal death following short-term cerebral ischaemia. Int. J. Biochem. Cell Biol. 27(6), 531–550 (1995).

74   M.D. Linnik, R.H. Zobrist and M.D. Hatfield: Evidence supporting a role for programmed cell death in focal cerebral ischaemia in rats. Stroke 24, 2002–2009 (1993).

75   J.M. MacManus, A.M. Buchan, I.E. Hill, I. Rasquinha and E. Preston: Global iscaemia can cause DNA fragmentation indicative of apoptosis in rat brain. Neurosci. Lett. 164(1–2), 89–92 (1993).

76   M. Okamoto, M. Matsumoto, T. Ontsuki, A. Taguichi, K. Mikoshita, T. Yanagihara and T. Kamada: Internucleosomal DNA cleavage involved in ischaemia-induced neuronal death. Biochem. Biophys. Res. Commun 196(3), 1356–1362 (1993).

77   E.M. Johnson, L.J.S. Greenlund, P.T. Akins and C.Y. Hsu: Neuronal apoptosis: current understanding of molecular mechanisms and potential role in ischaemic brain injury. J. Neurotrauma 12(5), 843–852 (1995).

78   S. Kure, T. Tominaga, T. Yoshimoto, K. Tada and K. Narisawa: Glutamate triggers internucleosomal DNA cleavage in neuronal cells. Biochem. Biophys. Res. Commun. 179(1), 39–45 (1991).

79   F. Dessi, C. Charriaut-Marlangue, M. Khrestchatisky, Y. Ben-Ari: Glutamate-induced neuronal death is not a programmed cell death in cerebellar cultures. J. Neurochem. 60(5), 1953–1955 (1993).

80   D.W. Choi, K. Koh, J.A. Demaro, H.S. Ying, M.F. Jaquin and V.J. Gwag: Even slowlytriggered neuronal death of cultured cortical neurons occurs by necrosis not apoptosis. 25th Soc. Neurosci. San Diego, USA 21, 1585 (1995).

81   M. Ankarcrona, J.M. Dypbukt, E. Bonfoco, B. Zhivotovsky, S. Orrenius, S.A. Lipton and P. Nicotera: Glutamate-induced neuronal death: a succession of necrosis or apoptosis depending on mitochondrial function. Neuron 15 (4), 961–973 (1995).

82 B.J. Gwag, D. Lobner, J.Y. Koh, M.B. Wie and D.W. Choi: Blockade of glutamate receptors unmasks neuronal apoptosis after oxygen-glucose deprivation *in vitro*. Neurosci. *68*(3), 615–619 (1995).

83 A. Copani, V.M.G. Bruno, V. Barresi, G. Battaglia, D.F. Condorelli and F. Nicoletti: Activation of metabatropic glutamate receptors prevents neuronal apotosis in culture. J. Neurochem. *64*(1), 101–108 (1995).

84 J.Y. Koh, E. Palmer and C.W. Cotman: Activation of the metabotropic glutamate receptor attenuates NMDA neurotoxicity in cortical cultures. Proc. Natl Acad. Sci. USA *88*, 9431–9435 (1991).

85 R.F. Regan and D.W. Choi: Excitotoxicity and central nervous system trauma. In: The Neurobiology of Central Nervous System Trauma. S.D. Salzman and A.L. (Eds.) Oxford University Press, New York 1994, 173–181.

86 T.K. McIntosh, R. Vink, L. Noble, I. Yamakami, S. Fernyak, H. Soares and L.H. Faden: Traumatic brain injury in the rat: characterisation of a lateral fluid-percussion model. Neurosci. *28*, 233–244 (1989).

87 A. Rink, K.-M. Fung, J.Q. Trojanowski, V.M.-Y. Lee, E. Neugebauer and T.K. McIntosh: Evidence of apototic cell death after experimental traumatic brain injury in the rat. Am J. Pathol. *147*(6), 1575–1583 (1995).

88 A. Conti, C.M. Hylton, R. Raghupathi, D.H. Smith, J.Q. Trojanowski, V.M.-Y. Lee and T.K. McIntosh: Magnesium deficiency decreases the occurrence of apoptosis after traumatic brain injury. 13th Annual Neurotrauma Symposium. San Diego, USA 1995.

89 G. Sinson, B. Perri, J.Q. Trojanowski, V.M.-Y. Lee and T.K. McIntosh: Apoptotic death in the septal nuclei after fluid percussion brain injury is attenuated by NGF infusion. 13th Annual Neurotrauma Symposium. San Diego, USA 1995.

90 W.I. McDonald and D.H. Silberberg: Multiple sclerosis Butterworths, London, 1986.

91 M. Dubois-Dalq and R. Armstrong: The cellular and molecular events of the central neurons remyelination. Bioessay *12*, 569–576 (1990).

92 B.A. Barres, I.K. Hart, H.S.R. Coles, J.F. Burne, J.T. Voyvodic, W.D. Richardson and M.C. Raff: Cell death and control of cell survival in the oligodendrocyte lineage. Cell *70*, 31–46 (1992).

93 P.E. Knapp, R.P. Skoff and W.R. Redstone: Oligodendroglial cell death in jimpy mice: an explanation for the myelin deficit. J. Neurosci. *6*(10), 2813–2822 (1986).

94 M.P. Pender, K.B. Nguyen, P.A. McCombe, and J.F.R. Kerr: Apoptosis in the nervous system in experimental allergic encephalomyelitis. J. Neurosci. *104*, 81–87 (1991).

95 K. Selmaj, C.S. Raine, M. Farooq, W.T. Norton and C.F. Brosnan: Cytokine toxicity against oligodendrocytes. Apoptosis induced by lymphotoxin. J. Immunol. *147*(5), 1522–1529 (1991).

96 S. Prabhakar, S. D'Souza, J.P. Antel, J.A. McLaurin, H.M. Schipper and E. Wang: Phenotypic and cell cycle properties of human oligodendrocytes *in vitro*. Brain Res. *195* 672, 159–169 (1995).

97 D. Muir and D.A.S. Compston: Growth factor stimulation triggers apoptotic cell death in mature rat oligodendrocytes. J. Neurosci. Res. *44* (1), 1–11 (1996).

98 N.J. Scolding and W.A.J. Houston, C. Linington, B.P. Morgan, A.K. Campbell and D.A.S. Compston: Oligodendrocytes activate complement but recover by vesicular removal of membrane attack complexes. Nature *338*, 620–622 (1989).

99 D.R. Wren and M. Noble: Oligodendrocytes and oligodendrocyte/type-2 astrocyte progenitor cells of adult rats are specifically susceptible to the lytic effects of complement in the absence of antibody. Proc. Natl Acad.Sci. USA *86*, 9025–9029 (1989).

100 A. Wood, M. Wing, C.D. Benham and D.A.S. Compston: Specific induction of intracellular oscillations by complement membrane attack on oligodendroglia. J. Neurosci. *13*, 3319–3332 (1993).

101 Z. Tabi, P.A. McCombe and M.P. Pender: Apoptotic elimation of V beta 8.2+ cells-from the central nervous system during recovery from EAE induced by the massive transfer of V beta 8.2 encepalitogenic T cells. Eur. J. Immunol. *24* (11), 2609–2617 (1994).

102 C.M. Pelfrey, L.R. Tranquill, S.A. Boehme, H.F. McFarland and M.J. Lenardo: Two mechanisms of antigen-specific apoptosis of myelin basic protein-specific T-lymphocytes derived from multiple sclerosis patients and normal individuals. J. Immunol. *154* (11), 6191–6202 (1995).

103 X. Mu, J. He, D.W. Anderson, J.Q. Trojanowski and J.E. Springer: Altered expression of bcl-2 and bax mRNA in amyotrophic lateral sclerosis motoneurons. 25th Soc. Neurosci. San Diego, USA *21*, 561 (1995).

104 M. Dubois-Dauphin, H. Frankowski, Y. Tsujimoto, J. Huarte and J.C. Martinou: Neonatal motoneurons overexpressing the bcl-2 proto-oncogene in transgenic mice are protected from axotomy-induced cell death. Proc. Natl Acad. Sci. USA *91*, 229–240 (1994).

105 C.M. Troy and M.L. Shelanski: Down regulation of copper/zinc superoxide dismutase causes apoptotic death in PC-12 neuronal cells. Proc. Acad. Natl Sci. USA *91*, 6384–6387 (1994).

106 L.S. Greenlund, T.L. Deckwerth, E.M. Johnson: Superoxide dismutase delays neuronal apoptosis: a role for reactive oxygen species in programmed neuronal death. Neuron *14*, 303–315 (1995).

107 J.D. Rothstein, L.A. Bristol, B. Hosler, R.H. Brown and R.W. Kuncl: Chronic inhibiton of superoxide dismutase produces apoptotic death of spinal neurons. Proc. Natl. Acad. Sci. USA *91*, 4155–4159 (1994).

108 S. Rabizadeh, E.B. Grallaeb, D.R. Borchelt, R. Gwinn, J.S. Valentine, S. Sisodia, P. Wong, M. Lee, H. Hahn and D.E. Bredesen: Mutations associated with amyotrophic lateral sclerosis convert superoxide dismutase from an antiapoptotic gene to a pro-apoptotic gene: studies in yeast and neural cells. Proc. Natl. Acad. Sci. USA *92*, 3024–3028 (1995).

109 J. Busciglio and B.A. Yankner: Apoptosis and increased generation of reactive oxygen species in Down's syndrome neurons *in vitro*. Nature *378*, 776–779 (1995).

110 P.J. Lucassen, A. Williams, W.C. Chung and H. Fraser: Dectection of apoptosis in murine scrapie. Neurosci. Lett. *198*(3), 185–188 (1995).

111 A. Giese, M.H. Groschup, B. Hess and H.A. Kretzschmar: Neuronal cell death in scrapie-infected mice is due to apoptosis. Brain Pathol. *5*(3), 213–221 (1995).

112 C. Portera-Cailliau, J.C. Hedreen, D.L. Price and V.E. Koliatos: Evidence for apoptotic cell death in Huntington's disease and excitotoxic animal models. J. Neurosci. *15*(5), 3775–3787 (1995).

113 Y.A. Lazebnik, S.H. Kaufmann, S. Desnoyers, G.G. Poirier, and W.C. Earnshaw: Cleavage of poly(ADP-ribose) polymerase by a proteinase with properties like ICE. Nature. *371*, 346–7 (1994).

114 L.A. Casciola-Rosen, D.K. Miller, G.J. Anhalt, and A. Rosen: Specific cleavage of the 70-kDa protein component of the U1 small nuclear ribonucleoprotein is a characteristic biochemical feature of apoptotic cell death. J. Biol. Chem. *269*, 30757–60 (1994).

115 S.J. Martin, G.A. O'Brien, W.K. Nishioka, A.J. McGahon, A. Mahboubi, T.C. Saido,

and D.R. Green: Proteolysis of fodrin (non-erythroid spectrin) during apoptosis. J Biol Chem. *270*, 6425–8 (1995).

116 M.J. Smyth and J.A. Trapani: Granzymes: exogenous proteinases that induce target cell apoptosis. Immunol Today. *16*, 202–6 (1995).

117 S. Kumar and N.L. Harvey: Role of multiple cellular proteases in the execution of programmed cell death. Febs Lett. *375*, 169–73 (1995).

118 M. Miura, H. Zhu, R. Rotello, E.A. Hartwieg, and J. Yuan: Induction of apoptosis in fibroblasts by IL-1 beta-converting enzyme, a mammalian homolog of the C. elegans cell death gene ced-3. Cell. *75*, 653–60 (1993).

119 V. Gagliardini, P.A. Fernandez, R.K. Lee, H.C. Drexler, R.J. Rotello, M.C. Fishman, and J. Yuan: Prevention of vertebrate neuronal death by the crmA gene [see comments] [published erratum appears in Science 1994 Jun 3264(5164):1388]. Science. *263*, 826–8 (1994).

120 I. Martinou, P.A. Fernandez, M. Missotten, E. White, B. Allet, R. Sadoul, and J.C. Martinou: Viral proteins E1B19K and p35 protect sympathetic neurons from cell death induced by NGF deprivation. J Cell Biol. *128*, 201–8 (1995).

121 P.A. Henkart: ICE family proteases: mediators of all apoptotic cell death? Immunity. *4*, 195–201 (1996).

122 A. Fraser and G. Evan: A license to kill. Cell *85*, 781–4 (1996).

123 M.K. Squier, A.C. Miller, A.M. Malkinson, and J.J. Cohen: Calpain activation in apoptosis. J Cell Physiol. *159*, 229–37 (1994).

124 K.K. Wang and P.W. Yuen: Calpain inhibition: an overview of its therapeutic potential. Trends Pharmacol Sci. *15*, 412–9 (1994).

125 J.M. Peters: Proteasomes: protein degradation machines of the cell. Trends Biochem Sci. *19*, 377–82 (1994).

126 A.L. Goldberg: ATP-dependent proteases in prokaryotic and eukaryotic cells. Semin Cell Biol. *1*, 423–32 (1990).

127 M. Pagano, S.W. Tam, A.M. Theodoras, P. Beer-Romero, G. Del-Sal, V. Chau, P.R. Yew, G.F. Draetta, and M. Rolfe: Role of the ubiquitin-proteasome pathway in regulating abundance of the cyclin-dependent kinase inhibitor p27 [see comments]. Science. *269*, 682–5 (1995).

128 S.J. Martin and D.R. Green: Apoptosis during HIV infection. A cytopathic effect of HIV or an important host-defense mechanism against viruses in general? Adv Exp Med Biol. *374*, 129–38 (1995).

129 G.J. Lees: The possible contribution of microglia and macrophages to delayed neuronal death after ischemia. J Neurol Sci. *114*, 119–22 (1993).

130 T. Morioka, A.N. Kalehua, and W.J. Streit: Characterization of microglial reaction after middle cerebral artery occlusion in rat brain. J Comp Neurol. *327*, 123–32 (1993).

131 J. Gehrmann, R. Gold, C. Linington, J. Lannes-Vieira, H. Wekerle, and G.W. Kreutzberg: Spinal cord microglia in experimental allergic neuritis. Evidence for fast and remote activation. Lab Invest. *67*, 100–13 (1992).

132 D. Giulian, M. Corpuz, S. Chapman, M. Mansouri, and C. Robertson: Reactive mononuclear phagocytes release neurotoxins after ischemic and traumatic injury to the central nervous system. J Neurosci Res. *36*, 681–93 (1993).

133 D. Giulian and C. Robertson: Inhibition of mononuclear phagocytes reduces ischemic injury in the spinal cord. Ann Neurol. *27*, 33–42 (1990).

134 R.A. Lang and J.M. Bishop: Macrophages are required for cell death and tissue remodeling in the developing mouse eye. Cell. *74*, 453–62 (1993).

135   E.J. Beilharz, C.E. Williams, M. Dragunow, E.S. Sirimanne, and P.D. Gluckman: Mechanisms of delayed cell death following hypoxic-ischemic injury in the immature rat: evidence for apoptosis during selective neuronal loss. Brain Res Mol Brain Res. *29*, 1–14 (1995).

136   B.A. Barres, R. Schmid, M. Sendnter, and M.C. Raff: Multiple extracellular signals are required for long-term oligodendrocyte survival. Development *118*, 283–95 (1993).

137   J. Guan, C. Williams, M. Gunning, C. Mallard, and P. Gluckman: The effects of IGF-1 treatment after hypoxic-ischemic brain injury in adult rats. J Cereb Blood Flow Metab. *13*, 609–16 (1993).

138   M. Oren: Relationship of p53 to the control of apoptotic cell death. Semin Cancer Biol. *5*, 221–7 (1994).

139   S. Sakhi, A. Bruce, N. Sun, G. Tocco, M. Baudry, and S.S. Schreiber: p53 induction is associated with neuronal damage in the central nervous system. Proc Natl Acad Sci USA *91*, 7525–9 (1994).

140   L.A. Donehower, M. Harvey, B.L. Slagle, M.J. McArthur, C. Montgomery Jr., J.S. Butel, and A. Bradley: Mice deficient for p53 are developmentally normal but susceptible to spontaneous tumours. Nature *356*, 215–21 (1992).

141   S.F. Dowdy, P.W. Hinds, K. Louie, S.I. Reed, A. Arnold, and R.A. Weinberg: Physical interaction of the retinoblastoma protein with human D cyclins. Cell *73*, 499–511 (1993).

142   V. Baldin, J. Lukas, M.J. Marcote, M. Pagano, and G. Draetta: Cyclin D1 is a nuclear protein required for cell cycle progression in G1. Genes Dev. *7*, 812–21 (1993).

143   R.S. Freeman, S. Estus, and E. Johnson Jr.: Analysis of cell cycle-related gene expression in postmitotic neurons: selective induction of Cyclin D1 during programmed cell death. Neuron *12*, 343–55 (1994).

144   O. Kranenburg, A.J. van-der-Eb, and A. Zantema: Cyclin D1 is an essential mediator of apoptotic neuronal cell death. Embo J. *15*, 46–54 (1996).

145   K. Herrup and J.C. Busser: The induction of multiple cell cycle events precedes target-related neuronal death. Development *121*, 2385–95 (1995).

146   K. Ando, F. Ajchenbaum-Cymbalista, and J.D. Griffin: Regulation of G1/S transition by cyclins D2 and D3 in hematopoietic cells. Proc Natl Acad Sci USA *90*, 9571–5 (1993).

147   T. Shimizu, P.M. O'Connor, K.W. Kohn, and Y. Pommier: Unscheduled activation of cyclin B1/Cdc2 kinase in human promyelocytic leukemia cell line HL60 cells undergoing apoptosis induced by DNA damage. Cancer Res. *55*, 228–31 (1995).

148   S.C. Chen, T. Curran, and J.I. Morgan: Apoptosis in the nervous system: new revelations. J Clin Pathol. *48*, 7–12 (1995).

149   Y. Gazitt and G.W. Erdos: Fluctuations and ultrastructural localization of oncoproteins and cell cycle regulatory proteins during growth and apoptosis of synchronized AGF cells. Cancer Res. *54*, 950–6 (1994).

150   L.H. Tsai, I. Delalle, V. Caviness Jr., T. Chae, and E. Harlow: p35 is a neural-specific regulatory subunit of cyclin-dependent kinase 5. Nature *371*, 419–23 (1994).

151   D. Tang, J. Yeung, K.Y. Lee, M. Matsushita, H. Matsui, K. Tomizawa, O. Hatase, and J.H. Wang: An isoform of the neuronal cyclin-dependent kinase 5 (Cdk5) activator. J Biol Chem. *270*, 26897–903 (1995).

152   J. Ham, C. Babij, J. Whitfield, C.M. Pfarr, D. Lallemand, M. Yaniv, and L.L. Rubin: A c-Jun dominant negative mutant protects sympathetic neurons against programmed cell death. Neuron *14*, 927–39 (1995).

153 Z. Xia, M. Dickens, J. Raingeaud, R.J. Davis, and M.E. Greenberg: Opposing effects of ERK and JNK-p38 MAP kinases on apoptosis. Science 270, 1326–31 (1995).

154 Z.N. Oltvai and S.J. Korsmeyer: Checkpoints of dueling dimers foil death wishes [comment]. Cell 79, 189–92 (1994).

155 G.A. Silverman, E. Yang, J.H. Proffitt, M. Zutter, and S.J. Korsmeyer: Genetic transfer and expression of reconstructed yeast artificial chromosomes containing normal and translocated BCL2 proto-oncogenes. Mol Cell Biol. 13, 5469–78 (1993).

156 C.M. Knudson, K.S. Tung, W.G. Tourtellotte, G.A. Brown, and S.J. Korsmeyer: Bax-deficient mice with lymphoid hyperplasia and male germ cell death. Science 270, 96–9 (1995).

157 E.H. Cheng, B. Levine, L.H. Boise, C.B. Thompson, and J.M. Hardwick: Bax-independent inhibition of apoptosis by Bcl-XL. Nature 379, 554–6 (1996).

158 H. Frankowski, M. Missotten, P.A. Fernandez, I. Martinou, P. Michel, R. Sadoul, and J.C. Martinou: Function and expression of the Bcl-x gene in the developing and adult nervous system. Neuroreport 6, 1917–21 (1995).

159 N. Motoyama, F. Wang, K.A. Roth, H. Sawa, K. Nakayama, K. Nakayama, I. Negishi, S. Senju, Q. Zhang, S. Fujii, et al.: Massive cell death of immature hematopoietic cells and neurons in Bcl-x-deficient mice. Science 267, 1506–10 (1995).

160 D.J. Veis, C.M. Sorenson, J.R. Shutter, and S.J. Korsmeyer: Bcl-2-deficient mice demonstrate fulminant lymphoid apoptosis, polycystic kidneys, and hypopigmented hair. Cell 75, 229–40 (1993).

161 E. Yang, J. Zha, J. Jockel, L.H. Boise, C.B. Thompson, and S.J. Korsmeyer: Bad, a heterodimeric partner for Bcl-XL and Bcl-2, displaces Bax and promotes cell death. Cell 80, 285–91 (1995).

162 S. Krajewski, S. Bodrug, M. Krajewska, A. Shabaik, R. Gascoyne, K. Berean, and J.C. Reed: Immunohistochemical analysis of Mcl-1 protein in human tissues. Differential regulation of Mcl-1 and Bcl-2 protein production suggests a unique role for Mcl-1 in control of programmed cell death in vivo. Am J Pathol. 146, 1309–19 (1995).

163 S.P. Jaw, D.D. Su, and D.D. Truong: Expression of Bcl-2 and Bax in the frontoparietal cortex of the rat following cardiac arrest. Brain Res Bull. 38, 577–80 (1995).

164 M.P. Mattson, S.W. Barger, J.G. Begley, and R.J. Mark: Calcium, free radicals, and excitotoxic neuronal death in primary cell culture. Methods Cell Biol. 46, 187–216 (1995).

165 D.W. Choi: Calcium: still center-stage in hypoxic-ischemic neuronal death. Trends Neurosci. 18, 58–60 (1995).

166 D.D. Friel and R.W. Tsien: An FCCP-sensitive Ca2+ store in bullfrog sympathetic neurons and its participation in stimulus-evoked changes in [Ca2+]i. J Neurosci. 14, 4007–24 (1994).

167 C. Giulivi, A. Boveris, and E. Cadenas: Hydroxyl radical generation during mitochondrial electron transfer and the formation of 8-hydroxydesoxyguanosine in mitochondrial DNA. Arch Biochem Biophys. 316, 909–16 (1995).

168 R.F. Castilho, A.J. Kowaltowski, A.R. Meinicke, and A.E. Vercesi: Oxidative damage of mitochondria induced by Fe(II)citrate or t-butyl hydroperoxide in the presence of Ca2+: effect of coenzyme Q redox state. Free Radic Biol Med. 18, 55–9 (1995).

169 L.L. Dugan, V.M. Bruno, S.M. Amagasu, and R.G. Giffard: Glia modulate the response of murine cortical neurons to excitotoxicity: glia exacerbate AMPA neurotoxicity. J Neurosci. 15, 4545–55 (1995).

170 I.J. Reynolds and T.G. Hastings: Glutamate induces the production of reactive oxy-

gen species in cultured forebrain neurons following NMDA recept
Neurosci. *15*, 3318–27 (1995).

171   M.A. Ator and R.E. Dolle: Interleukin-1β converting enzyme: biolc
try of inhibitors. Curr. Pharmaceutical Design *1*, 191–210 (1995).

172   J. Rotonda, D.W. Nicholson, K.M. Fazil, M. Gallant, Y. Gareau, M. Lat
son et al.: The three-dimensional structure of apopain/CPP-32, a k
apoptosis. Nat. Struct. Biol. *3*(7), 619–625 (1996).

Progress in Drug Research, Vol. 48 (E. Jucker, Ed.)
© 1997 Birkhäuser Verlag, Basel (Switzerland)

Viral quasispecies and the problem of vaccine-escape and drug-resistant mutants

By Esteban Domingo[1], Luis Menéndez-Arias[1], Miguel E. Quiñones-Mateu[1], Africa Holguín[1], Mónica Gutiérrez-Rivas[1], Miguel A. Martínez[1], Josep Quer[2], Isabel S. Novella[3] and John J. Holland[3]

[1]Centro de Biología Molecular «Severo Ochoa» (CSIC-UAM), Universidad Autónoma de Madrid, Cantoblanco, 28049 Madrid, Spain, [2]Recerca Medicina Interna, Hospital Vall d'Hebron, Pg. Vall d'Hebron 119-129, Barcelona, Spain, and [3]Department of Biology and Molecular Genetics, University of California, San Diego, 9500 Gilman Drive, La Jolla, California 92093-0116, USA
Correspondence to Esteban Domingo, Centro de Biología Molecular «Severo Ochoa» (CSIC-UAM), Universidad Autónoma de Madrid, Cantoblanco, 28049 Madrid, Spain, e-mail: edomingo@mvax.cbm.uam.es

Abbreviations
3TC, (-)-3'-thia-2'-deoxycytidine; α-APA, α-anilinophenylacetamide; AIDS, acquired immune deficiency syndrome; AZT, 3'-azido-2',3'-dideoxythymidine; BHAP, bis(heteroaryl)piperazine; d4T, 2',3'-didehydro-2',3'-dideoxythymidine; ddC, 2',3'-dideoxycytidine; ddI, 2',3'-dideoxyinosine; FMDV, foot-and-mouth disease virus; HBV, hepatitis B virus; HCV, hepatitis C virus; HEPT, 1-(2-hydroxyethoxymethyl)-6-(phenylthio)thymine; HIV, human immunodeficiency virus; HVR1, hypervariable region 1; MAb, monoclonal antibody; PETT, N-(2-phenylethyl)-N'-(2-thiazolyl)thiourea; TIBO, tetrahydroimidazo[4,5,1-jk][1,4]benzodiazepin-2(1H)-one and -thione; VSV, vesicular stomatitis virus.

1   Introduction: New data on viral quasispecies, and RNA genome evolution and adaptability

Since a first version of this article on the relevance of quasispecies to viral disease control was published by one of us [1], an explosion of information on viral quasispecies has been gathered by several groups. For many viruses, extreme complexity at the population level has been documented by direct copying into cDNA of viral RNA extracted from biological specimens using reverse transcriptase and amplification by thermostable polymerases (RT-PCR). Two systems relevant to human health for which extensive population heterogeneity has been revealed are hepatitis C virus (HCV) [2–4] and the human immunodeficiency viruses (HIV) [5–7, and references therein]. Particularly dramatic has been the inability to produce effective vaccines against any of these viruses [8–11] in spite of an urgent need to stop the progression of the AIDS pandemic. Also, the systematic selection of HIV-1 mutants resistant to antiretroviral inhibitors [12–14] has greatly limited the efficacy of antiretroviral treatments until the recent encouraging results with combination therapy.

Additional comparative studies have reinforced the early evidence of high mutation rates and mutation frequencies in animal and plant RNA viruses, and these data have been reviewed in several books and articles [15–19, and references therein]. Pertinent to the mechanism of high mutation rates in viral enzymes have been further biochemical [20] and structural [21, 22] studies that support the absence of proofreading activities associated with viral RNA-dependent RNA polymerases and reverse transcriptases. Recently, a high rate of mutation has also been quantitated for the retrotransposon Ty*1* of yeast [23] extending to cellular elements the great genetic flexibility which is the norm for RNA replicons [1–10, 15–19, 24]. Finally, considerable new information has been obtained regarding fitness variation and the effect of population size on virus adaptability. This review is an update of concepts of RNA virus evolution as they influence current disease control strategies, with emphasis on mechanisms of drug-resistance in HIV-1.

2   Genetic bottlenecks, massive infections, and heterogeneous environments in the evolution of viral quasispecies

The main feature that distinguishes the evolution of RNA viruses from that of differentiated DNA-based organisms is that RNA viruses replicate with high mutation rates, in the range of 10^{-3} to 10^{-5} misincorporations per nucleotide and round of copying [25–28], and produce many progeny genomes in a short time. RNA viruses are subjected to a continuous process of mutation, competition and selection of those genomes best adapted to the environment [1, 8–10, 29]. The adaptive response to an environmental change is not driven by a single, defined genomic type, but by a swarm of non-identical but related genomes termed viral quasispecies [1, 8–10, 26, 29–32].

The degree of adaptation of an RNA virus to an environment can be estimated from the ability of the virus to produce infectious progeny in that environment. This parameter has been termed viral fitness, and it is necessarily a relative value. In cell culture, relative fitness values have been obtained by growth-competition experiments. Cells are coinfected with the virus to be tested together with a genetically or phenotypically marked reference virus. The viral progeny is then used to infect additional monolayers, and the process of infection is repeated serially to determine the proportion of the two competing viruses as a function of passage number [33, 34]. A convenient marker is resistance to neutralization by a monoclonal antibody (MAb). If the reference virus has been selected for such a resistance, the plating of virus in the presence and the absence of MAb provides a quantitation of the two competing viruses in the course of the infection series [33, 34].

By measuring relative fitness values of several RNA viruses under different experimental conditions it has been observed that fitness variations are extremely dependent on the population size of the evolving RNA virus population. In particular, it has been shown that massive infections of cells with large numbers of infectious viruses lead to rapid fitness gains [35]. As the population size of an RNA virus increases, the repertoire of multiple mutants that may be subjected to positive selection increases also. New types of viral variants are often selected when very large numbers of infectious particles are employed for serial infections [36, 37]. The extremely large population size (viral load) of HIV-1 in many infected patients together with the rapid turnover of virions [38–42] is a determinant factor in the systematic selection of HIV-1 mutants resistant to antiretroviral inhibitors [12–14] (section 4).

In contrast to massive infections, repeated bottleneck events such as those occurring upon plaque-to-plaque transfers of RNA viruses result in fitness losses. Stochastic decreases in fitness were first documented with the RNA bacteriophage ø6 [43], then with vesicular stomatitis virus (VSV) [44–46] and, more recently, with foot- and-mouth disease virus (FMDV) [47]. In a plaque-to-plaque passage regime the number of genomes that enter into a competition to gain in replicative ability is very restricted, and competition is limited to the step of plaque development on the cell monolayer. The accumulation of deleterious mutations when compensatory mechanisms – such as competitive selection, true reversions, or recombination – cannot act, was first proposed by Muller [48] and it is known as Muller's ratchet. In addition to Muller's ratchet, other important principles of population genetics have been shown to operate during the evolution of RNA viruses. The Red Queen hypothesis [49] and the Competitive Exclusion principle [50] were documented by studying competitive passages of two VSV clones with similar initial fitness [51]. Although the two populations could coexist for many generations, eventually one of them suddenly and rapidly displaced the other [51]. This exclusion of one viral quasispecies by the other was undoubtedly hastened by the high mutation rates operating during VSV replication and the stochastic nature of mutagenesis. When a strongly advantageous mutation occurred in a genome of one of the competing populations, the modified quasispecies rapidly became dominant. However, both the winners and the losers in the competition gained fitness, an observation in agreement with the Red Queen hypothesis [49, 51, 52]. Interestingly, and in spite of the generally unpredictable evolution of viral quasispecies, recent results of competition among VSV clones of similar fitness have documented a reproducible nonlinear behavior [53]. Thus, on occasions, it may be possible to predict winners and losers in competitions among some types of neutral genetic variants of viruses.

These series of experiments on fitness losses and gains have documented a surprising ability of RNA viruses to abandon profound nonadaptive pits and to reach high fitness peaks. Relevant to the adaptability of RNA viruses *in vivo* are fitness variations in changing environments. Selection of FMDV variants resistant to neutralization by site-specific polyclonal antibodies resulted in viral populations with very low fitness when the latter was measured in the absence of antibodies [54]. Fitness loss was accompanied by fixation of amino acid replacements at several capsid sites, including antibody-binding sites [54]. In agreement with the results with VSV [35] serial passage of the debilitated FMDV populations in the absence of anti-FMDV antibodies resulted in dramatic fitness gains. However, and most relevant to the antigenic evolution of RNA viruses, the fitness gains occurred without reversion of any of the antigenically critical amino acid substitutions [54]. That is, the net result of passages under strong antibody pressure, followed by passages in the absence of antibodies, was an antigenically altered but biologically competent FMDV.

A related observation with VSV was that persistent infections of the virus in insect cells for prolonged time periods resulted in variant populations with fitness over two million-fold greater in sandfly cells than in mammalian cells [55]. This paralleled a similar decrease in neurovirulence for mice. The great adaptive capacity of VSV was documented by an enormous fitness increase for mammalian cells and mice neurovirulence upon a single passage of the virus in BHK-21 cells [55]. An entire organism offers a variety of cell types and of microenvironments to an infecting virus, with conflicting selective constraints of the type seen in the model studies with VSV. It has been suggested that viruses which alternate between different hosts during their life cycle (such as between insect and mammals in the case of arboviruses) have an added restriction to genetic variation [56]. Viruses may not be able to cope with all types of selective constraints. For example, passage of VSV in cells treated with α-interferon showed only a minor increase in fitness and little adaptation of the virus to growing in cells treated with α-interferon [57]. It is likely that because of the pleiotropic effects of α-interferon on viral replication and gene expression, VSV variation could not cope with the multiple selective pressures, at least within the number of viral generations tested. Difficulties met by RNA viruses to overcome multiple inhibitory activities reinforces the concept expressed earlier [1, 8–10] that multivalent vaccines and combination therapy with antiviral inhibitors are the most efficient approaches to control viral quasispecies. Recent results with HIV-1 multidrug therapy have amply confirmed this suggestion.

3　　Multivalent versus monovalent vaccines and virus-escape variants

One of the most important principles for the design of a new vaccine is that to be protective a vaccine must generally induce an immune response similar to the response induced by the pathogen as it causes natural infections [58, 59]. In the case of vaccines intended to protect against viral quasispecies this is particularly important due to the possibility of the virus escaping because of highly directed selective pressures [1, 8–10 and references therein]. An optimal vaccine must stimulate all branches of the immune response [58–60]. In addition to several problems related to efficacy of synthetic vaccines reviewed earlier [1, 8–10], recent results have documented the occurrence of vaccine-escape mutants of hepatitis B virus (HBV) [61–64]. A single amino acid substitution at an important epitope of the surface antigen was associated with antibody-escape [62–64], and, consequently, with failures of immunoprophalaxis in chronically infected newborns [62]. Passive immunoprophalaxis with anti-HBV surface immunoglobulin has been used to prevent graft reinfection after orthotopic liver transplantation. Circulating antigen and viral replication reappeared in 29% of the treated patients [65, 66]. Again, escape-mutants were selected as a result of treatment with MAbs or polyclonal antibodies following liver transplantation [67, 68]. It is still too early to evaluate whether these HBV-escape mutants will become epidemiologically significant as the use of current vaccines is extended.

Efforts to produce anti-hepatitis C virus (HCV) vaccines meet with difficulty due to the extreme heterogeneity and diversity of HCV populations [2–4]. Antibodies directed to the hypervariable region 1 (HVR1) of the envelope glycoprotein can block the attachment of virus to target cells [69–71]. However, antibodies directed to the surface glycoprotein are not sufficient to clear the infection. Chimpanzees treated with anti-HVR1 antibodies are reinfected upon challenge with either homologous or heterologous HCV [72, 73]. Vaccination of chimpanzees with recombinant multimeric envelope glycoproteins E1 and E2 induced an effective immune response [74]. The response protected partially against challenge with homologous virus [74] but not with heterologous virus [72, 73]. Nine CD8+ T cell epitopes in HCV have been described [75] and some of them appear to be well conserved among HCV isolates [76]. These recent results provide the possibility of attempting to engineer vaccines based on multiple B-cell and T-cell epitopes. However, it is suspected that the high frequency of chronic HCV infections may reflect an inherent ability of HCV quasispecies to escape from B-cell and T-cell responses.

An even more formidable task faces the preparation of vaccines for the prevention of AIDS [11, 77–80]. Early efforts were directed towards peptide-based synthetic vaccines, the least likely to afford solid protection in view of the extreme heterogeneity of HIV-1 populations [1, 8, 11, 77–80]. Recently a consensus towards the need to design multivalent, whole-virus vaccines has been manifested among many experts [78, 79], and this may tip the balance in future research toward the more promising complex anti-HIV-1 vaccines.

4   Drug-resistant variants of RNA viruses

Although the literature has been dominated by reports of systematic isolation of HIV-1 mutants resistant to antiretroviral inhibitors [12–14; sections 4.1, 4.2 and 4.3], selection of drug-resistant mutants is by no means unique to HIV-1 since the phenomenon is inherent to the population dynamics of cells and viruses [81–84]. In several cases of drug-resistance of viruses which were reviewed earlier [1], it was shown that one or few amino acid substitutions affecting viral gene products were often sufficient to confer the resistance phenotype. More recent studies have provided further support to this suggestion. For example, the resistance of influenza virus to 4-guanidino-Neu5Ac2en is associated with the replacement Glu119Gly at the active site of the neuraminidase [85, 86]. A more complex cluster of mutations appears to be required to confer resistance of viruses to interferon. Individual patients with chronic hepatitis B or C infections respond very differently to interferon, and it has been suggested that a poor response may be associated with a higher complexity of the quasispecies replicating in infected individuals [87–92]. Mutations at a specific region of gene 5A of HCV appear to correlate with interferon sensitivity [93].

All retroviruses contain reverse transcriptase, protease and integrase. Since the discovery of HIV-1 as the etiological agent causing AIDS, these enzymes have been widely studied as potential targets of antiviral drugs. Many inhibitors have been synthesized and tested *in vitro*, and some of them have been subjected to clinical evaluation. As of December 1996, the Food and Drug Administration has approved the use of seven inhibitors of the HIV-1 reverse transcriptase and three inhibitors of the protease (Table 1). Others are likely to be appoved in the near future. However, the effectiveness of all these drugs is limited by the emergence of drug-resistant viral variants. Here, we will focus on the molecular basis of resistance to reverse transcriptase and protease inhibitors.

4.1 Resistance to HIV-1 reverse transcriptase inhibitors

The HIV-1 reverse transcriptase plays a pivotal role in the retrovirus life cycle since it catalyzes the synthesis of proviral DNA using the viral RNA as template. It is a multifunctional enzyme with RNA-dependent and DNA-dependent DNA polymerase activity, and a ribonuclease activity termed RNase H. In the virus, the enzyme is composed of two subunits of 66 and 51 kDa [94], respectively. Both polypeptides derive from a 66kDa homodimer, which is cleaved to the 66kDa/51kDa heterodimer by an aspartyl-protease encoded within the viral genome. Crystal structures of reverse transcriptase were initially reported by Kohlstaedt et al. [95] and Jacobo-Molina et al. [96], and revealed a different folding for each subunit. Both subunits contain four common subdomains termed fingers, palm, thumb and connection for their resemblance to a right hand. In the 66 kDa subunit these subdomains form a nucleic acid binding cleft, which is absent in the 51 kDa subunit. Aspartic acid residues at positions 110,

Table 1.
Reverse transcriptase and protease inhibitors approved by the U.S. Food and Drug
Administration for the treatment of HIV infection.

Drugs	Commercial name	Company	Date of approval
Reverse transcriptase inhibitors			
AZT (Zidovudine)	Retrovir	Glaxo Wellcome	March 1987
ddI (Didanosine)	Videx	Bristol Myers-Squibb	October 1991
ddC (Zalcitabine)	Hivid	Hoffmann-La Roche	June 1992
d4T (Stavudine)	Zerit	Bristol Myers-Squibb	June 1994
3TC (Lamivudine)	Epivir	Glaxo Wellcome	November 1995
Nevirapine	Viramune	Boehringer Ingelheim Pharm. & Roxane Labs.	June 1996
Foscarnet	Foscavir	Astra Pharmaceutical	September 1991[a]
Protease inhibitors			
Saquinavir	Invirase	Hoffmann-La Roche	December 1995
Ritonavir	Norvir	Abbott Laboratories	March 1996
Indinavir	Crixivan	Merck & Co. Inc.	March 1996

[a] Foscarnet has been approved only for treatment of cytomegalovirus retinitis (September 1991) and acyclovir-resistant herpes simplex virus infections (June 1995), which are both AIDS-related illnesses.

185 and 186 define the polymerase active site in the palm subdomain of the 66 kDa subunit, which also contains the RNase H domain, located at its C-terminus.

The inhibitors of the reverse transcriptase can be classified into two groups: nucleoside analogs which compete with natural substrates and function as chain terminators, and nonnucleoside inhibitors which bind to an allosteric site on the enzyme. Nucleoside analogs include the licensed drugs AZT, ddI, ddC, d4T and 3TC, whose structural formulae are given in Figure 1. These compounds have to be phosphorylated by cellular nucleoside kinases in order to function as competitive inhibitors of reverse transcriptase. The best-known compound in this group is AZT (or zidovudine), which has constituted the main therapy for HIV-1 infection since its approval in March 1987. Apart from undesirable side effects, such as anemia, leukopenia or myopathy, a major limitation to its use results from

---

Fig. 1
Structural formulae of inhibitors of the reverse transcriptase and the protease of HIV-1.

Reverse transcriptase inhibitors

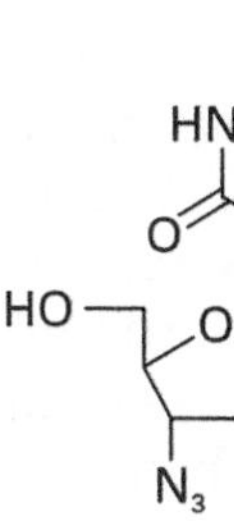

AZT 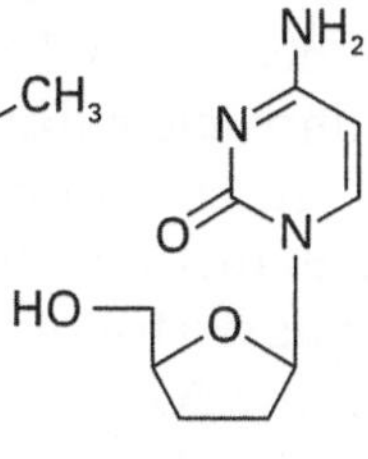   ddC 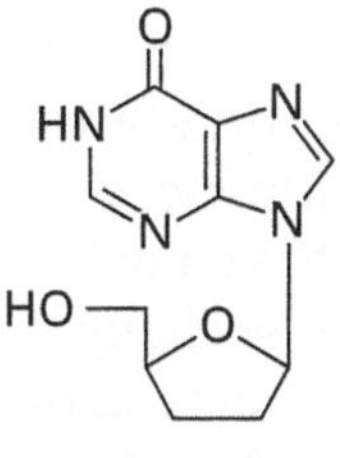   ddI 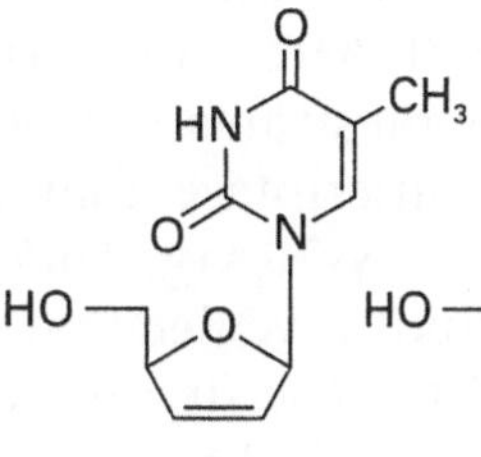   d4T 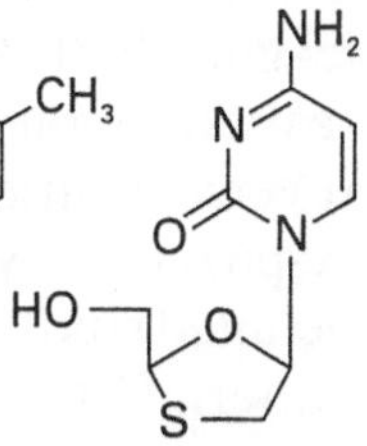   3TC

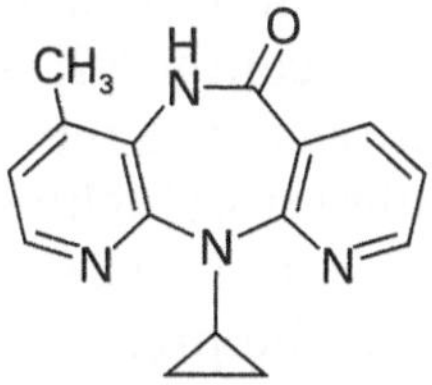

Nevirapine

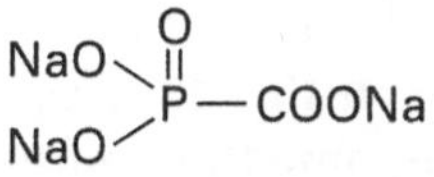

Sodium Foscarnet

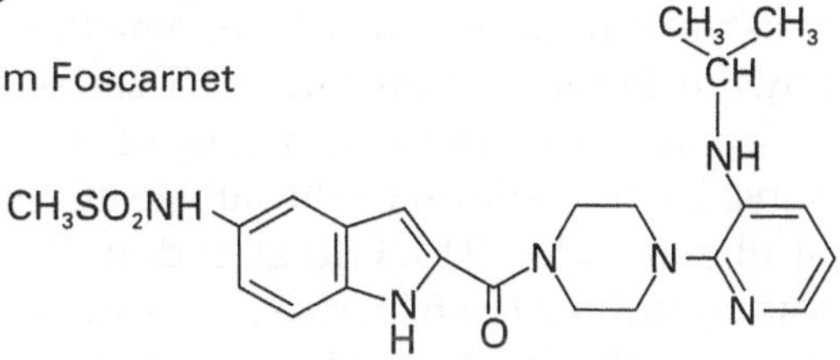

Deavirdine

Protease Inhibitors

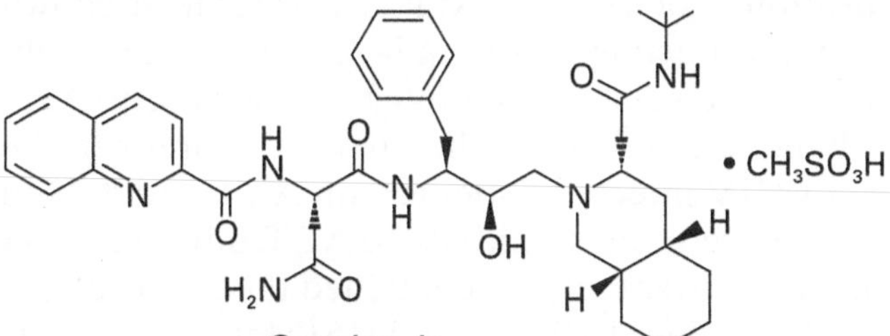

Saquinavir

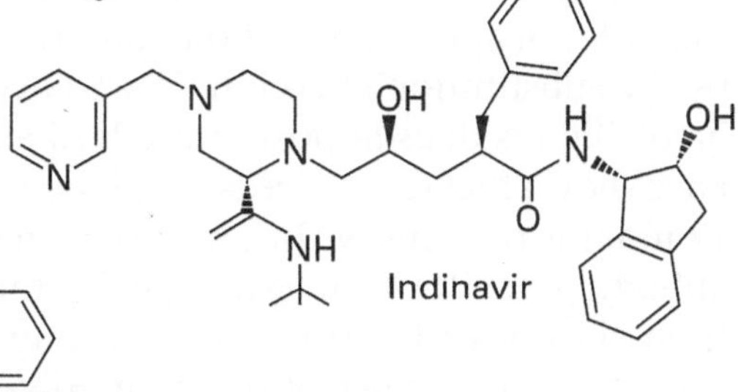

• CH_3SO_3H

Indinavir

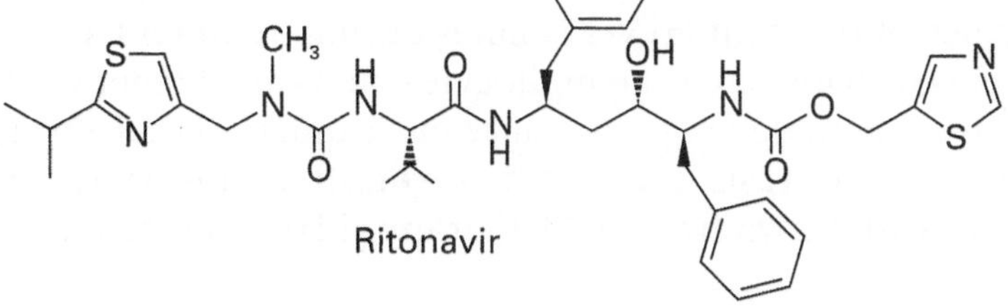

Ritonavir

the appearance of AZT-resistant viral strains [97; and references therein]. Evidence of this phenomenon was initially reported by Larder and colleagues [98]. After comparison of the sequences of AZT-sensitive and resistant viral strains, they identified five amino acid substitutions in the reverse transcriptase that influenced AZT susceptibility (Met41Leu, Asp67Asn, Lys70Arg, Thr215Tyr and Lys219Gln) [99, 100]. A further detailed study revealed that these changes appeared following an ordered pattern [101]. The first mutations to arise during AZT therapy result in the amino acid change Lys70Arg, followed by Thr215Tyr. Then, the Lys70Arg population declines with a simultaneous emergence of variants with the substitution Met41Leu. Genetic linkage of Met41Leu and Thr215Tyr is the cornerstone in the development of significantly AZT-resistant viral strains, which become the dominant population during therapy. Further treatment with AZT can result in the accumulation of highly-resistant virus strains with four of five of the resistance mutations (see Table 2). In addition to the substitutions mentioned above, the presence of Phe at codon 215, Glu at codon 219 and Trp instead of Leu-210, can also contribute to an increased resistance to AZT [101, 103, 104]. Although these are the most commonly found amino acid changes in natural resistant isolates, we cannot exclude the possibility of acquiring resistance through different substitutions. For example, Kim et al. [115] have shown that many amino acid changes affecting residues 67–78 in the 'fingers' subdomain of the reverse transcriptase can confer *in vitro* resistance to AZT without altering the polymerase activity of the enzyme. Moreover, the simultaneous treatment of HIV-infected patients with AZT and ddI led to the isolation of clones with reduced sensitivity to AZT, ddC, ddI, ddG and d4T [113, 116–118]. The resistant viruses contained the substitutions Ala62Val, Val75Ile, Phe77Leu, Phe116Tyr and Gln151Met. In this case, the order of appearance of the mutations starts with codon 151, followed by the substitution at codon 77, and at a later stage, amino acid changes involving residues at positions 62, 75 and 116 [116, 118]. Clinical studies have shown that resistance is developed in most AZT-treated patients after 12 months of therapy. It has also been shown that AZT-resistant clones already preexist in the quasispecies found in individuals who were not treated with AZT [119], demonstrating that natural selection plays a key role in the emergence of resistant HIV-1 isolates during treatment. Consequently, individuals with lower CD4 lymphocyte counts and higher viral load at the start of treatment develop resistance more quickly [120]. Over a period of months to years, resistance can be reversed in most (but not all) patients who are withdrawn from AZT therapy [121, and references therein].

Table 2.
Mutations in the HIV-1 reverse transcriptase coding region that confer resistance to nucleoside analogs, as confirmed by site-directed mutagenesis.[a]

Drug	Mutations of the following wild-type codon[b]													
	41 Met	50 Ile	65 Lys	67 Lys	69 Thr	70 Lys	74 Leu	75 Val	89 Glu	115 Tyr	184 Met	210 Leu	215 Thr	219 Lys
AZT (Zidovudine)	Leu			<u>Asn</u>		Arg						<u>Trp</u>	Tyr Phe	<u>Gln</u> <u>Glu</u>
ddI (Didanosine)			Arg				Val	Thr			Val			
ddC (Zalcitabine)			Arg		Asp		Val	Thr			Val		Cys	
d4T (Stavudine)		Thr						Thr						
3TC (Lamivudine)			Arg			Glu					Val Ile			
L-ddC and L-FddC											Val			
1592U89			Arg				Val			Phe	Val			
ddATP			Arg			Arg	Val							
ddGTP									Gly					
MDL 74968			Arg											
Adefovir (PMEA) and PMEA diphosphate			Arg			Glu								

[a] Data shown in this table have been taken from [102] and updated with information coming from the following references: AZT [103, 104], ddI [105], 3TC [105, 106], L-ddC and L-FddC [107], ddATP [105, 108], ddGTP [109, 110], MDL 74968 [111], and adefovir (9-(2-phosphonylmethoxyethyl)adenine, PMEA) and PMEA diphosphate [106, 112]. Multidrug resistance to AZT and nucleoside analogs occurs with mutations at codons 62, 75, 77, 116 and 151 (see text). The significance of other mutations (at codons 44, 60, 68, 118, 210, 228 and 369) emerging with antiretroviral therapy with AZT alone or in combination with other drugs [113, 114] awaits further investigation.
[b] Substitutions whose contribution to resistance has been shown only in combination with other resistance mutations are shown underlined.

In Table 2 we summarize the amino acid changes that confer resistance to several nucleoside analog inhibitors of HIV-1 reverse transcriptase. Most of these substitutions are found dispersed through the 'fingers' subdomain of the 66 kDa subunit [110, 122, 123], or at the putative dNTP-binding site of the HIV-1 reverse transcriptase (e.g., Tyr-115, Met-184 or Lys-219). The molecular basis of resistance to nucleoside analogs is still not well understood [reviewed in ref. 124], due in part to the lack of a three-dimensional structure of HIV-1 reverse transcriptase complexed to a template-primer and a nucleoside analog or dNTP. Modeling studies suggest that substitutions at the 'fingers' subdomain, such as Leu74Val, could interfere with the correct positioning or conformation of the template-primer, during interaction with the reverse transcriptase [125, 126]. In those cases where substitutions involve residues in the vicinity of the catalytic site (e.g. Met184Val), dNTP binding could be affected, albeit not necessarily through a direct interaction. A certain degree of cross-resistance is observed between nucleoside analog inhibitors of the reverse transcriptase. For example, Leu74Val, Val75Thr and Met184Val confer resistance to ddI and ddC. 3TC resistance is also achieved through the substitution of Met-184 by Val. On the other hand, resistance to nucleoside analog inhibitors can be suppressed by substitutions conferring resistance to other drugs. For example, Leu74Val which arises after treatment with ddI, and Met184Val which appears quickly after initiation of 3TC therapy [127] are responsible for the suppression of AZT resistance [128, 129].

Nonnucleoside reverse transcriptase inhibitors are represented by compounds such as nevirapine, delavirdine and other piperazines, pyridinones, benzodiazepinones, HEPT-derivatives, thiocarboxanilides, or α-APA derivatives. A detailed review on this class of inhibitors of HIV-1 reverse transcriptase has been recently published [130]. These compounds do not require intracellular metabolism (i.e., phosphorylation), their action is not compromised by cellular dNTP pool levels, and they bind to a site which is not present in other polymerases. Nonnucleoside inhibitors are highly specific for HIV-1 group M isolates and do not bind to HIV-2 reverse transcriptase. Nevirapine and other compounds of this group are effective without toxicity at relatively high concentrations (0.1–1 mM). However, drug-resistant strains appear quickly [127, 131]. Nonnucleoside inhibitors of the reverse transcriptase show a higher binding affinity for the enzyme-substrate complex than for the free enzyme [132–134]. Nevertheless, the rate of incorporation of the dNTPs decreases upon binding of the inhibitor [132]. Crystal structures of HIV-1 reverse transcriptase complexed to nonnucleoside inhibitors such as nevirapine [96], benzodiazepinones (TIBO derivatives) [135, 136], α-APA derivative R 95845 [137], and HEPT-derivatives [138, 139] revealed that all bind at a common site in the 66 kDa subunit. This binding site is a hydrophobic cavity, located close to the polymerase active site. The side chains of Tyr-181, Tyr-188, Phe-227 and Trp-229 make a significant contribution to the formation of the cavity which is not observed in the native enzyme [140]. Most of the drug-resistant mutations affect Tyr-181, Tyr-188 or other amino acids located in the vicinity of the binding site, including Glu-138 which is located in the 51 kDa subunit [141] (Table 3). Several mechanisms leading to drug resistance have been proposed: (i) loss of favorable interactions between the inhibitor and the reverse transcriptase, as occurs with the substitution Tyr181Cys or Val106Ala, (ii) creation of steric hindrances between inhibitor and protein as in Gly190Ala, or (iii) induction of conformational changes in the binding pocket as the result of any of the mutations. Resistance to nonnucleoside inhibitors of HIV-1 reverse transcriptase is usually achieved by single point mutations, although it may be increased by additional substitutions. Thus, high-level resistance due to a mutation at codon 181 may appear within the first two weeks of treatment with nevirapine, although accompanying mutations at codons 103, 106, 108, 188 and 190 have been detected within 8 weeks of nevirapine monotherapy [131]. As shown in Table 3, the substitution Tyr181Cys confers resistance to most nonnucleoside inhibitors of HIV-1 reverse transcriptase. As in the case of nucleoside analogs, suppression of resistance to nonnucleoside inhibitors can be achieved by mutations arising after treatment with another drug. The Pro236Leu substitution which confers resistance to BHAP- and HEPT-derivatives restores partially the sensitivity of Tyr181Cys mutant strains to TIBO derivatives, nevirapine or pyridinones [164]. This effect has been also shown for combinations of nonnucleoside inhibitors with nucleoside analogs. Thus, the AZT resistance mutation at codon 215 (Thr215Tyr/Phe) is suppressed by Tyr181Cys [165], and this substitution, which is present in nevirapine-treated patients can also be suppressed if AZT is coadministered with nevirapine [131]. Despite these antagonizing effects, combination of mutations in HIV-1 reverse transcriptase can confer multidrug resistance as well. For example, the mutant Met41Leu/Thr215Tyr/Leu74 Val/Val106Ala shows resistance to AZT, ddI and nevirapine [166]. These observations reinforce the need for careful assessment of the status of the viral infection in the individual before therapy.

Apart from the specific inhibitors of the reverse transcriptase described above, foscarnet (phosphonoformic acid) has also been licensed for treatment of cytomegalovirus retinitis and acyclovir-resistant herpes simplex virus infection, arising during the course of AIDS. Foscarnet is a broad spectrum antiviral agent which inhibits DNA polymerases including the HIV-1 reverse transcriptase. It is a pyrophosphate analog that prevents chain elongation upon binding to the putative pyrophosphate binding site of those enzymes. Site-directed mutagenesis studies have shown that mutations at codons 72, 115, 151 and 183 of HIV-1 reverse transcriptase can lead to resistance to foscarnet [167–169]. However, in vitro selection in the presence of this inhibitor allowed the identification of foscarnet-resistant viruses with the following substitutions: Trp88Ser, Glu89Gly/Lys, Leu92Ile, Ser156Ala, Gln161Leu and His208Tyr [170, 171]. The mechanism leading to foscarnet resistance is not clear for these mutants, since the affected residues are away from the putative binding site. An indirect mechanism involving changes in the geometry of the polymerase active site, similar to that described for nucleoside analogs, has been proposed [170, 171]. Interestingly, the introduction of the mutations Trp88Gly, Glu89Lys, Leu92Ile and Gln161Leu into an HIV-1 strain having the AZT

Table 3
Mutations in the HIV-1 reverse transcriptase coding region that confer resistance to nonnucleoside inhibitors.[a]

Mutations of the following wild-type codons[b]

Drug	98	100	101	103	106	108	138	141	179	181	188	190	230	233	236	238
(wild type)	Ala	Leu	Lys	Lys	Val	Val	Glu	Gly	Val	Tyr	Tyr	Gly	Met	Glu	Pro	Lys
Dipyridodiazepinones																
Nevirapine (BI-RG-587)	Gly	Ile	Ile	Asn	Ala	Ile		Glu	Asp	Cys,Ile	Cys,His	Ala,Glu				
Benzodiazepinones																
TIBO R82150		Ile					Lys			Cys	*His*	Glu				
TIBO R82913		Ile			Ala		Lys		Asp	Cys,Ile	His,Leu	Glu				
TIBO R86183		Ile	Glu	Asn,Thr	Ala		Lys			Ile	Leu	Glu				
Pyridinones																
L-697,593	Gly			Asn						Cys						
L-697,661	Gly	Ile	Glu	Asn,Gln,Thr	Ile	Ile	Lys	Glu	Asp,Glu	Cys,Ile	His	Glu				
Piperazines																
BHAP U90,152 (delavirdine)		Ile		Asn,Thr				Glu	Asp	Cys,Ile	Leu	Glu	Leu		Leu	
BHAP U87,201 (atevirdine)			*Glu*							Cys	*His*			Val	Leu,Thr,His	*Thr*
BHAP U88,204		Ile		Asn	Ala					Cys,Ile	His	Glu	Leu		Leu,Thr,His	
AAP-BHAP U104,489		Ile	Glu							Cys		Glu	Leu		Leu	
AAP-BHAP U95,133		Ile								Cys		Glu	Leu		Leu	
HEPT-derivatives																
HEPT				Asn					Asp	Cys,Ile	Leu				Leu	
E-BPU										Cys,Ile	His				Leu	
E-EBU-dM		Ile		Asn	Ala		Lys			Cys						
I-EBU (MKC-442)		Ile	Ile	Asn,Thr	Ile,Ala		Lys	Glu		Cys						
E-BPTU (NSC 648400)			Glu	Asn,Arg	Ile				Asp	Cys	Cys				Leu	
E-EPU and E-EPSeU			Glu	Asn	Ile	Ile	Lys			Cys	Cys					
Quinoxaline derivatives																
HBY 097		Ile			Ala				Asp	Cys,Ile	Leu	Glu,Ala,Ser	Leu			
S-2720		Ile			Ala				Asp	Cys,Ile	His	Glu,Gln				
TSAO-derivatives																
TSAO-m^{3}T		Ile	Glu	Asn,Thr	Ala		Lys			Cys,Ile,Phe	His,Leu	Glu				
TSAO-T		Ile		Asn			Lys			Cys,Ile,Phe	His					
TSAO-e^{3}T		Ile		Asn			Lys			Cys,Ile	His					

Thiocarboxanilides												
UC10	Gly	Ile	Glu	Asn,Thr	Ala				Asp	Cys		Glu
UC16		Ile	Ile	Asn	Ala					Cys		
UC25		Ile	Glu	Asn	Ala			Glu	Asp	Cys		
UC33	Gly	Ile	Glu	Asn	Ala	Ile				Cys	His	
UC38	Gly	Ile	Glu	Asn	Ala				Asp	Cys		Glu
UC40	Gly	Ile	Glu	Asn	Ala	Ile			Asp	Cys		
UC42		Ile	Ile	Asn,Thr	Ala		Lys			Cys		
UC57	Gly	Ile	Glu	Asn,Thr	Ala	Ile			Asp	Cys		
UC68		Ile	Ile	Asn,Thr	Ala		Lys			Cys	His	
UC70		Ile	Glu	Asn,Thr	Ala				Asp	Cys		
UC81		Ile	Ile	Asn,Thr	Ala		Lys			Cys		
UC84		Ile	Glu	Asn	Ala		Lys		Asp	Cys		
PETT derivatives												
Trovirdine (LY 300046 HCl)		Ile								Cys	His	
Benzoxazinones												
L-743,726 (DMP-266)		Ile	Glu	Asn	Ala					Cys		
α-anilinophenylacetamides												
α-APA R 89439 (loviride)										Cys		
α-APA R 88703		Ile								Cys		Leu
α-APA R 18893										Cys		
Other compounds												
BM + 51.0836										Cys		
1H,3H-thiazolo[3,4-a]benzimidazole(4i), or TBA		Ile		Asn						Ile	Leu	
Calanolide A		Ile		Asn						Ile	Leu	
Halogenated Gomisin J derivatives 1506, 1580 and 1689										Cys	Leu	

a Data shown in this table have been taken from [102] and updated with the following compounds and references: Nevirapine [142, 143], benzodiazepinones [122, 142, 144–146], pyridinones [142, 146, 147], piperazines [142, 143, 148–151], HEPT-derivatives [122, 130, 146, 152–154], quinoxaline derivatives [142, 143, 146, 155], TSAO derivatives [122, 142, 145–147], thiocarboxanilides [146, 153, 156, 157], trovirdine and other PETT derivatives [158, 158a], L-743,726 [159], α-anilinophenylacetamides [151, 160], 1H,3H-thiazolo[3,4-a]benzimidazole(4i) [161], Calanolide A [161], and Gomisin J derivatives [162]. The substitutions of Leu-74 by Val or Ile, and Val-75 by Leu or Ile appeared after prolonged cell culture treatment with HBY 097, but their contribution to HBY 097 resistance has not been demonstrated [143]. The effects of the Glu138Lys substitution on resistance were relatively mild in all cases, except for TSAO-derivatives [162a]. Regions determining the susceptibility to calanolide are localized at residues 94-157 and 225-427 [163].

b Substitutions that contribute to resistance only in the presence of other resistance mutations are underlined. Other drug-related substitutions whose contributions to resistance have not been demonstrated by site-directed mutagenesis are shown in italics.

resistance mutations at codons 41, 67, 70 and 215 completely reversed high-level AZT resistance [172], while various foscarnet-resistant strains were hypersensitive to the nonnucleoside inhibitors TIBO R82150 and nevirapine [171].

4.2   Resistance to HIV-1 protease inhibitors

The HIV-1 protease is the enzyme responsible for the cleavage of the viral *gag* and *gag-pol* polyprotein gene products, which yields the structural proteins and the enzymes of the viral particle. The HIV-1 protease is a dimeric enzyme formed by two noncovalently associated, identical polypeptides. Each monomer has 99 amino acids and contains the conserved sequence Asp-Thr-Gly, which provides the aspartyl group necessary for catalysis. The active site of the enzyme is located at the dimer interface. Knowledge of the structure and function of the HIV-1 protease led to development of many inhibitors, which in some cases are currently being used in AIDS therapy (Table 1 and Figure 1). Most of these drugs are substrate-based inhibitors, whose design has been facilitated by the wealth of crystallographic data, available for the enzyme in its native form or complexed with inhibitors [173, and references therein]. As observed for reverse transcriptase inhibitors, *in vitro* selection of drug-resistant HIV-1 strains can be also achieved using specific protease inhibitors [174–177]. Sequence analysis of these mutants revealed a set of amino acid substitutions whose contribution to the resistance phenotype was analyzed *in vitro* by site-directed mutagenesis. A compilation of amino acid substitutions which lead to resistant phenotypes after exposing the virus to different protease inhibitors is shown in Table 4. Resistance mutations are usually found at codons 32, 82 and 84, and are often responsible for the observed cross-resistance to protease inhibitors. Cross-resistance may also appear during treatment with a single protease inhibitor, after accumulation of several resistance mutations, as shown in the case of indinavir [179]. This finding is not unexpected, since protease inhibitors have been optimized to bind to a well-defined pocket of the protease. The substrate binding pocket of the protease is formed by a series of subsites (termed S3, S2, S1, S1´, S2' and S3'), which correspond to binding sites of the inhibitor. The S1 and S1' subsites are the closest to the conserved catalytic aspartic acid residues of the protease. Mutations conferring a drug-resistant phenotype usually affect residues involved in protease-inhibitor interactions. Examples are the replacement of Arg-8 by Gln or Lys at subsite S3, the substitutions Val32Ile, Ile47Val and Ile84Val at S2, or the substitution of Val82 by Ala, Ile, Phe or Thr at subsite S1. The mechanisms leading to drug resis-

Table 4
Mutations in the HIV-1 protease coding region that confer resistance to protease inhibitors. [a]

Drug	8 Arg	10 Leu	23 Leu	24 Leu	32 Val	45 Lys	46 Met	47 Ile	48 Gly	50 Ile	54 Ile	63 Leu	71 Ala	75 Val	81 Pro	82 Val/Ile	84 Ile	88 Asn	90 Leu	97 Leu
Hydroxyethylamine derivatives (R'-cyclic)																				
Saquinavir (Ro-31-8959)	Gln	Arg			Ile	Ile	Ile		Val		Val	Pro				Ile,Ala,Thr	Val		Met	
Nelfinavir (AG-1343)	Arg,Gln	Phe			Ile	Ile	Ile		Val							Ile,Ala,Thr	Val		Met	
BILA 1906 BS		Ile			Ile	Ile	Leu						Val				Val			
BILA 2185 BS		Ile	Ile		Ile	Ile	Ile	Val			Met		Val				Val			
Symmetry-based derivatives																				
Ritonavir (ABT-538, A-84538)	Gln	Arg		Val	Ile		Ile		Val		Val	Pro	Val			Phe,Ala,Ser,Thr	Val			
A-77003	Gln,Lys				Ile		Leu,Phe,Ile		Val				Val			Phe,Ile,Ala,Thr				
A-75925					Ile															
A-80987		Arg					Ile,Leu				Met	Pro				Ala,Thr	Val			
MP-134																	Ile			
MP-167									Val							Phe,Ala	Val			
P9941																				
Hydroxyethylene derivatives																				
Indinavir (MK639 or L-735524)	Gln	Arg		Val	Ile		Ile,Leu	Leu			Val	Pro	Val			Phe,Ile,Ala,Thr	Val			
L-689502					Ile															
L-731723					Ile															
SB203386						Glu		Val	His,Tyr											
U-89360E and derivatives																Ile Glu,Asp				
Hydroxyethylsulfonamide derivatives																				
VB-11,328 and VX-478		Arg,Phe			Ile		Ile	Val	Val	Val	Val	Pro				Thr	Val			
Norstatine derivatives																				
KNI-272	Gln				Ile		Ile									Ile,Ala	Val			
RPI 312													Thr				Val			
Aminodiol derivatives																				
BMS-186,318																Ala				
Hydroxyethylurea derivatives																				
SC-52151		Arg,Phe		Val		Ile	Ile		Val			Pro	Val	Ile	Thr	Ala,Thr	Val	Asp		
SC-55389a		Phe																Ser		
Cyclic urea																				
XM-323		Phe,Arg				Ile	Ile					Pro				Phe,Ala,Thr	Val			Val

a Data shown in this table have been taken from [102], and updated with information taken from the following references: Saquinavir [178–180], Nelfinavir [181], BILA 1906 BS and 2185 BS [182], Ritonavir [180, 183, 184], A-77003 [180, 185, 186], A-80987 [179, 187], MP-134 and MP-167 [188], P9941 [187], Indinavir and related hydroxyethylene derivatives [179, 180, 183, 189–191], VX-478 [179, 192, 193], KNI-272 [180], BMS-186,318 [186], SC-52151 [179, 194], and XM-323 [179, 187, 195]. Drug resistance to U-89360E and other similar inhibitors (U-71038, U-76088, U-85548, U-88566, U-93840 and U-93965) was assigned, assuming the kinetic model proposed by Tang and Hartsuck [196]. Additional substitutions (Lys20Arg, Glu35Asp and Met36Ile) have been reported to occur *in vivo* after treatment with ritonavir [184], and amino acid changes at codons 10, 24, 48 and 90 appear to correlate with the loss of viral susceptibility to indinavir as selected *in vitro* [184a, 184b]. In all these cases, the significance of the substitutions awaits further investigation.

b Substitutions that contribute to resistance only in the presence of other resistance mutations are underlined. Other drug-related substitutions whose contributions to resistance have not been demonstrated by site-directed mutagenesis are shown in italics.

tance can be diverse for these mutants. Several mutations, like Ile84Val or Val82Ala, can affect hydrophobic and van der Waals interactions between the enzyme and the inhibitor [197]. Others, such as Arg8Gln can affect electrostatic contacts, leading to the loss of the intersubunit salt bridge between Arg-8 and Asp-29' which may decrease the stability of the enzyme [176, 197]. In addition to the active-site mutants described, there are other substitutions that map outside the substrate binding region. Some of them appear in combination with active-site mutations, as occurs with Met46Ile which is found almost exclusively in combination with the defective Arg8Gln. Other non-active-site mutants, such as Leu90Met which is located far from the active site, may indirectly alter the structure of the active site loop that contains the catalytic aspartic acid residues [178]. In addition, the effect of several substitutions (e.g., Ala71Thr, Leu63Pro) is almost negligible when present alone, but may provide some selective growth advantage to viral strains having other resistance mutations [183]. For example, a recent report showed that an HIV-1 RF clone carrying the mutations Gly48Val, Ala71Thr and Val82Ala grew well in culture and displayed cross-resistance to four protease inhibitors, unlike the corresponding defective NL4-3 triple mutant which was nonviable [198]. The presence of Ile instead of Leu at position 10 of the protease of HIV-1 RF was apparently responsible for the observed growth differences between both clones. A third mechanism for resistance to HIV-1 protease inhibitors relates to mutation of cleavage sites in Gag or Gag-Pol which may lead to better substrates. Resistant viruses with mutations at the NC(p7)-p1 and p1-p6 maturation sites of Gag and Gag-Pol have been obtained after *in vitro* selection in the presence of hydroxyethylamine derivatives such as BILA 1906 BS and BILA 2185 BS. Those mutations can synergize with substitutions found in the protease gene, compensating for impaired protease activity [182].

4.3   Combination therapy

A large number of compounds including nucleoside analogs and non-nucleoside inhibitors of the reverse transcriptase, as well as protease inhibitors have been tested in combination. The synergistic activity of several drug combinations has been also demonstrated. Theoretically, an initial consideration for the choice of inhibitors for use in combination therapy should be the lack of cross-resistance between drugs. The resistance patterns observed in the three major groups of inhibitors (nucleoside analogs, nonnucleoside inhibitors of reverse transcriptase and protease inhibitors) are different. From this point of view, the combination of drugs targeting different viral proteins or different sites within the same protein should be beneficial. Suppression of drug resistance by mutations appearing after treatment with other drugs is also important for the selection of drug combinations. Apart from the examples discussed above (i.e., AZT/ddI), several combinations of nonnucleoside inhibitors of reverse transcriptase can also produce mutually antagonizing mutations [130, and references therein]. Triple combinations of AZT, ddC and saquinavir have been shown to be effective against HIV infection, and are currently approved for AIDS therapy. Another important aspect relates to the amount of drug used. Low levels of drug can lead to the acquisition of cross-resistance. This phenomenon has been observed with monotherapy [179] and also with convergent combination therapy [131, 166]. Thus, viruses having the mutations Leu74Val, Lys103Asn, Thr215Tyr and Lys219Gln are resistant to nevirapine, AZT and ddI, and arise after combination therapy with the three drugs [166]. On the other hand, high doses of these compounds can completely suppress virus replication in cell culture for months [130]. In clinical studies, a drastic reduction of plasma viremia can be achieved after treatment with certain protease inhibitors, such as indinavir or ritonavir [39, 40]. Clinical studies in which any of these inhibitors is used in combination with AZT and 3TC have shown that viral load, measured as HIV-1 RNA copies per ml, remains at baseline levels for at least one year in 90% of patients receiving therapy. Nevertheless, resistance mutations may still emerge in the long run. Recombination between strains resistant to reverse transcriptase inhibitors and to protease inhibitors has been demonstrated *in vitro* as a source for dual resistance [194]. All these data indicate that a detailed knowledge of the resistance patterns and the evolution of the HIV-1 quasispecies upon drug treatment is essential for the therapeutic management of HIV infection.

4.4   The preexistence of inhibitor-resistant substitutions in reverse transcriptase of HIV-1 quasispecies of infected patients: An update

Mutations related to resistance to reverse transcriptase or protease inhibitors preexist in the HIV-1 quasispecies of patients undergoing no therapy with the relevant inhibitors [109, 119, 199, 200]. Since the time of publication of this observation for reverse transcriptase [119], additional inhibitors of this enzyme have been used in clinical trials, and additional drug-resistance mutations have been identified. Figure 2 shows an update of amino acid substitutions related to resistance to inhibitors found in patients untreated with the inhibitors. It is based on a set of 81 sequences previously analyzed by our group [7, 119]. The results confirm our previous conclusions, and suggest again that the high mutation frequencies in *pol* [7,119] render inevitable the occasional appearance of mutations associated with resistance to inhibitors. This finding illustrates the biological relevance of the quasispecies structure of RNA viruses as a reservoir of phenotypic variants. Overall, the totality of findings reviewed have emphasized the impact of RNA virus quasispecies on antiviral drug therapy, and the need to deal with quasispecies complexity to achieve rational therapeutic regimens.

Acknowledgments

We are indebted to many colleagues for providing information before publication. We thank D. Clarke, E. Duarte, C. Escarmís, M.G. Mateu, N. Sevilla, and S. Wain-Hobson for valuable information and discussions. We also thank J.M. Galán for preparation of Fig. 1 and L. Horrillo for manuscript preparation. Work in Madrid supported by grants DGICYT PB94-0034-C02-01 and FIS 95/0034-1, Fundación Rodríguez Pascual, Comunidad Autónoma de Madrid, and Fundación Ramón Areces. Work in La Jolla supported by grant AI-14627 from the National Institute of Allergy and Infectious Diseases. A visit of ED to La Jolla was supported by a fellowship from NATO.

Fig. 2

Summary of amino acid replacements found at the codons specifying amino acids related to resistance to reverse transcriptase inhibitors. The single-letter amino acid code is used. The consensus amino acid sequence was obtained from a series of samples collected from untreated HIV-infected individuals, and previously described [119]. The sequence is identical to the HIV-1 CAM-1 sequence [201]. Above the consensus, amino acid replacements related to resistance to reverse transcriptase inhibitors (taken from Tables 2 and 3) are indicated. NNRTIs stands for nonnucleoside reverse transcriptase inhibitors. Below the consensus sequence, the amino acid replacements found in the HIV-1 quasispecies of patients which were not subjected to antiretroviral therapy (untreated) or were treated with AZT or ddI, are indicated. Clones 137, 49 and V75-5 represent samples of the first group of patients which were analyzed for the mutant spectra of individual quasispecies. Clone D17/+20 represents the identified mutant spectrum of the quasispecies of an AZT-treated individual.

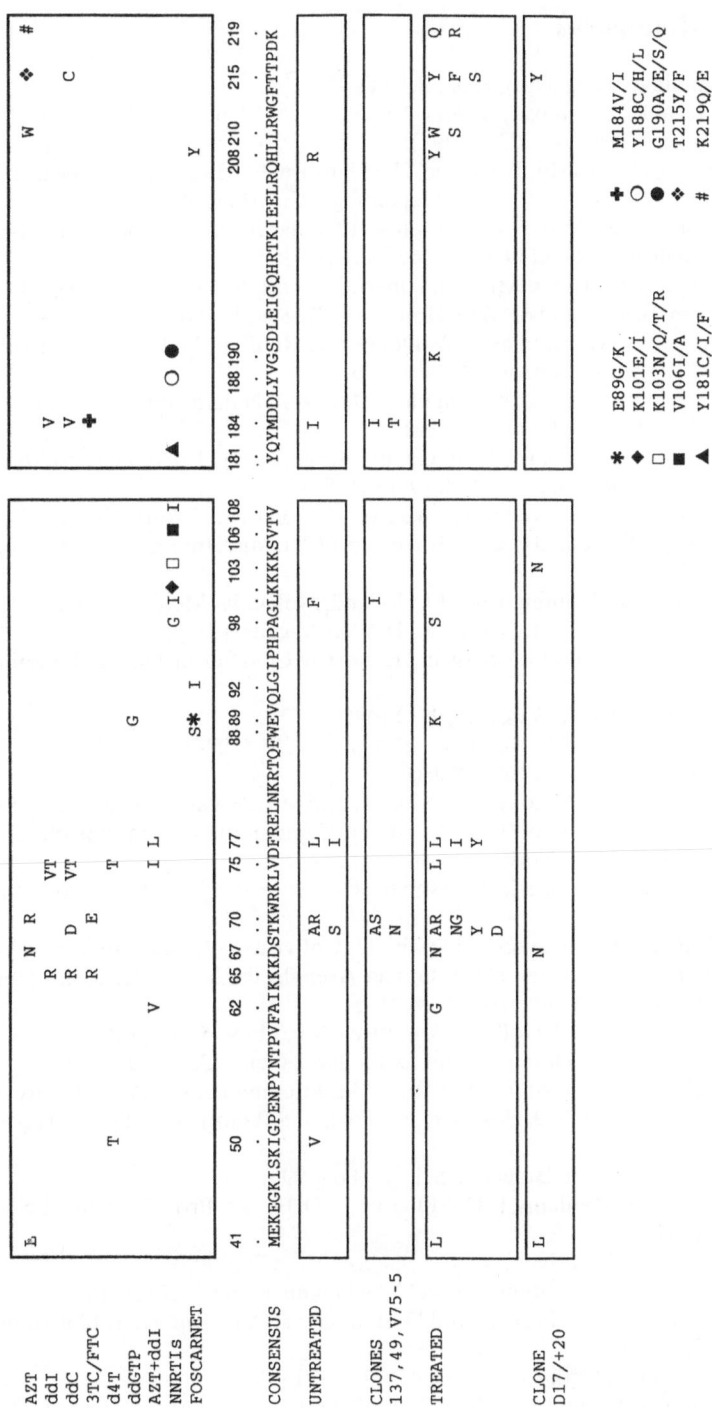

Fig. 2

References

1   E. Domingo: Prog. Drug Res. *33*, 93 (1989).
2   M. Martell, J.I. Esteban, J. Quer, J. Genesce, A. Weiner, R. Esteban, J. Guardia and J. Gómez:J. Virol. *66*, 3225 (1992).
3   M. Naito, N. Hayashi, T. Moribe, H. Hagiwara, E. Mita, Y. Kanazawa, A. Kasahara, H. Fusamoto and T. Kamada: Hepatology *22*, 407 (1995).
4   J. I. Esteban, J. Gómez, M. Martell and J. Guardia: Viral hepatitis, pp. 147–216, Ed. R. A. Willson. Marcel Dekker, Inc., New York, 1997.
5   A. Meyerhans, R. Cheynier, J. Albert, M. Seth, S. Kwok, J. Sninsky, L. Morfeldt-Månson, B. Asjo and S. Wain-Hobson: Cell *58*, 901 (1989).
6   M. A. Penny, S.J. Thomas, N.W. Douglas, S. Ranjbar, H. Holmes and R.S. Daniels: AIDS Res. Hum. Retrov. *13*, 741 (1996).
7   M.E. Quiñones-Mateu, A. Holguín, J. Dopazo, I. Nájera and E. Domingo: AIDS Res. and Hum. Retrov. *12*, 1117 (1996).
8   E. Domingo and J.J. Holland: Genetic Engineering, Principles and Methods, J. K. Setlow, ed., Plenum Press, Vol. *14*, 13 (1992).
9   E.A. Duarte, I.S. Novella, S.C. Weaver, E. Domingo, S Wain-Hobson, D.K. Clarke, A. Moya, S.F. Elena, J.C. de la Torre and J.J. Holland: Infectious Agents and Disease *3*, 201 (1994).
10   I.S. Novella, E. Domingo and J.J. Holland: Molecular Medicine Today *1*, 248 (1995).
11   R. Wagner, L. Deml, T. Fitzon and H. Wolf: Vaccines 95, pp. 347–356, Eds. R.M. Chanock, F. Brown, H.S. Ginsberg and E. Norrby. Cold Spring Harbor Laboratory Press, 1995.
12   B.A. Larder: J. Gen. Virol. *75*, 951 (1994).
13   D.D. Richman: AIDS Res. Hum. Retrov. *10*, 901 (1994).
14   G.J. Moyle: Drugs *52*, 168 (1996).
15   E. Kurstak, R.G. Marusyk, F. A. Murphy and M.H.V. Van Regenmortel, eds.: Applied Virology Research, vol. 2, Virus variability, epidemiology, and control. Plenum Medical Book Co, New York and London 1989.
16   J.J. Holland, ed.: Genetic diversity of RNA viruses. Current Top. Microbiol. Immunol. *176*.
17   S.S. Morse, ed.: The evolutionary biology of viruses. Raven Press, New York, 1994.
18   A. Gibbs, C.H. Calisher and F. García-Arenal, eds.: Molecular basis of virus evolution. Cambridge University Press, 1995.
19   E. Domingo and J.J. Holland: Annu Rev. Microbiol. *51*, in press, 1997.
20   D. Steinhauer, E. Domingo, and J.J. Holland: Gene *122*, 281 (1992).
21   L.A. Kohlstaedt, J. Wang, P.A. Rice, J.M. Friedman and T.A. Steitz: Reverse transcriptase, pp. 223–249, Eds. A.M. Skalka and S.P. Goff. Cold Spring Harbor Laboratory Press, 1993.
22   R. Sousa: Trends in Biochem. Sci. *21*, 186 (1996).
23   A. Gabriel, M. Willems, E.H. Mules and J.D. Boeke: Proc. Natl. Acad. Sci. USA *93*, 7767 (1996).
24   B.D. Preston: Proc. Natl. Acad. Sci. USA *93*, 7427 (1996).
25   E. Batschelet, E. Domingo and C. Weissmann: Gene *1*, 27 (1976).
26   J.J. Holland, J.C. de la Torre and D. Steinhauer: Curr. Top. Microbiol. Immunol. *176*, 1 (1992).
27   J. Drake: Proc. Natl. Acad. Sci. USA *90*, 4171 (1993).
28   E. Domingo, E. and J.J. Holland: Mutation rates and rapid evolution of RNA viruses.

Evolutionary Biology of viruses, pp. 161–184, Ed. S. S. Morse, Raven Press, New York, 1994.

29 M. Eigen and C. Biebricher: RNA Genetics, vol. 3 pp. 211–245. Eds. E. Domingo, J.J. Holland and P. Ahlquist. CRC Press Inc., Boca Raton, Florida, 1988.

30 E. Domingo, D.L. Sabo, T. Taniguchi and C. Weissmann: Cell *13*, 735 (1978).

31 M. Eigen: Gene *135*, 37 (1993).

32 M. Eigen: Trends in Microbiol. *4*, 212 (1996).

33 J.J. Holland, J.C. de la Torre, D.K. Clarke and E. Duarte: J. Virol. *65*, 2960 (1991).

34 M.A. Martínez, C. Carrillo, F. González-Candelas, A. Moya, E. Domingo and F. Sobrino: J. Virol. *65*, 3954 (1991).

35 I.S. Novella, E.A. Duarte, S.F. Elena, A. Moya, E. Domingo and J.J. Holland: Proc. Natl. Acad. Sci. USA *92*, 5841 (1995).

36 N. Sevilla and E. Domingo: J. Virol. *70*, 6617 (1996).

37 N. Sevilla, N. Verdaguer and E. Domingo: Virology *225*, 400 (1996).

38 S. Wain-Hobson: The Evolutionary Biology of Viruses, pp. 185–209. Ed. S.S. Morse. Raven Press, New York, 1994.

39 X. Wei, S.K. Ghosh, M.E. Taylor, V.A. Johnson, E.A. Emini, P. Deutsch, J. D. Lifson, S. Bonhoeffer, M.A. Nowak, B.H. Hahn, M.S. Saag and G.M. Shaw: Nature *373*, 117 (1995).

40 D.D. Ho, A.U. Neuman, A.S. Perelson, W. Chen, J.M. Leonard and M. Markowitz: Nature *373*, 123 (1995).

41 J.M. Coffin: Science *267*, 483 (1995).

42 A.S. Perelson, A.U. Neumann, M. Markowitz, J. M. Lenard and D.D. Ho: Science *271*, 1582 (1996).

43 L. Chao: Nature *348*, 454 (1990).

44 E. Duarte, D. Clarke, A. Moya, E. Domingo and J. J. Holland: Proc. Natl. Acad. Sci. USA *89*, 6015 (1992).

45 D.K. Clarke, E.A. Duarte, A. Moya, S.F. Elena, E. Domingo and J.J. Holland: J. Virol. *67*, 222 (1993).

46 E.A. Duarte, D.K. Clarke, A. Moya, S.F. Elena, E. Domingo and J.J. Holland: J. Virol. *67*, 3620 (1993).

47 C. Escarmís, M. Dávila, N. Charpentier, A. Bracho, A. Moya and E. Domingo: J. Mol. Biol. *264*, 255 (1996).

48 H.J. Muller: Mutat. Res. *1*, 2 (1964).

49 L. van Valen: Evol. Theory *1*, 1 (1973).

50 G.F. Gause: The Struggle for Existence. Dover, New York, 1971.

51 D.K. Clarke, E.A. Duarte, S.F. Elena, A. Moya, E. Domingo and J.J. Holland: Proc. Natl. Acad. Sci. USA *91*, 4821 (1994).

52 E. Domingo, C. Escarmís, N. Sevilla, A. Moya, S.F. Elena, J. Quer, I.S. Novella and J.J. Holland: FASEB J. *10*, 859 (1996).

53 J. Quer, R. Huerta, I.S. Novella, L. Tsimring, E. Domingo and J.J. Holland: J. Mol. Biol. *264*, 465 (1996).

54 B. Borrego, I.S. Novella, E. Giralt, D. Andreu and E. Domingo: J. Virol. *67*, 6071 (1993).

55 I.S. Novella, D.K. Clarke, J. Quer, E.A. Duarte, C.H. Lee, S.C. Weaver, S.F. Elena, A. Moya, E. Domingo and J.J. Holland: J. Virol. *69*, 6805 (1995).

56 T.W. Scott, S.C. Weaver and V.L. Mallampalli: The Evolutionary Biology of Viruses, pp. 293–324, Ed. S.S. Morse, Raven Press, New York, 1994.

57 I.S. Novella, M. Cilnis, S.F. Elena, J. Kohn, A. Moya, E. Domingo and J.J. Holland: J. Virol. *70*, 6414 (1996).

58   A.S. Evans: Viral Infections of Humans: Epidemiology and Control. Plenum Medical Book Co., New York, 1984.

59   J.J. Whitton and M.B.A. Oldstone: Fields Virology, pp. 345–374, Eds. B.N. Fields, D.M. Knipe, P.M. Howley, R.M. Chanock, J.L. Melnick, T.P. Monath, B. Roizman and S.E. Straus. Lippincott-Raven Publishers, Philadelphia, New York, 1996.

60   P.J. Delves: Synthetic Vaccines, pp. 1–25. Ed. B.H. Nicholson. Blackwell Scientific Publications, 1994.

61   A.R. Zanetti, E. Tanzi, G. Manzillo, G. Maio, C. Sbreglia, N. Caporaso, H. Thomas and A.J. Zuckerman: Lancet *ii*, 1132 (1988).

62   W.F. Carman, A.R. Zanetti, P. Karayianni, J. Waters, G. Manzillo, E. Tanzi, A.J. Zuckerman and H.C. Thomas: Lancet *336*, 325 (1990).

63   W.F. Carman, H.C. Thomas and E. Domingo: Lancet *341*, 349 (1993).

64   K. Murray: Synthetic vaccines, pp. 433–452. Ed. B.H. Nicholson. Blackwell Scientific Publications, Oxford, 1994.

65   D. Samuel, A. Bismuth, D. Mathien, J.L. Arulnaden, M. Reynes, J.P. Behamou, C. Brechot and H. Bismuth: Lancet *337*, 813 (1991).

66   R. Muller, G. Gubernatis, M. Farie, G. Niehoff, H. Klein, C. Wittekind, G. Tusch, H.U. Lantz, K. Boker, W. Stangel and R. Pichlmayr: J. Hepatol. *13*, 90 (1991).

67   A.E. Hawkins, R.J.C. Gilson, N. Gilbert, T.G. Wreghitt, J.J. Gray, I. Ahlers-de Boer, R.S. Tedder and G.J.M. Alexander: J. Hepatol. *24*, 8 (1996).

68   W.F. Carman, C. Trautwein, F.J. Van Deursen, K. Colman, E. Doman, G. McIntyre, J. Waters, V. Kliem, R. Müller, H.C. Thomas and M.P. Manns: Hepatology *24*, 489 (1996).

69   Y.K. Shimizu, M. Hijikata, A. Iwamoto, J.J. Alter, R.H. Purcell and H. Yoshikura: J. Virol. *68*, 1494 (1994).

70   Y.K. Shimizu, H. Igarashi, T. Kiyohara, T. Cabezon, P. Farci, R.H. Purcell and H. Yoshikura: Virology *223*, 409 (1996).

71   A. Zibert, E. Schreir and M. Roggendorf: Virology *208*, 653 (1995).

72   P. Farci, H.J. Alter, S. Govindarajan, D.C. Wong, R. Engle, R.R. Lesniewski, I.K. Muehahwar, S.M. Dosai, S.H. Miller, N. Ogata and R.H. Purcell: Science *258*, 135 (1992)

73   H. Okamoto, S. Mishiro, H. Tokita, F. Tsuda, Y. Miyakawa and M. Mayumi: Hepatology *20*, 1131 (1994).

74   Q.L. Choo, G. Kuo, R. Ralston, A. Weiner, D. Chien, G. Van Nest, J. Han, K. Berger, K. Thudium, C. Kuo, J. Kansopon, J. McFarland, A. Tabrizi, K. Ching, B. Moss, L.B. Cummins, M. Houghton and E. Muchmore: Proc. Natl. Acad. Sci. USA *91*, 1294 (1994).

75   A. Cemy, J.G. McHutchison, C. Pasquinelli, M.E. Brown, M.A. Brothers, B. Grabscheld, P. Fowler, H. Houghton and F.V. Chisari: J. Clin. Invest. *95*, 521 (1995).

76   P.A. Wentworth, A. Sette, E. Celis, J. Sidney, S. Southwood, C. Crimi, S. Stitely, E. Keogh, N.C. Wong, B. Livingston, D. Alazard, A. Vitiello, H.M. Grey, F.V. Chisari, R.W. Chesnut and J. Fikes: International Immunology *8*, 651 (1995).

77   E.J. Scott and G.C. Schild: Synthetic vaccines, pp. 453–470, Ed. B.H. Nicholson, Blackwell Scientific Publications, Oxford, 1994.

78   Summary report and recommendations of an international ad hoc scientific committee: The Rockefeller Foundation and the Fondation Mérieux, Paris, France, 1994.

79   B.F. Haynes: Lancet *348*, 933 (1996).

80   B.R. Bloom: Science *272*, 1888 (1996).

81   H. Temin: Cancer Res. *48*, 1697 (1988).

82   M. Mamman, G. Gettinby, N.B. Murphy, S. Kemei and A. S. Peregrine: Antimicrob. Agents and Chemother. *39*, 1107 (1995).

83   S. Gassis and P.K. Rathod: Antimicrob. Agents and Chemother. *40*, 914 (1996).

84   M. Taylor and R. Feyereisen: Mol. Biol. Evol. *13*, 719 (1996).

85   T.J. Blick, T. Tiong, A. Sahasrabudhe, J.N. Varghese, P.M. Colman, G.J. Hart, R.C. Bethelland, J.L. McKimm-Breschkin: Virology *214*, 475 (1995).

86   K.A. Stadschke, J.M. Colacino, A.J. Baxter, G.M. Air, A. Bansal, W.J. Hornback, J.E. Munroe and W.G. Lover: Virology *214*, 642 (1995).

87   J.R. Wands, T.J. Liang, H.E. Blum and D.A. Schafritz: Seminars in Liver Disease *12*, 252 (1992).

88   N.V. Naoumov, M.G. Thomas, A.L. Mason, S. Chokshi, G.J. Bodicky, F. Farzaneh, R. Williams and R.P. Perrillo: Gastroenterology *108*, 505 (1995).

89   S.I. Okada, Y. Akahane, H. Suzuki, H. Okamoto and S. Mishiro: Hepatology *15*, 619 (1992).

90   K. Koizumi, M. Enomots, M. Kurosaki, T. Murakami, N. Izumi, F. Marumo and C. Sato: Hepatology *22*, 30 (1995).

91   Y. Kanazawa, N. Hayashi, E. Mita, T. Li, H. Hagiwara, A. Kasahara, H. Fusamoto and T. Kamada: Hepatology *20*, 1121 (1994).

92   N. Enomoto, M. Kurosaki, Y. Tanaka, F. Marumo and C. Sato: J. Gen. Virol. *75*, 1361 (1995).

93   N. Enomoto, I. Sakuma, Y. Asahina, M. Kurosaki, T. Murakami, C. Yamamoto, Y. Ogura, N. Izumi, F. Marumo and C. Sato: N. Engl. J. Med. *334*, 77 (1996).

94   F. Di Marzo Veronese, T.D. Copeland, A.L. DeVico, R. Rahman, S. Oroszlan, R.C. Gallo and M.G. Sarngadharan: Science *231*, 1289 (1986).

95   A. Jacobo-Molina, J. Ding, R.G. Nanni, A.D. Clark Jr., X. Lu, C. Tantillo, R.L. Williams, G. Kamer, A.L. Ferris, P. Clark, A. Hizi, S.H. Hughes and E. Arnold: Proc. Natl. Acad. Sci. USA *90*, 6320 (1993).

96   L.A. Kohlstaedt, J. Wang, J.M. Friedman, P.A. Rice and T.A. Steitz: Science *256*, 1783 (1992).

97   G.X. McLeod and S.M. Hammer: Ann. Internal Medicine *117*, 487 (1992).

98   B.A. Larder, G. Darby and D.D. Richman: Science *243*, 1731 (1989).

99   B.A. Larder and S.D. Kemp: Science *246*, 1155 (1989).

100 B.A. Larder, P. Kellam and S.D. Kemp: AIDS *5*, 137 (1991).

101 P. Kellam, C.A.B. Boucher and B.A. Larder: Proc. Natl. Acad. Sci. USA *89*, 1934 (1992).

102 J.W. Mellors, B.A. Larder and R.F. Schinazi: Int. Antivir. News *3*, 8 (1995).

103 P.R. Harrigan, I. Kinghorn, S. Bloor, S.D. Kemp, I. Nájera, A. Kohli and B.A. Larder: J. Virol. *70*, 5930 (1996).

104 D.J. Hooker, G. Tachedjian, A.E. Solomon, A.D. Gurusinghe, S. Land, C. Birch, J.L. Anderson, B.M. Roy, E. Arnold and N.J. Deacon: J. Virol. *70*, 8010 (1996).

105 Z. Gu, R.S. Fletcher, E.J. Arts, M.A. Wainberg and M.A. Parniak: J. Biol. Chem. *269*, 28118 (1994).

106 J.M. Cherrington, A.S. Mulato, M.D. Fuller and M.S. Chen: Antimicrob. Agents Chemother. *40*, 2212 (1996).

107 A. Faraj, L.A. Agrofoglio, J.K. Wakefield, S. McPherson, C.D. Morrow, G. Gosselin, C. Mathe, J.L. Imbach, R.F. Schinazi and J.P. Sommadossi: Antimicrob. Agents Chemother. *38*, 2300 (1994).

108 P.L. Sharma, P.A. Chatis, A.L. Dogon, D.L. Mayers, F.E. McCutchan, C. Page and C.S. Crumpacker: Virology *223*, 365 (1996).

124   Esteban Domingo et al.

109   V.R. Prasad, I. Lowy, T. De los Santos, L. Chiang and S.P. Goff: Proc. Natl. Acad. Sci. USA *88*, 11363 (1991).
110   Y. Kew, S. Qingbin and V.R. Prasad: J. Biol. Chem. *269*, 15331 (1994).
111   D.L. Taylor, S.P. Ahmed, T.M. Brennan, J.F. Nave, P. Casara and A.S. Tyms: Antivir. Chem. Chemother. *7*, 253 (1996).
112   Z. Gu, H. Salomon, J.M. Cherrington, A.S. Mulato, M.S. Chen, R. Yarchoan, A. Foli, K.M. Sogocio and M.A. Wainberg: Antimicrob. Agents Chemother. *39*, 1888 (1995)
113   R.W. Shafer, A.K.N. Iversen, M.A. Winters, E. Aguiniga, D.A. Katzenstein and T.C. Merigan: J. Infect. Dis. *172*, 70 (1995).
114   A.D. Gurusinghe, S.A. Land, C. Birch, C. McGavin, D.J. Hooker, G. Tachedjian, R. Doherty and N.J. Deacon: J. Med. Virol. *46*, 238 (1995).
115   B. Kim, T.R. Hathaway and L.A. Loeb: J. Biol. Chem. *271*, 4872 (1996).
116   T. Shirasaka, M.F. Kavlick, T. Ueno, W.-Y. Gao, E. Kojima, M.L. Alcaide, S. Choke-kijchai, B.M. Roy, E. Arnold, R. Yarchoan and H. Mitsuya: Proc. Natl. Acad. Sci. USA *92*, 2398 (1995).
117   T. Ueno, T. Shirasaka and H. Mitsuya: J. Biol. Chem. *270*, 23605 (1995).
118   A.K.N. Iversen, R.W. Shafer, K. Wehrly, M.A. Winters, J.I. Mullins, B. Chesebro and T.C. Merigan: J. Virol. *70*, 1086 (1996).
119   I. Nájera, A. Holguín, M.E. Quiñones-Mateu, M.A. Muñoz-Fernández, R. Nájera, C. López-Galíndez and E. Domingo: J. Virol. *69*, 23 (1995).
120   D.D. Richman, J.M. Grimes and S.W. Lagakos: J. Acquired Immune Defic. Syndr. *3*, 743 (1990).
121   D.D. Richman: Antimicrob. Agents Chemother. *37*, 1207 (1993).
122   P.L. Boyer, J. Ding, E. Arnold and S.H. Hughes: Antimicrob. Agents Chemother. *38*, 1909 (1994).
123   P.L. Boyer and S.H. Hughes: Nature Struct. Biol. *3*, 579 (1996).
124   E.J. Arts and M.A. Wainberg: Antimicrob. Agents Chemother. *40*, 527 (1996).
125   P.L. Boyer, C. Tantillo, A. Jacobo-Molina, R.G. Nanni, J. Ding, E. Arnold and S.H. Hughes: Proc. Natl. Acad. Sci. USA *91*, 4882 (1994).
126   C. Tantillo, J. Ding, A. Jacobo-Molina, R.G. Nanni, P.L. Boyer, S.H. Hughes, R. Pauwels, K. Andries, P.A.J. Janssen and E. Arnold: J. Mol. Biol. *243*, 369 (1994).
127   R. Schuurman, M. Nijhuis, R. van Leeuwen, P. Schipper, D. de Jong, P. Collis, S.A. Danner, J. Mulder, C. Loveday, C. Christopherson, S. Kwok, J. Sninsky and C.A.B. Boucher: J. Infect. Dis. *171*, 1411 (1995).
128   M.H. St. Clair, J.L. Martin, G. Tudor-Williams, M.C. Bach, C.L. Vavro, D.M. King, P. Kellam, S.D. Kemp and B.A. Larder: Science *253*, 1557 (1991).
129   M. Tisdale, S.D. Kemp, N.R. Parry and B.A. Larder: Proc. Natl. Acad. Sci. USA *90*, 5653 (1993).
130   E. De Clercq: Med. Res. Reviews *16*, 125 (1996).
131   D.D. Richman, D. Havlir, J. Corbeil, D. Looney, C. Ignacio, S.A. Spector, J. Sullivan, S. Cheeseman, K. Barringer, D. Pauletti, C.-K. Shih, M. Myers and J. Griffin: J. Virol. *68*, 1660 (1994).
132   R.A. Spence, W.M. Kati, K.S. Anderson and K.A. Johnson: Science *267*, 988 (1995).
133   K. Rittinger, G. Divita and R.S. Goody: Proc. Natl. Acad. Sci. USA *92*, 8046 (1995).
134   R.A. Spence, K.S. Anderson and K.A. Johnson: Biochemistry *35*, 1054 (1996).
135   J.S. Ren, R. Esnouf, A. Hopkins, C. Ross, Y. Jones, D. Stammers and D. Stuart: Structure *3*, 915 (1995).
136   J. Ding, K. Das, H. Moereels, L. Koymans, K. Andries, P.A.J. Janssen, S.H. Hughes and E. Arnold: Nature Struct. Biol. *2*, 407 (1995).

137   J. Ding, K. Das, C. Tantillo, W. Zhang, A.D. Clark Jr., S. Jessen, X. Lu, Y. Hsiou, A. Jacobo-Molina, K. Andries, R. Pauwels, H. Moereels, L. Koymans, P.A.J. Janssen, R.H. Smith Jr., M. Kroeger Koepke, C.J. Michejda, S.H. Hughes and E. Arnold: Structure *3*, 365 (1995).

138   R. Esnouf, J. Ren, C. Ross, Y. Jones, D. Stammers and D. Stuart: Nature Struct. Biol. *2*, 303 (1995).

139   A.L. Hopkins, J. Ren, R.M. Esnouf, B.E. Willcox, E.Y. Jones, C. Ross, T. Miyasaka, R.T. Walker, H. Tanaka, D.K. Stammers and D.I. Stuart: J. Med. Chem. *39*, 1589 (1996).

140   D.W. Rodgers, S.J. Gamblin, B.A. Harris, S. Ray, J.S. Culp, B. Hellmig, D.J. Woolf, C. Debouck and S.C. Harrison: Proc. Natl. Acad. Sci. USA *92*, 1222 (1995).

141   H. Jonckheere, J.-M. Taymans, J. Balzarini, S. Velázquez, M.-J. Camarasa, J. Desmyter, E. De Clercq and J. Anné: J. Biol. Chem. *269*, 25255 (1994).

142   J. Balzarini, A. Karlsson, C. Meichsner, A. Paessens, G. Riess, E. De Clercq and J.-P. Kleim: J. Virol. *68*, 7986 (1994).

143   J.-P. Kleim, M. Rösner, I. Winkler, A. Paessens, R. Kirsch, Y. Hsiou, E. Arnold and G. Riess: Proc. Natl. Acad. Sci. USA *93*, 34 (1996).

144   R. Pauwels, K. Andries, Z. Debyser, M.J. Kukla, D. Schols, H.J. Breslin, R. Woestenborghs, J. Desmyter, M.A.C. Janssen, E. De Clercq and P.A.J. Janssen: Antimicrob. Agents Chemother. *38*, 2863 (1994).

145   J. Balzarini, A. Karlsson, M.-J. Pérez-Pérez, L. Vrang, J. Walbers, H. Zhang, B. Öberg, A.-M. Vandamme, M.-J. Camarasa and E. De Clercq: Virology *192*, 246 (1993).

146   J. Balzarini, M.-J. Pérez-Pérez, S. Velázquez, A. San-Félix, M.-J. Camarasa, E. De Clercq and A. Karlsson: Proc. Natl. Acad. Sci. USA *92*, 5470 (1995).

147   J. Balzarini, A. Karlsson, V.V. Sardana, E.A. Emini, M.-J. Camarasa and E. De Clercq: Proc. Natl. Acad. Sci. USA *91*, 6599 (1994).

148   N. Fan, D.B. Evans, K.B. Rank, R.C. Thomas, W.G. Tarpley and S.K. Sharma: FEBS Lett. *359*, 233 (1995).

149   N. Fan, K.B. Rank, D.E. Slade, S.M. Poppe, D.B. Evans, L.A. Kopta, R.A. Olmsted, R.C. Thomas, W.G. Tarpley and S.K. Sharma: Biochemistry *35*, 9737 (1996).

150   N. Fan, K.B. Rank, D.B. Evans, R.C. Thomas, W.G. Tarpley and S.K. Sharma: FEBS Lett. *370*, 59 (1995).

151   R.A. Olmsted, D.E. Slade, L.A. Kopta, S.M. Poppe, T.J. Poel, S.W. Newport, K.B. Rank, C. Biles, R.A. Morge, T.J. Dueweke, Y. Yagi, D.L. Romero, R.C. Thomas, S.K. Sharma and W.G. Tarpley: J. Virol. *70*, 3698 (1996).

152   R.W. Buckheit, T.L. Kinjerski, V. Fliakas-Boltz, J.D. Russell, T.L. Stup, L.A. Pallansch, W.G. Brouwer, D.C. Dao, W.A. Harrison, R.J. Schultz, J.P. Bader and S.S. Yang: Antimicrob. Agents Chemother. *39*, 2718 (1995).

153   R.W. Buckheit Jr., V. Fliakas-Boltz, S. Yeagy-Bargo, O. Weislow, D.L. Mayers, P.L. Boyer, S.H. Hughes, B.-C. Pan, S.-H. Chu and J.P. Bader: Virology *210*, 186 (1995).

154   M. Seki, Y. Sadakata, S. Yuasa and M. Baba: Antivir. Chem. Chemother. *6*, 73 (1995).

155   J.-P. Kleim, R. Bender, R. Kirsch, C. Meichsner, A. Paessens, M. Rösner, H. Rübsamen-Waigmann, R. Kaiser, M. Wichers, K.E. Schneweis, I. Winkler and G. Riess: Antimicrob. Agents Chemother. *39*, 2253 (1995).

156   J. Balzarini, H. Jonckheere, W.A. Harrison, D.C. Dao, J. Anne, E. De Clercq and A. Karlsson: Antivir. Chem. Chemother. *6*, 169 (1995).

157   J. Balzarini, W.G. Brouwer, E.E. Felauer, E. De Clercq and A. Karlsson: Antivir. Res. *27*, 219 (1995).

158   H. Zhang, L. Vrang, K. Bäckbro, P. Lind, C. Sahlberg, T. Unge and B. Öberg: Antivir. Res. *28*, 331 (1995).

158a A.S. Cantrell, P. Engelhardt, M. Högberg, S.R. Jaskunas, N.G. Johansson, C.L. Jordan, J. Kangasmetsä, M.D. Kinnick, P. Lind, J.M. Morin, Jr., M.A. Muesing, R. Noreén, B. Öberg, P. Pranc, C. Sahlberg, R.J. Ternansky, R.T. Vasileff, L. Vrang, S.J. West and H. Zhang: J. Med. Chem. *39*, 4261 (1996).

159 S.D. Young, S.F. Britcher, L.O. Tran, L.S. Payne, W.C. Lumma, T.A. Lyle, J.R. Huff, P.S. Anderson, D.B. Olsen, S.S. Carroll, D.J. Pettibone, J.A. O'Brien, R.G. Ball, S.K. Balani, J.H. Lin, I.-W. Chen, W.A. Schleif, V.V. Sardana, W.J. Long, V.W. Byrnes and E.A. Emini: Antimicrob. Agents Chemother. *39*, 2602 (1995).

160 R. Pauwels, K. Andries, Z. Debyser, P. Van Daele, D. Schols, P. Stoffels, K. De Vreese, R. Woestenborghs, A.-M. Vandamme, C.G.M. Janssen, J. Anne, G. Cauwenbergh, J. Desmyter, J. Heykants, M.A.C. Janssen, E. De Clercq and P.A.J. Janssen: Proc. Natl. Acad. Sci. USA *90*, 1711 (1993).

161 P.L. Boyer, M.J. Currens, J.B. McMahon, M.R. Boyd and S.H. Hughes: J. Virol. *67*, 2412 (1993).

162 T. Fujihashi, H. Hara, T. Sakata, K. Mori, H. Higuchi, A. Tanaka, H. Kaji and A. Kaji: Antimicrob. Agents Chemother. *39*, 2000 (1995).

162a J. Balzarini, J.-P. Kleim, G. Riess, M.-J. Camarasa, E. De Clerq and A. Karlsson: Biochem. Biophys. Res. Commun. *201*, 1305 (1994).

163 A. Hizi, R. Tal, M. Shaharabany, M.J. Currens, M.R. Boyd, S.H. Hughes and J.B. McMahon: Antimicrob. Agents Chemother. *37*, 1037 (1993).

164 T.J. Dueweke, T. Pushkarskaya, S.M. Poppe, S.M. Swaney, J.Q. Zhao, I.S.Y. Chen, M. Stevenson and W.G. Tarpley: Proc. Natl. Acad. Sci. USA *90*, 4713 (1993).

165 B.A. Larder: Antimicrob. Agents Chemother. *36*, 2664 (1992).

166 B.A. Larder, P. Kellam and S.D. Kemp: Nature *365*, 451 (1993).

167 B.A. Larder, S.D. Kemp and D.J.M. Purifoy: Proc. Natl. Acad. Sci. USA *86*, 4803 (1989).

168 D.M. Lowe, V. Parmar, S.D. Kemp and B.A. Larder: FEBS Lett. *282*, 231 (1991).

169 S. Sarafianos, V.N. Pandey, N. Kaushik and M.J. Modak: J. Biol. Chem. *270*, 19729 (1995).

170 J.W. Mellors, H.Z. Bazmi, R.F. Schinazi, B.M. Roy, Y. Hsiou, E. Arnold, J. Weir and D.L. Mayers: Antimicrob. Agents Chemother. *39*, 1087 (1995).

171 G. Tachedjian, D.J. Hooker, A.D. Gurusinghe, H. Bazmi, N.J. Deacon, J. Mellors, C. Birch and J. Mills: Virology *212*, 58 (1995).

172 G. Tachedjian, J. Mellors, H. Bazmi, C. Birch and J. Mills: J. Virol. *70*, 7171 (1996).

173 A. Wlodawer and J.W. Erickson: Ann. Rev. Biochem. *62*, 543 (1993).

174 M.J. Otto, S. Garber, D.L. Winslow, C.D. Reid, P. Aldrich, P.K. Jadhav, C.E. Patterson, C.N. Hodge and Y.-S.E. Cheng: Proc. Natl. Acad. Sci. USA *90*, 7543 (1993).

175 M.A. El-Farrash, M.J. Kuroda, T. Kitazaki, T. Masuda, K. Kato, M. Hatanaka and S. Harada: J. Virol. *68*, 233 (1994).

176 D.D. Ho, T. Toyoshima, H. Mo, D.J. Kempf, D. Norbeck, C.-M. Chen, N.E. Wideburg, S.K. Burt, J.W. Erickson and M.K. Singh: J. Virol. *68*, 2016 (1994).

177 A.H. Kaplan, S.F. Michael, R.S. Wehbie, M.F. Knigge, D.A. Paul, L. Everitt, D.J. Kempf, D.W. Norbeck, J.W. Erickson and R. Swanstrom: Proc. Natl. Acad. Sci. USA *91*, 5597 (1994).

178 H. Jacobsen, K. Yasargil, D.L. Winslow, J.C. Craig, A. Kröhn, I.B. Duncan and J. Mous: Virology *206*, 527 (1995).

179 J.H. Condra, W.A. Schleif, O.M. Blahy, L.J. Gabryelski, D.J. Graham, J.C. Quintero, A. Rhodes, H.L. Robbins, E. Roth, M. Shivaprakash, D. Titus, T. Yang, H. Teppler, K.E. Squires, P.J. Deutsch and E.A. Emini: Nature *374*, 569 (1995).

180 S.V. Gulnik, L.I. Suvorov, B. Liu, B. Yu, B. Anderson, H. Mitsuya and J.W. Erickson: Biochemistry *34*, 9282 (1995).

181 A.K. Patick, H. Mo, M. Markowitz, K. Appelt, B. Wu, L. Musick, V. Kalish, S. Kaldor, S. Reich, D. Ho and S. Webber: Antimicrob. Agents Chemother. *40*, 292 (1996).

182 L. Doyon, G. Croteau, D. Thibeault, F. Poulin, L. Pilote and D. Lamarre: J. Virol. *70*, 3763 (1996).

183 M. Markowitz, H. Mo, D.J. Kempf, D.W. Norbeck, T.N. Bhat, J.W. Erickson and D.D. Ho: J. Virol. *69*, 701 (1995).

184 A. Molla, M. Korneyeva, Q. Gao, S. Vasavanonda, P.J. Schipper, H.-M. Mo, M. Markowitz, T. Chernyavskiy, P. Niu, N. Lyons, A. Hsu, R. Granneman, D.D. Ho, C.A.B. Boucher, J.M. Leonard, D.W. Norbeck and D.J. Kempf: Nature Med. *2*, 760 (1996).

184a J.H. Condra, D.J. Holder, W.A. Schleif, O.M. Blahy, R.M. Danovich, L.J. Gabryelski, D.J. Graham, D. Laird, J.C. Quintero, A. Rhodes, H.L. Robbins, E. Roth, M. Shivaprakash, T. Yang, J.A. Chodakewitz, P.J. Deutsch, R.Y. Leavitt, F.E. Massari, J.W. Mellors, K.E. Squires, R.T. Steigbigel, H. Teppler and E.A. Emini: J. Virol. *70*, 8270 (1996).

184b M.B. Vasudevachari, Y.-M. Zhang, H. Imamichi, T. Imamichi, J. Falloon and N.P. Salzman: Antimicrob. Agents Chemother. *40*, 2535 (1996).

185 A.M. Borman, S. Paulous and F. Clavel: J. Gen. Virol. *77*, 419 (1996).

186 A.K. Patick, R. Rose, J. Greytok, C.M. Bechtold, M.A. Hermsmeier, P.T. Chen, J.C. Barrish, R. Zahler, R.J. Colonno and P.-F. Lin: J. Virol. *69*, 2148 (1995).

187 R.W. King, S. Garber, D.L. Winslow, C. Reid, L.T. Bacheler, E. Anton and M.J. Otto: Antivir. Chem. Chemother. *6*, 80 (1995).

188 H.M. Mo, M. Markowitz, P. Majer, S.K. Burt, S.V. Gulnik, L.I. Suvorov, J.W. Erickson and D.D. Ho: AIDS Res. Human Retrovir. *12*, 55 (1996).

189 V.V. Sardana, A.J. Schlabach, P. Graham, B.L. Bush, J.H. Condra, J.C. Culberson, L. Gotlib, D.J. Graham, N.E. Kohl, R.L. LaFemina, C.L. Schneider, B.S. Wolanski, J.A. Wolfgang and E.A. Emini: Biochemistry *33*, 2004 (1994).

190 J.P. Vacca, B.D. Dorsey, W.A. Schleif, R.B. Levin, S.L. McDaniel, P.L. Darke, J. Zugay, J.C. Quintero, O.M. Blahy, E. Roth, V.V. Sardana, A.J. Schlabach, P.I. Graham, J.H. Condra, L. Gotlib, M.K. Holloway, J. Lin, I.-W. Chen, K. Vastag, D. Ostovic, P.S. Anderson, E.A. Emini and J.R. Huff: Proc. Natl. Acad. Sci. USA *91*, 4096 (1994).

191 S.S. Hoog, E.M. Towler, B. Zhao, M.L. Doyle, C. Debouck and S.S. Abdel-Meguid: Biochemistry *35*, 10279 (1996).

192 J.A. Partaledis, K. Yamaguchi, M. Tisdale, E.E. Blair, C. Falcione, B. Maschera, R.E. Myers, S. Pazhanisamy, O. Futer, A.B. Cullinan, C.M. Stuver, R.A. Byrn and D.J. Livingston: J. Virol. *69*, 5228 (1995).

193 S. Pazhanisamy, C.M. Stuver, A.B. Cullinan, N. Margolin, B.G. Rao and D.J. Livingston: J. Biol. Chem. *271*, 17979 (1996).

194 L. Moutouh, J. Corbeil and D.D. Richman: Proc. Natl. Acad. Sci. USA *93*, 6106 (1996).

195 M. Tisdale, R.E. Myers, B. Maschera, N.R. Parry, N.M. Oliver and E.D. Blair: Antimicrob. Agents Chemother. *39*, 1704 (1995).

196 J. Tang and J.A. Hartsuck: FEBS Lett. *367*, 112 (1995).

197 J.W. Erickson: Nature Struct. Biol. *2*, 523 (1995).

198 R.E. Rose, Y.-F. Gong, J.A. Greytok, C.M. Bechtold, B.J. Terry, B.S. Robinson, M. Alam, R.J. Colonno and P.-F. Lin: Proc. Natl. Acad. Sci. USA *93*, 1648 (1996).

199 W.J. Lech, G. Wang, Y.L. Yang, Y. Chee, K. Dorman, D. McCrae, L.C. Lazzeroni, J.W. Erickson, J.S. Sinsheimer and A.H. Kaplan: J. Virol. *70*, 2038 (1996).

200 D.V. Havlir, S. Eastman, A. Gamst and D.D. Richman: J. Virol. *70*, 7894 (1996).

201 G.M. Myers, B. Korber, J.A. Berzofsky, R.F. Smith and G.N. Paulakis: Human retro-
     viruses and AIDS 1994: A compilation and analysis of nucleic acid and amino acid
     sequences. Theoretical Biology and Biophysics Group, Los Alamos National Labor-
     atory, Los Alamos, New Mexico, 1994.

Progress in Drug Research, Vol. 48 (E. Jucker, Ed.)
© 1997 Birkhäuser Verlag, Basel (Switzerland)

Immunotherapy for brain diseases and mental illnesses

By Vijendra K. Singh

Department of Pharmaceutics, College of Pharmacy, The University of Michigan, Ann Arbor, MI 48109-1065, USA

1   Introduction

In recent years, research on molecular and cellular phenomena has alluded to a reciprocal interrelationship between the nervous system and immune system [1–4]. The central nervous system (CNS) as well as the peripheral nervous system (PNS) have been shown to interact with the immune system. Often, these interactions are referred to as «neuroimmune interactions» and they exist virtually at all levels: cellular, molecular, structural, physiological, and pathological [2]. Human behavior can be modified by immune factors; for instance stressful events are generally associated with immune suppression [5] and stress reduces natural resistance to wound-healing [6]. In some theoretical sense perhaps the immune system might function as a sensory organ, which has the ability to recognize and respond to environmental stimuli. Fundamentally, the dysfunction of neuroimmunological interactions could induce pathological conditions of the nervous system and several examples indeed confirm this statement [1–4]. Conceptually speaking, the diseases of the nervous system can be divided into three categories: neurodevelopmental diseases that result from abnormal development of the brain; neurodegenerative diseases that show a progressive downward course of a neurologic function such as cognition; and neuropsychiatric diseases which affect behavior or psyche. The immune system greatly impacts CNS diseases, both pathogenetically as well as therapeutically. While autoimmunity appears to be a critical pathogenic factor, other cellular immune factors such as cytokines also contribute to the disease. Moreover, just about all CNS diseases respond to treatment with immunotherapies. Thus, it is quite reasonable to postulate that most, if not all, CNS diseases are systemic diseases with the clinical manifestations confined centrally to the brain. This line of thinking may also explain why patients with CNS diseases respond to systemically-administered immunotherapies. The present paper summarizes immune factors such as autoimmunity as a cornerstone of current therapies for CNS diseases, in particular multiple sclerosis (MS), Alzheimer's disease (AD), Guillain-Barre syndrome (GBS), obsessive-compulsive disorder (OCD), and autistic syndrome (AS).

2   ·   Rationale for immunotherapy in brain diseases

The field of neuroimmunology almost exclusively evolved from the earlier immune studies of multiple sclerosis (MS) and myathenia gravis (MG) and animal models thereof. Immunologic evaluation of patients revealed abnormalities of immune parameters and therefore the connection was made between immunity and MS or MG. Both of these diseases are now believed to be the outcome of an autoimmune pathogenesis. As the topic of neuroimmunology became more generally acceptable, researchers worldwide began to examine the role of immune factors in other CNS diseases also. Immunologic assessment of patients with virtually all CNS diseases has clearly demonstrated aberrations of both cellular and humoral immunity; the impact of immune factors in some diseases being stronger than in others. Abnormality of immune function implies that these diseases may be amenable to treatment with immunotherapies. Thus, the existence of bidirectional neuroimmune interactions and immune abnormalities in patients should be a strong rationale for immunotherapy in CNS diseases.

Therapeutic effects of immunotherapies have been investigated in some CNS diseases. In each case, therapy and response depend on the nature of immune abnormality; whether it is cellular or humoral or a combination of the two. Thus the identification of potential targets for immunotherapy is absolutely essential (Table 1). For autoimmune diseases, three main targets are commonly experimented: immune activation (antigen-presenting cells); immunoregulation (CD4+ and CD8+ T lymphocytes and their cytokines); and oral tolerance induction (antigen-specific).

3   Multiple sclerosis

Multiple sclerosis (MS) is a demyelinating disease of the human CNS. It damages the sheath of myelin that protects nerves and ultimately blocks the ability of nerves to send messages to muscles, resulting in debilitating disabilities in patients. The clinical symptoms vary largely depending on the location of lesions and the disease is either a remitting-relapsing or a chronic-progressive disease. In spite of extensive research, the etiology and pathogenesis of MS remains poorly understood. It is generally believed that immunological factors such as autoimmunity are involved [7–9]. The autoimmune basis of MS, to a greater degree, is supported by an animal model known as experimental autoimmune encephalomyelitis (EAE) [10, 11]. Indeed, the EAE models and human MS are probably the most extensively studied diseases of autoimmune origin, which also respond to immunotherapies. While the precise nature of autoantigen(s) remains elusive, myelin basic protein (MBP) has been extensively implicated. To that end, an altered form of MBP may be involved in MS [12–13].

Table 1.
Potential targets of immunotherapies for CNS disorders

1. Antigen-presentation cells:	Processing (Proteinase inhibitor) MHC II presentation (Blocking antibodies to MHC II; modified epitopes such as Copolymer-1)
2. T cell:	Antibody to T-cell receptor (TCR) Antibody to CD3 and/or CD4 Vaccination with T cells Immunization with TCR peptides Generate antiidiotype
3. Cytokines and cytokine receptors:	Cytokines (IL-12, IL,-10, IFN-α, IFN-β, TNF-α, etc.) Naturally-occurring antagonists Antibodies to cytokines or cytokine receptors Cytokine soluble receptors
4. Costimulatory pathways:	CD28/B7 CTLA-4
5. Oral tolerance:	Antigen-specific, e.g. MBP
6. Miscellaneous:	Lymphoid cell trafficking (Anti-adhesion molecules) Anti-neuronal antibodies (Plasmapheresis; IV-Ig) Immune reconstitution (Bone marrow transplantation) Immune suppression (Steroids; Thiopurines; Cyclosporine A) Inflammation (Glucocorticoids; Indomethacin) Blood-brain barrier (Prazosin)

Therapeutic strategies for MS rely heavily on the nature of immune abnormality, which may be targeted for immunotherapy. Earlier studies included non-specific immunosuppressants (steroids, azathiopurine, and 6-mecaptopurine), antiinflammatories (glucocorticoids), copolymer-1, plasmapheresis, and IV-Ig. Cyclosporine A, a well-known immunosuppressant [14], may also have therapeutic effects in MS. This suggestion is based on some indirect studies. Axonal regeneration does not occur in the central nervous system although it is well known to occur in the peripheral nervous system. Immune factors such as autoimmunity may be the reason for inability of axonal regeneration in the CNS [15]. Recently, a connection between autoimmunity and abortive axonal regeneration has been demonstrated after the administration of cyclosporine A. The cyclosporine A treatment of rats, who had completely transverse-sectioned spinal cords, caused a significant recovery of morphological as well as functional characteristics of spinal fibers [16]. In these studies, it was suggested that cyclosporine A, owing to its immunosuppressive properties, blocked an autoimmune reaction that was presumably involved in the mechanism of abortive axonal regeneration. Thus, cyclosporine A might be a good immunosuppressant for treating MS and other CNS disorders involving autoimmunity.

For treatment of MS, copolymer 1 (COP-1) was developed shortly after steroid therapy in the early 1970s. COP-1 is composed of random polymers of approximately 7 kD molecular weight. It contains four amino acids (L-alanine, L-glutamic acid, L-lysine, and L-tyrosine) that are also found in MBP. COP-1 is quite safe for human consumption and a subcutaneously administered therapeutic dose of 20 mg daily is generally recommended. Based on EAE animal studies, COP-1 has been shown to modify immunity by either the induction of antigen-specific suppressor function or inhibition of antigen-specific helper function; antigen being MBP. The ability of various copolymers to suppress EAE correlates positively with their ability to react with MBP. First series of trials showed clinical improvement on COP-1 therapy in MS patients [17]. While new designs are currently underway, its therapeutic efficacy was assessed alone or in conjunction with interferon-beta [18]. The trade name for COP-1 is Copaxone (Teva Pharmaceutical Industries, Tel Aviv, Israel), which is expected to be approved shortly by the Food and Drug Administration of the United States.

The clinical manifestations of MS have also been treated with aminopyridines, in particular with 4-aminopyridine (4-AP) and 3,4-diaminopyridine (DAP) [19, 20]. They are potassium ion-channel blockers [21], neurotransmitter release inducers [22], and short-term memory enhancers [23]. Regarding MS, the aminopyridine treatment relied on ion-channel blocker activity and influenced the physiology of conduction failure in demyelinated fibers [24]. And a double-blind placebo-controlled trial showed significant improvements in neurologic deficits [24]. This trial pointed to a new approach of treating MS patients. It should be mentioned that potassium ion-channel blockers may have immunomodulating properties; for example phencyclidine (PCP), a potassium ion-channel blocker, is also an immunosuppressor [25]. In addition, we recently found that 4-AP stimulates lymphocyte proliferation. Moreover, 4-AP stimulated PHA-induced lymphocyte proliferation but it had no effect on the PWM- or Con A-

Table 2.
Stimulatory effect of 4-aminopyridine on lymphocyte proliferation

4-Aminopyridine (4-AP) concentration	Incorporation of [3H]-Methyl-Thymidine into DNA*	
	(cpm)	(% of Control)
(a) Without mitogen		
0	1,872	(100)
10^{-9} M	2,897	156
10^{-8} M	3,728	200
10^{-7} M	2,402	129
(b) With mitogen		
PHA	80,017	(100)
PHA + 10^{-7} M 4-AP	151,625	190
PWM	91,353	(100)
PWM + 10^{-7} M 4-AP	92,500	101
Con A	54,308	(100)
Con A + 10^{-7} M 4-AP	55,405	102

* All other assay conditions were the same as described elsewhere [V.K. Singh, et al: Mech. Age. Develop. 37, 257 (1987)]. Lymphocytes were separated from human blood.

induced proliferation of lymphocytes (Table 2). Since PHA is a well-known mitogen of T lymphocytes [2] and 4-AP stimulated this response, therefore 4-AP activated T lymphocytes. Based on these observations, it is implied that the therapeutic effects of 4-AP in MS patients may be related to its immunomodulating property, in addition to or in lieu of potassium ion-channel blocking activity.

Based on increasing knowledge of immunomodulatory networks, novel immune modulators are being developed. One such synthetic immuno-modulator is Linomide, a quinoline-3-carboxamide. While Linomide is known to stimulate T cell-mediated immune responses [26], it dramatically suppresses induction of several experimental autoimmune diseases, including acute as well as chronic EAE [27, 28]. The Linomide-induced suppression of EAE suggested that it may potentially be used for treating MS. Indeed, Linomide has produced promising results in two studies: First, it suppressed neurologic symptoms in a phase II trial of secondary progressive MS [29]; and second, it significantly reduced the development of MS-related active MRI lesions in a double-blind study [30]. Thus, Linomide may be a novel immunomodulator for treating relapsing-remitting MS and other CNS disorders.

Recently, intravenous immunoglobulin (IV-Ig) has been suggested as an immunotherapy for MS [31]. This treatment indeed promotes remyelination and is being investigated in detail. In addition, bone marrow transplantation (BMT) has been used successfully for about 30 years to treat a number of immunodeficiency diseases, e.g. severe acquired immunodeficiency (SCID) and certain cancers, e.g. acute lymphoblastic leukemia (ALA). Recently, BMT has shown initial success for treating autoimmune diseases such as rheumatoid arthritis, psoriasis or ulcerative colitis. Syngeneic BMT has been used for treating EAE in rats [32, 33]. Based on these animal studies, BMT has been suggested as a treatment for MS [34]. Some 15 transplants were completed in Europe last year while a few cases of MS have been treated in the U.S. and patients are in remission [unpublished reports].

Lately, evidence is accumulating to suggest that oral feeding or administration of putative autoantigen(s) can be used to treat autoimmune diseases. In this regard, the current major focus is on oral tolerance. Indeed, oral tolerance is a viable approach to alleviating autoimmune diseases, including MS [35, 36]. Oral tolerance utilizes natural immune mechanisms of the gut (small intestine). Through these mechanisms, the body accepts orally-ingested autoantigen(s) by suppressing the immune response that would otherwise develop against a foreign substance. This suppression can be directed toward an organ (or tissue) under attack by the body's own immune system, which occurs during an autoimmune process. Thus, organ-specific immunosuppression can be induced by appropriate selection and dosing of the autoantigen [36]. The mechanisms by which orally given antigens induce tolerance include immune suppression [36], clonal anergy [37], and clonal deletion [38]. These mechanisms are primarily dependent on the dose of antigen administered: low doses induce immunosuppression [36] whereas high doses favor clonal anergy [37] or clonal deletion [38]. These fundamental principles have been used to treat MS [35] and EAE [39, 40]. The phase I clinical trial of oral myelin showed promising results; low-dose feeding of myelin reduced the number of exacerbations in the remitting-relapsing MS patients [35]. This study is being expanded to a two-year multicenter phase III trial, in which Myoral (Oral Myelin) treatment of 515 patients is currently under investigation (Autoimmune Inc., Boston, MA).

Another form of therapy for MS includes cytokine-based immunotherapy. Fundamentally, this strategy depends on blocking or neutralizing the expression and function of cytokines or their receptors. The target may either be a pro-inflammatory cytokine or an immunomodulatory cytokine. The latter controls Th1- and Th2-cell-mediated immune responses. One such target may be TNF-α based on its presumed pathogenic role in EAE and MS [9, 41]. Indeed, the treatment with agents that inhibit the production or action of TNF-α suppressed development of EAE: agents tested were anti-TNF antibodies [42, 43], pentoxyfylline (PTX) [44, 45], and phosphatidylserine [46]. Based on these studies in animals, a pilot study of PTX was recently conducted in 20 MS patients; none responded to PTX therapy, precluding the importance of TNF-α inhibitors for treating MS [47]. By contrast, interferon-beta (IFNB) is a very important target for controlling progression of the disease. Indeed, INFB-based therapy is the first approved treatment for MS in the United States. And two commercial products, namely Betaseron (Berlex Laboratories Inc.) and Avonex (Biogen Inc.), have been approved by the Food and Drug Administration of the United States. Approximately 40,000 MS patients have been treated with IFNB and the outcome is quite dramatic. The IFNB treatment significantly reduced a number of exacerbations and decreased new lesions as revealed by serial MRI scans [38]. This is a very important new development in the treatment of MS, in particular because no other treatment produces both clinical as well as MRI improvements simultaneously. Thus, IFNB is an effective therapy for a majority of MS patients [48, 49], especially those in the early stages of the disease.

4   Guillain-Barre syndrome

This syndrome is considered to be an immune-mediated disorder of the peripheral nerves. The affliction occurs in children as well as adults. Histologically, a lymphocytic infiltrate is present surrounding peripheral nerve lesion. Most probably preceded by an infection, T lymphocytes [50] and other humoral factors such as antiganglioside antibodies [51, 52] are involved in causing demyelination of the peripheral nerves. Thus, GBS is an autoimmune inflammatory disease and patients are responsive to immunotherapies. Although initially steroid and plasma exchange therapies were administered, disorder is now commonly treated with IV-Ig. Recently, a retrospective multicenter study of GBS children considered natural history and immunomodulating treatment effects [53]. It showed that corticosteroids were weak and plasmapheresis could not be properly assessed. However, IV-Ig treatment was able to overcome clinical symptoms, especially in children who were unable to walk unaided.

5   Rasmussen's encephalitis

Rasmussen's encephalitis (RE) is a rare form of encephalitis with devastating manifestations. It is a progressive neurological disorder characterized by intractable focal seizures, progressive hemiplegia, and cognitive decline. RE usually affects children but can occur in adults also. Pathological examinations have shown that an early active phase of pronounced perivascular inflammation and reactive microglia is followed by a more chronic phase of microglial nodules, gliosis, and tissue destruction. Although the etio-pathogenetic factors and treatment of RE are not well known, some progress has been made. The role of autoimmunity has been investigated. The autoimmune hypothesis stemmed from an animal study. Immunization of rabbits with glutamate receptor subunit 3 (GluR3) produced seizures and pathological changes characteristic of RE, and the animals had circulating autoantibodies to GluR3 [54]. The autoantibodies also modified electrophysiological responses of cultured cortical neurons [55]. Based on a possible link between autoimmunity and RE, an open-label clinical trial of immunotherapy has been conducted. Plasmapheresis caused dramatic clinical improvement, as evaluated by lower seizure frequency and enhanced neurologic function, in 3 out of 4 patients aged 6 to 15 years [56]. The improvement persisted for up to 9 weeks and the longer term effects are not known. In this study, the effects on anti-GluR3 titers could not be clearly resolved, presumably because of a very small number of subjects studied. Additional multicenter trials will be necessary to evaluate therapeutic effects of this immunotherapy in RE. Recently, CMV genome has been detected in the brain of RE patients [57, 58]. McLachlan and coworkers [59] showed significant improvement of EEG, cognitive function, and neurologic signs in RE patients treated with ganciclovir, a potent anti-CMV drug. This response to antiviral therapy and evidence of CMV in patient's brain suggested a viral etiology for chronic RE. It is possible that a viral-induced autoimmune mechanism may be involved in the pathogenesis of this syndrome. Thus, anti-viral and immunomodulating agents may potentially be used to treat RE patients.

6   Obsessive-compulsive disorder

The movement disorders such as obsessive-compulsive disorder (OCD) are some of the prevalent chronic conditions in psychiatry. Although the neuroanatomical substrate may involve basal ganglia, the pathogenesis of these disorders is poorly understood. On the basis of therapeutic

responses to serotonergic antidepressants, a dysfunction of the serotonin system has been implicated in OCD [60]. Accumulating evidence suggest that some cases of OCD may be immunologically-derived, involving an autoimmune mechanism. In early-onset OCD, the patients have
high titers of antineuronal antibodies [61], antibodies to somatostatin and
prodynorphin [62], and blocking antibodies to brain serotonin receptor
[63]. Recently, it has been suggested that antineuronal antibodies in a significant number of early-onset OCD may result from group A [beta]-
hemolytic streptococcal (GABHS) infections [61]. These researchers also
described that immunotherapy with plasmapheresis dramatically reduced
OCD symptoms and clinical improvement was related to the antineuronal antibody titers. The patients also showed multiple remission-relapse
episodes of OCD symptoms depending on antineuronal antibody titers
[61]. More recently, OCD patients after IV-IG therapy showed about 30%
decrease in OCD symptoms and about 45% reduction in movement disorders [64].

Since plasmapheresis and IV-IG are treatments for autoimmune diseases,
their therapeutic effects would imply a pathogenic role for autoimmunity
in OCD. In this paper, it is postulated that antibodies to brain serotonin
receptor may also be pathogenetically-relevant to early-onset OCD. If
serotonin receptor antibodies [63] are the same antibodies as the antineuronal antibodies [61], they may induce an immune assault to serotonergic neurons in basal ganglia, the most consistently affected brain region
in OCD. In our double-blind study, we found that OCD patients on serotonergic antidepressants did not have serotonin receptor antibodies but
those without the medication did [63]. Thus, it is quite possible that the
antidepressants commonly used to treat OCD patients may indeed help
them by suppressing the autoimmune reaction. Although this possibility
remains to be investigated, there is reason to believe that this indeed might
happen since serotonin is known to induce proliferation of antibody-pro-
ducing B lymphocytes [65].

7   Alzheimer's disease

Alzheimer's disease (AD) is a degenerative disease of the CNS. The disease is diagnosed according to psychiatric symptoms and brain autopsies.
The hallmark of AD is the loss of higher mental functions, memory loss
especially of recent events. There is no known cause, no definitive diag-
nostic test, and no cure or treatment for the disease. Many studies suggest that AD is a very complex and heterogeneous disorder involving mul-

tiple factors: genetic factors, immune factors, neurochemical factors, and environmental factors. Several lines of investigations suggest that immune factors may be involved in the pathogenesis of AD or a subset thereof. We recently proposed a "Neuroautoimmunity (NAI) Model" that may explain the immune basis of the disease [66]. It was suggested that neurodegeneration may result from a suppressor/cytotoxic cell-mediated autoimmune reaction, in which antigen-specific autoantibodies may direct immune assault to affected neurons [66, 67]. The credence to this model comes from numerous observations of autoimmune factors in AD (Table 3).

Recently, inflammation of the brain has been linked to AD. This association relied on retrospective studies of rheumatoid arthritis and frequency of the AD-type dementia [68] and an inverse relationship between anti-inflammatory treatments and frequency of AD [69, 70]. On the basis of these considerations, preliminary trials of anti-inflammatory drugs have been conducted. In one clinical trial, the non-steroidal anti-inflammatory drug (NSAID) indomethacin prevented the decline of cognitive functions when compared to placebo-control [71]. This prompted a clinical trial of prednisone, which is not quite complete as yet but the preliminary indications are that this drug is of limited or no value in AD [72]. In spite of the lack of a typical inflammatory response in AD, two points should be noted: (i) anti-inflammatory drugs such as ACTH and prednisone are well-known immunosuppressive agents [73] whereas indomethacin enhances cellular immunity (NK cell) in the immuosuppressed host [74]; and (ii) inflammation is typically an immune-mechanism reaction. Thus, therapy should be directed toward more appropriate immune targets. Although there are several potential targets for immunotherapy (i.e. immune activation, immunoregulation, anti-neuronal antibodies, and cytokines) in AD, none has been investigated except for a pilot study of transfer factor and piracetam with minor cognitive improvements [75]. Therefore, it should be possible to treat AD patients with immunotherapies such as plasmapheresis, IV-Ig, antigen-specific oral tolerance, 4-aminopyridine, and Linomide.

8 Autistic syndrome

Autism or autistic syndrome (AS) is an early-onset disorder of behavioral manifestations: limited or no language and communication skills; abnormal responses to sensations, people, events, and objects; and self-injurious and repetitive rocking behaviors. The causation may be multifactorial: environmental factors, immune factors, genetic susceptibility, and neurochem-

Table 3.
Immunologic dysfunction in Alzheimer's disease

Immune Parameter:	Modification
1. Immunogenetics:	Increased frequency of HLA-BW15; Prevalence of HLA haplotypes and Gm allotypes; Association of HLA-linked C4B2 allele.
2. Serum Ig:	No significant change of IgM, IgG, and IgA; Normal IgG and IgA but decreased IgM; IgG3 isotype increased.
3. Blood lymphocytes:	Normal levels of T and B lymphocytes; No change of T subsets (CD4+ and CD8+); Increased activated T cells (IL-2R+ and HLA-DR+); Increased CD4/CD8 ratios; Increased CD8+ T cells but slight decrease of CD4+ cells; Increased expression of S100 (CD8+ cells).
4. Lymphocyte functions:	Decreased AMLR, a helper T-cell function; Suppressed lymphocyte proliferation to T cell mitogens; Diminished Ca2+ uptake in mitogen-activated lymphocytes; No change in PWM-induced IgG synthesis; Enhanced Con A-induced T suppressor (Ts) cell function; Deficiency of lymphocyte proliferation by beta-amyloid protein.
5. Cytokine production:	Normal IFN production after Con A-stimulation; Enhanced production of IL-1, IL-2, and IL-6.
6. Serum immune acti- vation antigens:	Increased TNF, sCD8, and sICAM-1; Increased level of IL-6 but normal levels of IFN-α, IFN-γ, and IL-12; Enhanced levels of S100α and S100β proteins.
7. Autoantibodies:	Anti-brain cells; Anti-astrocytes; Anti-cholinergic cells; Anti-pituitary cells; Anti-microglial cells; Anti-thymic cells; Anti-myelin basic protein; Anti-neuritic plaques; Anti-neurofibrillary tangles; Antineuron-axon filament protein (200 kD); Anti-beta-amyloid protein.

* Modified from Singh [66].

ical imbalance. The treatment modalities generally include behavior modification and pharmacotherapy, without any significant therapeutic value. Immunology is probably the most extensively studied topic of research in autism, possibly because of faulty immunoregulation and autoimmunity [76–79]. Immunologic evaluation of autistic patients showed depressed lymphocyte proliferation to mitogens [76, 80], impaired cellular immunity of macrophages [81] and NK cells [82], circulating autoantibodies to brain proteins [76, 78, 83, 84], elevation of T-cell activation antigens soluble interleukin-2 and soluble CD8 [77], increased activated T cells expressing DR antigen [85, 86], and elevated levels of circulating IL-12 and IFN-γ [79]. Based on these observations, we hypothesized that autism in a subset may be caused by an organ-specific autoimmune response [78, 79]. We postulated that the positive titers of anti-MBP antibodies and increase of IL-12 and IFN-γ are related to autoimmune process in autism [79]. Autistic children have impaired myelin function [87] and they respond inappropriately to MBP in cellular immunity assays, for instance macrophage-migration-inhibition-factor production and lymphocyte proliferation [81, 88]. Moreover, autistic-like symptoms are found in about 75% of children with Landau-Kleffner syndrome (LKS), in which autoimmunity to myelin has been implicated [89]. The IL-12 is produced by macrophages and it induces IFN-γ in helper T cells, promoting development of Th-1 cells. Since these cells are known to induce organ-specific autoimmune diseases in animals [90–92], they may initiate an autoimmune reaction in autism as well.

On the basis of the above considerations, it is suggested that selective immunotherapy may be of considerable therapeutic importance in autism. Initially, treatment based on immunostimulators such as transfer factor and isoprinosine produced some clinical improvement [93]. Moreover, improvement of autistic-like symptoms was found when autistic children were treated with immunosuppressant ACTH [94]. Of late, IV-Ig treatment showed improvement of some of the autistic symptoms [95]. Plasmapheresis, which recently showed improvement in the quality of behavioral symptoms in children with Rasmussen's encephalitis [54] and obsessive-compulsive disorder [61], has not been used to treat autistic patients. In these cases, benefit was derived from the lowering of antineuronal antibodies titers in patients due to autoimmune process. Since autistic children have positive titers of brain autoantibodies [78], they should also respond to plasma exchange therapy. The identification of autoantigen(s) such as MBP should also permit clinical trials of antigen-specific oral tolerance. Thus, for reasons outlined, immunotherapy has a strong prospect for treating patients with autistic syndrome.

9   Concluding remarks

The concept of immunotherapies for brain disorders has a short history but it is already at the threshold of a new era of therapeutic strategies for neurodegenerative as well as neuropsychiatric diseases. The hallmark example is that of MS, for which IFNB immunotherapy has gained tremendous approval worldwide. Based on lessons learned from the immunology of MS, immune mechanisms and immunotherapies are currently being explored in other CNS disorders. Plasmapheresis and IV-Ig treatments are the topics of clinical trials, which in some cases demonstrate significant improvement of clinical symptoms. This is particularly true of MS, GBS, RE, and OCD. Although IV-Ig treatment is used more frequently [31], some caution should be exercised with this therapy, especially when it is administered to children and adolescents. This concern is raised because the long-term effects of IV-Ig are virtually unknown and complications resulting from it could be quite dramatic in CNS patients [96, 97]. The therapeutic strategies for CNS diseases encounter blood-brain barrier, which precludes entry of circulating immune factors into the CNS. However, viral or microbial infection, activated T lymphocytes, and MHC class I and II expression are known to increase permeability across the blood-brain barrier [3, 98, 99]. The MHC class I expression in brain is upregulated by IFN-γ [100], which may activate or disrupt blood-brain barrier. It is possible that pretreatment with IFN-γ may serve as a tool to modify blood-brain barrier, allowing systemically-administered drugs to reach targets in the brain. Another point of interest is that the majority of brain diseases seemed to involve autoimmunity and/or inflammation. This implies the need for novel immunotherapies. Treatment with non-specific immunomodulators such as Linomide and oral tolerance after autoantigen feeding may be quite effective but the nature of immune abnormality and autoantigen(s) should be identified. To conclude, the emerging field of neuroimmunology or psychoimmunology is witnessing a modern era of immunotherapies for CNS disorders. This evolution of our 'mind and body' should not come as a surprise – after all they are interconnected.

References

1   G.F. Solomon: Brain Behav. Immunity 7, 352 (1993).
2   V.K. Singh: Prog. Drug Res. 45, 9 (1995).
3   Z. Fabry, C.S. Raine and M.N. Hart: Immunol. Today 15, 218 (1994).
4   R.L. Wilder: Annu. Rev. Immunol. 13, 307 (1995).
5   J.E. Hillhouse, J.K. Kiecolt-Glaser and R. Glaser: In: Plotnikoff, N., Murgo, A., Faith,

R. and Wybran, J. (eds.): Stress and Immunity, pp. 3, CRC Press, Inc., Boca Raton, Florida, USA 1991.

6   J.K. Kiecolt-Glaser, P.T. Marucha, W.B. Malarkey, A.M. Mercado and R. Glaser: Lancet *346*, 1194 (1995).

7   R. Martin, H.F. McFarland and D.E. McFarlin: Annu. Rev. Immunol. *10*, 153 (1992).

8   C.S. Raine: Ann. Neurol. *36*, S61 (1994).

9   V. Navikas and H. Link: J. Neurosci. Res. *45*, 322 (1996).

10   S.S. Zamvil and L. Steinman: Annu. Rev. Immunol. *8*, 579 (1992).

11   R.H. Swanborg: Clin. Immunol. Immunopathol. 77, 4 (1995).

12   D.D. Wood, J.M. Bilbao, P. O'Connors and M.A. Moscarello: Ann. Neurol. *40*, 18 (1996).

13   J.N. Whitaker and G.W. Mitchell: Ann. Neurol. *40*, 3 (1996).

14   N.H. Sigal and F.J. Dumont: Annu. Rev. Immunol. *10*, 519 (1992).

15   G.M. Lauro, V. Margotta, G. Venturini, A. Teichner, B. Caronti and G. Palldini: Boll. Zool. *59*, 215 (1992).

16   G. Palladini, B. Caronti, G. Pozzessere, A. Teichner, F.R. Buttarelli, E. Morselli, E. Valle, G. Venturini, A. Fortuna and F.E. Pontier: J. Brain Res. *37*, 145 (1996).

17   M.B. Bornstein, A. Miller, S. Slagle, M. Weitzman, H. Crystal, E. Drexler, M. Keilson, A. Merriam, S. Wassertheil-Smoller, V. Spada, W. Weiss, R. Arnon, I. Jacobson, D. Teitelbaum and M. Sela: N. Engl. J. Med. *317*, 408 (1987).

18   K.P. Johnson: Ann. Neurol. *36*, S115 (1994).

19   C.H. Polman, F.W. Bertelsmann, A.C. van Loenen and J.C. Koetsier: Arch. Neurol. *51*, 292 (1994).

20   C.T. Bever: Ann. Neurol. *36*, S118 (1994).

21   J.F. Storm: Prog. Brain Res. *83*, 161 (1990).

22   R. Tapia and M. Sitges: Brain Res. *250*, 291 (1982).

23   C. Peterson and G.E. Gibson: Neurobiol. Aging *4*, 25 (1983).

24   C.M. Bowe, J.D. Kocsis, E.F. Targ and S.G. Waxman: Ann. Neurol. *22*, 264 (1987).

25   V.K. Singh and H.H. Fudenberg: In: Domino, E.F. and Kamenka, J.M. (eds.): Sigma Phencyclidine-like Compounds as Molecular Probes in Biology, pp. 653, NPP Books, Ann Arbor, Michigan, USA 1988.

26   E. Larsson, A. Joki and T. Stalhandske: Int. J. Immunopharmacol. *9*, 425 (1987).

27   D.M. Karussis, D. Lehmann, S. Slavin, U. Vourka-Karussis, R. Mizrachi-Koll, H. Ovadia, A. Ben-Nun, T. Kalland and O. Abramsky: Ann. Neurol. *34*, 654 (1993).

28   D.M. Karussis, D. Lehmann, S. Slavin, U. Vourka-Karussis, R. Mizrachi-Koll, H. Ovadia, T. Kallard and O. Abramsky: Proc. Natl. Acad. Sci. USA *90*, 6400 (1993).

29   D.M. Karussis, Z. Meiner, D. Lehman, J.M. Gomori, A. Schwarz, A. Linde and O. Abramsky: Neurology *47*, 341 (1996).

30   O. Andersen, J. Lycke, P.O. Tollesson, A. Svenningsson, B. Runmarker, A.S. Linde, M. Astrom, P. Gjorstrup and S. Ekholm: Neurology *47*, 895 (1996).

31   A. Otten, M. Vermeulen, P.M.M. Bossuyt and A. Otten: J. Neurol. Neurosug. Neuropsychiat. *59*, 359 (1995).

32   M. van Gelder, E.P. Kinwel-Bohre and D.W. van Bekkum: Bone Marrow Transplant. *11*, 233 (1993).

33   R.K. Burt, W. Burns, P. Ruvolo, A.Fischer, C. Shiao, A. Guimaraes, J. Barrett and A. Hess: J. Neurosci. Res. *41*, 526 (1995).

34   R.K. Burt, W. Burns and A. Hess: Bone Marrow Transplant. *16*, 1 (1995).

35   H.L. Weiner, G.A. Macklin, M. Matsui, E.J. Orav, S.J. Khoury, D.M. Dawson and D.A. Hafler: Science *259*, 1321 (1993).

36 H.L. Weiner, A. Friedman, A. Miller, S.J. Khoury, A. Al-Sabbagh, L.M.B. Santos, M. Sayegh, R.B. Nussenblatt, D.E. Trentham and D.A. Hafler: Annu. Rev. Immunol. *12*, 809 (1994).

37 C.C. Whitacre I.E. Gienapp, C.G. Orosz and D. Bitar: J. Immunol. *147*, 2155 (1991).

38 J.M. Critchfield, M.K. Racke, J.C. Zuniga-Pflucker, B. Cannella, C.S. Raine, J. Goverman and M.J. Lenardo: Science *263*, 1139 (1994).

39 Y. Chen, V.K. Kuchroo, J.I. Inobe, D.A. Hafler and H.L. Weiner: Science *265*, 237 (1994).

40 A.L. Meyer, J.M. Benson, I.E. Gienapp, K.L. Cox and C.C. Whitacre: J. Immunol. *157*, 4230 (1996).

41 P. Reickmann, M. Albrecht, B. Kitze, T. Weber, H. Tumani, A. Broocks, W. Luer, A. Helwig and S. Poser: Ann. Neurol. *37*, 82 (1995).

42 N.H. Ruddle, C.M. Bergman, K.M. McGrath, E.G. Lingenheld, M.L. Grunnet, S.J. Padula and R.B. Clark: J. Exp. Med. *172*, 1193 (1990).

43 D. Baker, D. Butler, B.J. Scallon, J.K. O'Neill, J.L. Turk and M. Feldman: Eur. J. Immunol. *24*, 2040 (1994).

44 S. Nataf, J.P. Louboutin, D. Chabannes, J.R. Feve and J.Y. Muller: Acta Neurol. Scand. *88*, 97 (1993).

45 O. Rott, E. Cash and B. Fleischer: Eur. J. Immunol. *23*, 1745 (1993).

46 G. Monastra, A.H. Cross, A. Bruni and C.S. Raine: Neurology *43*, 153 (1994).

47 B.W. van Oosten, M.H.G. Rep, R.A.W. van Lier, P.E.T. Scholten, B.M.E. von Blomberg, K.W. Pflughaupt, H.P. Hartung, H.J. Ader and C.H. Polman: J. Neuroimmunol. *66*, 49 (1996).

48 IFNB Multiple Sclerosis Study Group: Neurology *43*, 665 (1993).

49 D. Paty: Ann. Neurol. *36*, S113 (1994).

50 A. Ben-Smith, J.S.H. Gaston, P.C. Barber and J.B. Winer: J. Neurol. Neurosurg. Psychiatry *61*, 362 (1996).

51 A.F. Hahn, T.E. Feasby, C. Wilkie and D. Lovgren: Muscle Nerve *16*, 1174 (1993)

52 I. Illa, N. Ortiz, E. Gallard, C. Juarez and M.C. Dalakas: Ann. Neurol. *38*, 218 (1995)

53 R. Korinthenberg and J. Schulte Monting: Arch. Dis. Child. *74*, 281 (1996).

54 S.W. Rogers, P.I. Andrews, L.C. Gahring, T. Whisehand, K. Cauley, B. Crain, T.E. Hughes, S.F. Heinmann and J.O. McNamara: Science *265*, 648 (1994).

55 R.E. Twyman, L.C. Gahring, J. Spiess and S.W. Rogers: Neuron *14*, 755 (1995).

56 J.M. Andrews, J.A. Thompson, T.J. Pysher, M.L. Walker and M.E. Hammond: Ann. Neurol. *28*, 88 (1990).

57 C. Power, S.D. Poland, W.T. Blume, J.P. Girvin and G.P.A. Rice: Lancet *336*, 1282 (1990).

58 V. Jay, L.E. Becker, H. Ostubo, M. Cortez, P. Hwang, H.J. Hoffman and M. Zielenska: Neurology *45*, 108 (1995).

59 R.S. McLachlan, S. Levin and W.T. Blume: Neurology *47*, 925 (1996).

60 D.L. Murphy, J. Zohar, C. Benkelfat, M.T. Pato, T.A. Pigott and T.R. Insel: Br. J. Psychiatry *155*, 15 (1989).

61 S.E. Sowedo, H.L. Leonard and L.S. Kiessling: Pediatrics *93*, 323 (1994).

62 B.F. Roy, C. Benkelfat, J.L. Hill, P.F. Pierce, M.M. Dauphin, T.M. Kelly, T. Sunderland, D.R. Weinberger and N. Breslin: Biol. Psychiatry *35*, 335 (1994).

63 G. Hanna, V.K. Singh, G. Curtis, J. Himle, E. Weidmer-Mikhail and D. Koram: Proceedings of the 43rd Annual Meeting of the American Academy of Child and Adolescent Psychiatry, Philadelphia, Pennsylvania; pp. 109, Abstract #NR-80 (1996).

64 S.E. Swedo: Brown University Child and Adolescent Behavior Letter *11*, 3 (1995).

65 K. Iken, S. Chheng, A. Fargin, A.C. Goulet and E. Kouassi: Cell. Immunol. *163*, 1 (1995).

66   V.K. Singh: Gerontology *43*, 79 (1997).
67   V.K. Singh: Mol. Chem. Neurochem. *28*, 105 (1996).
68   P.L. McGeer and J. Rogers: Neurology *42*, 447 (1992).
69   J.C.S. Breiter, B.A. Gau, K.A. Welch, B.L. Plassman, W.M. McDonald, M.J. Helms and J.C. Anthony: Neurology *44*, 227 (1994).
70   J.B. Rich, D.X. Rasmusson, M.F. Folstein, K.A. Carson, C. Kawas and J. Brandt: Neurology *45*, 51 (1995).
71   J. Rogers, L.C. Kirby, S.R. Hempelman, D.L. Berry, P.L. McGeer, A.W. Kaszniak, J. Zalinski, M. Cofield, L. Mansukhani, P. Wilson and F. Kogan: Neurology *43*, 1609 (1993).
72   P.S. Aisen: Gerontology *43*, 143 (1997).
73   T.R. Copps and A.S. Fauci: Immunol. Rev. *65*, 133 (1982).
74   B.K. Pedersen, N. Tvede, K. Klarlund, L.D. Christensen, F.R. Hansen, H. Galbo, A. Kharazmi and J. Halkjaer-Kristensen: Int. J. Sports Med. *11*, 127 (1990).
75   V.K. Singh and H.H. Fudenberg: Prog. Drug Res. *32*, 21 (1988).
76   V.K. Singh, H.H. Fudenberg, D. Emerson and M. Coleman: Ann. N.Y. Acad. Sci. *540*, 602 (1988).
77   V.K. Singh, R.P. Warren, J.D. Odell and P. Cole: Clin. Immunol. Immunopathol. *61*, 448 (1991).
78   V.K. Singh, R.P. Warren, J.D. Odell, L. Warren and P. Cole: Brain, Behav. Immunity *7*, 97 (1993).
79   V.K. Singh: J. Neuroimmunol. *66*, 143 (1996).
80   E.G. Stubbs, M.L. Crawford, D.R. Burger and A.A. Vanderbark: J. Autism Childh. Schizophr. *7*, 49 (1977).
81   A. Weizman, R. Weizman, G.A. Szekely, H. Wijsenbeek and E. Livni: Am. J. Psychiat. *139*, 1462 (1982).
82   R.P. Warren, A. Foster and N.C. Margaretten: J. Am. Acad. Child Adol. Psychol. *26*, 333 (1987).
83   R.D. Todd, J.M. Hickok, G.M. Anderson and D.J. Cohen: Biol. Psychiatry *23*, 644 (1988).
84   A.V. Plioplys, A. Greaves, K. Kazemi and E. Silverman: Neuropsychobiology *29*, 12 (1994).
85   A.V. Plioplys, A. Greaves, K. Kazemi and E. Silverman: Dev. Brain Dysfunct. *7*, 12 (1994).
86   R.P. Warren, J. Yonk, R.P. Burger and D. Odell: Neuropsychobiology *31*, 53 (1995)
87   R.J. McClelland, D.G. Eyre, D. Watson, G.J. Calvert and E. Sherrad: Brit. J. Psychiatry *160*, 659 (1992).
88   V.K. Singh: Presented at the Annual Conference of the Greater Long Beach South Bay Chapter of the Autism Society of America, Long Beach, California, USA, October 13–14, 1995.
89   S. Nevsimalova, A. Tauberova, S. Doutlik, V. Kucera and O. Dlouha: Brain Dev. *14*, 34 (1992).
90   G. Trinchieri: Immunol. Today *14*, 335 (1993).
91   A.J. McNight, G.J. Zimmer, I. Fogelman, S.F. Wolf and A.K. Abbas: J. Immunol. *152*, 2172 (1994).
92   R.S. Liblau, S.M. Singer and H.O. McDevitt: Immunol. Today *16*, 58 (1995).
93   H.H. Fudenberg, V.K. Singh, D. Emerson and M. Coleman: J. Neuroimmunol. *16*, 58 (1987).
94   J.K. Buitelaar, H. van Engeland, K.H. de Kogel, H. de Vries, J.A. van Hooff and J.A. van Ree: Biol. Psychiatry *31*, 1119 (1992).

95   S. Gupta, S. Aggawal and C. Heads: J. Autism Dev. Disord. *26*, 439 (1996).
96   R. Voltz, F.V. Rosen, T. Yousry, J. Beck and R. Hohlfeld: Neurology *46*, 250 (1996)
97   D.A. Tam, L.D. Morton, D.F. Stroncek and R.T. Leshner: J. Neuroimmunol. *64*, 175 (1996).
98   H.F. Cserr and P.M. Knopf: Immunol. Today *13*, 507 (1992).
99   J.M. Spies, K.W. Westland, J.G. Bonner and J.D. Pollard: Brain *118*, 857 (1995).
100 H. Neumann, A. Cavalie, D.E. Jenne and H. Wekerle: Science *269*, 549 (1995).

Progress in Drug Research, Vol. 48 (E. Jucker, Ed.)
© 1997 Birkhäuser Verlag, Basel (Switzerland)

Natural products and their derivatives as cancer chemopreventive agents

By Shijun Ren and Eric J. Lien[1]

Department of Pharmaceutical Sciences, School of Pharmacy, University of Southern California, 1985 Zonal Ave., Los Angeles, CA 90033, USA

Abbreviations
AOM: azoxymethane; BPDE-2: *anti-trans*-benzo(α)pyrene-7,8-diol-9,10-epoxide; B(α)P: benzo(α)pyrene; DBA: dibutylamine; DMBA: 7,12-dimethylbenz(α)anthracene; DMH: dimethylhydrazine; ENNG: N-ethyl-N'-nitro-N-nitrosoguanidine; 3-MCA: 3-methylcholanthrene; NBOA: N-nitroso-bis(2-oxopropyl)amine; NDEA: N-nitrosodiethylamine; NMBA: N-nitrosomethybenzylamine; NMU: N-nitrosomethylurea; NNK: 4-(methylnitrosamino)-1-(3-pyridyl)-1-butanone; 4-NQO: 4-nitroquinoline-N-oxide; NS: nitrososarcosine; PMA: phorbol myristate acetate; TPA: 12-O-tetradecanoylphorbol-13-acetate; UVB: ultraviolet B radiation.

---

[1] To whom correspondence should be addressed.

1   Summary

This review summarizes currently available data on the chemopreventive efficacies, proposed mechanisms of action and relationships between activities and structures of natural products like vitamin D, calcium, dehydro-epidandrosterone, coenzyme Q_{10}, celery seed oil, parsley leaf oil, sulforaphane, isoflavonoids, lignans, protease inhibitors, tea polyphenols, curcumin, and polysaccharides from *Acanthopanax* genus.

2   Introduction

Cancer chemoprevention is an emerging field with great potential for impacting on cancer incidence rates in defined high-risk groups and the general population. To search for chemopreventive agents, hundreds of compounds with chemopreventive efficacies have been isolated from human body, foods and plants. Among these compounds, vitamins A, C, and E, selenium, organic sulfur compounds, ellagic acid, flavonoids, tannic acid, indoles, unsaturated fatty acids, etc. have been reviewed by Gao and Lien [1]. In this review, emphasis is placed upon the chemopreventive efficacies, proposed mechanisms of action and relationships between the activities and the structures of compounds not included in the previous report, e.g. vitamin D, calcium, dehydroepidandrosterone, coenzyme Q_{10}, celery seed oil, parsley leaf oil, sulforaphane, isoflavonoids, lignans, protease inhibitors, tea polyphenols, curcumin, and polysaccharides from *Acanthopanax* genus.

3   Natural products from the human body

3.1   Vitamin D

The possibility that vitamin D (**1**) (see Figure 1 for the structure) deficiency might increase the risk of prostate cancer and colorectal cancer has been suggested by Schwartz and Garland [2–4]. A recent report by Corder et al. [5] analyzed levels of vitamin D and metabolites in stored serum in a population of 181 men who subsequently developed prostate cancer. Mean serum levels of 1,25-dihydroxyvitamin D_3 (**2**) (1,25-D_3 or calcitriol, the active form of the hormone), were slightly but significantly lower in the cancer patients as compared to the controls. Risk of prostate cancer decreased with higher levels of 1,25-D_3, especially in men with low

25-hydroxyvitamin D_3, the inactive precursor which serves as the major reservoir for 1,25-D_3 in the body. Braun's findings are somewhat conflicting [6, 7]. One ecological study supports the hypothesis that vitamin D produced in the skin from sunlight exposure may be a protective factor for ovarian cancer mortality [8].

1,25-D_3, exerts its action *via* a specific intracellular vitamin D receptor (VDR) to modulate gene expression in a fashion analogous to the classical steroid hormones [9, 10]. The list of tissues containing the VDR includes pancreatic B cells, pituitary gland, breast tissue, placenta, lymphocytes, keratinocytes, colon, prostate, intestine, bone, kidney, as well as many cancer cell lines [11]. The human malignant cell lines that were shown to possess VDR and to be differentiated and/or growth-inhibited by 1,25-D_3 treatment included HL-60 leukemic cells [12], breast cancer cells [13, 14], malignant melanoma cells [15], rectal mucosa [16], colon carcinoma cells [17, 18], and prostate cancer cells [19]. 1,25-D_3 also suppresses the proliferation and promotes the differentiation of a number of non-malignant tissues *in vitro* [20] including normal osteoblasts [21], myoblasts [22], keratinocytes [23], and intestinal cells [18, 24].

The antiproliferative effects of 1,25-D_3 have also been demonstrated *in vivo*. 1,25-D_3 inhibited the growth of xenografts of human melanoma and colonic cancers in immunosuppressed mice [14]. Moderately elevated plasma concentrations of vitamin D were associated with a large reduction in the incidence of colorectal cancer in the recent studies of Garland et al. [4, 5, 25]. Mammary tumors induced by NMU in rats have also been shown to be inhibited by 1,25-D_3 [13].

Over the past decade at least 400 analogs of 1,25-D_3 have been designed that have actions similar to vitamin D in calcemic effects, inhibiting cell growth and stimulating cellular differentiation and with a reduced tendency to cause hypercalcemia, a major side-effect following the use of vitamin D preparations in patients [11]. Their structure-activity relationship has been studied by Bikle [26] and Norman et al. [27]. EB-1089 [1(S), 3(R)-dihydroxy-20(R)-(5'-ethyl-5'-hydroxy-hepta-1'(E), 3'(E)-dien-1'-yl)-9,10-secopregna-5(Z),7(E), 10(19)-tiene] (**3**), one analog of 1,25-D_3, exhibits greater binding potency for the VDR than 1,25-D_3. EB-1089 also inhibits breast cancer cell growth *in vitro* [28]. It also causes a significant dose-dependent inhibition and even regression of the N-methylnitrosourea-induced rat mammary tumor *in vivo* [29]. The ability of EB-1089 to affect calcium metabolism *in vivo* is lower as compared to that of 1,25-D_3. This low calcemic effect combined with the strong cancer prevention effect with a potency of 50 to 100 times that of 1,25-D_3 on cancer cells *in vitro* makes EB-1089 an interesting candidate for the prevention of cancer [30]. In a

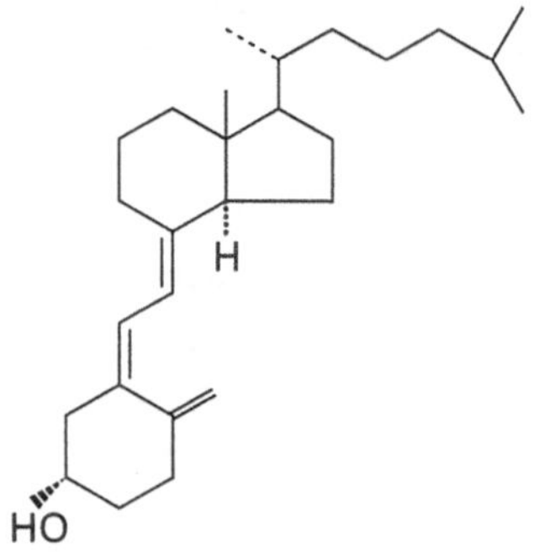

1. Vitamin D₃   **2.** 1,25-D₃   **3.** EB-1098

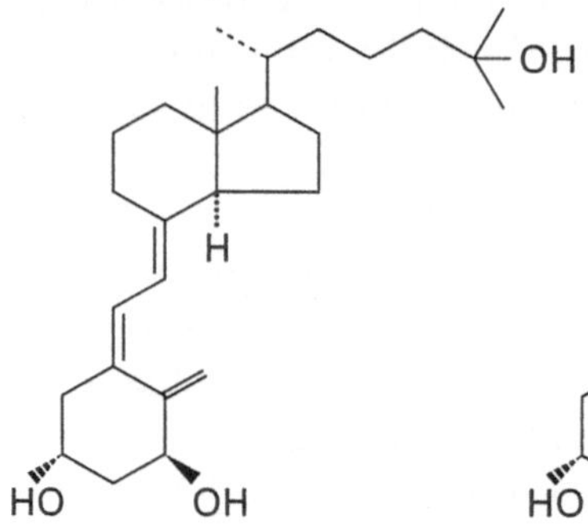

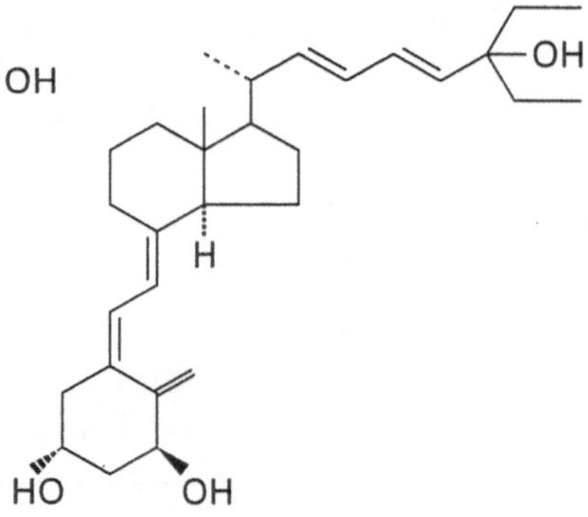

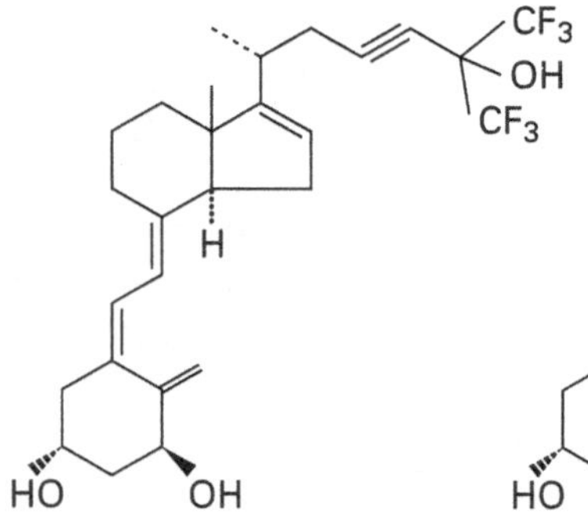

4. Ro24-5531 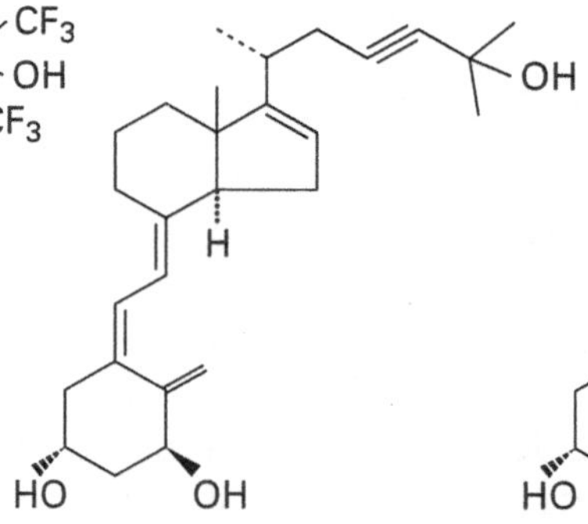   **5.** Ro23-7553 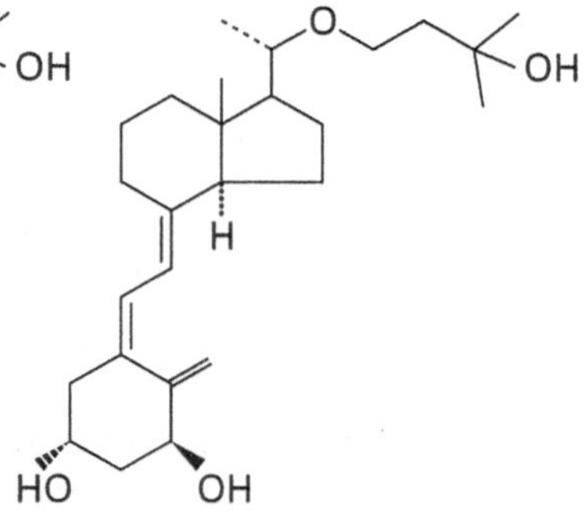   **6.** OCT

Fig. 1
Vitamin D and its derivatives

recent study, use of vitamin D analog Ro24-5531 [1,25(OH)$_2$-16-ene-23-yne-26,27-hexafluorocholecalciferol] (**4**) lessened tumor incidence and extended tumor latency in a rat breast cancer study [31]. Ro24-5531 was also significantly effective at reducing the incidence of invasive carcinomas of the siminal vesicle, and anterior prostate [32]. Ro23-7553 [1,25(OH)$_2$-16-ene-23-yne-D$_3$] (**5**) was discovered to be more potent than 1,25-D$_3$ in inhibiting clonal proliferation of HL-60, EM-2, U937, and patient's myeloid leukemic cells, and in inducing differentiation of HL-60 promyelocytes, as well as in stimulating clonal growth of normal human myeloid stem cells. This compound appears to be significantly less toxic than 1,25-D$_3$ [33]. OCT [1,25(OH)$_2$-22-oxa-D$_3$] (**6**), a newly developed noncalcemic analog, suppresses the growth of estrogen receptor-negative as well as estrogen receptor-positive breast carcinoma *in vivo* without causing hypercalcemia in athymic mice implanted with human breast carcinoma [34].

Based on examples in many different malignant cells, vitamin D appears to be antiproliferative and promotes cellular maturation. It must be viewed as an important cellular modulator of growth and differentiation in addition to its classical role as a regulator of calcium homeostasis. 1,25-D$_3$ and its analogs may prove useful in cancer chemoprevention. The data currently available provide the basis for an optimistic view on the possible use of vitamin D as a cancer chemopreventive agent, although further investigation is clearly warranted to better define its potential chemopreventive utility in humans.

3.2   Calcium

An enormous amount of variation in calcium intake exists. The epidemiologic studies that have analyzed the association between calcium and malignancies have mainly been studied in colon cancer. Most of the nineteen studies have shown an inverse relationship between the consumption of calcium and colon cancer incidence in both cohort and case-control studies [35]. Among these studies, a 19-year prospective study of 1965 men in Chicago by Garland et al. [36] demonstrated a significant protective effect of dietary calcium and vitamin D against colorectal cancer. Slattery et al. [37] also found that increased dietary calcium intake reduced the risk of colonic cancer, particularly in men. An inverse geographic relationship between latitude and colon cancer incidence suggested that increased exposure to sunlight reduced the risk of colorectal cancer presumably through mechanisms that involve vitamin D formation and calcium [38]. Other studies, however, have not shown positive correlation between dietary calcium intake and colon cancer risk [39, 40].

Increasing calcium concentration in cell and organ culture media decreased cell proliferation and induced cell differentiation in rat esophageal epithelial cells, murine epidermal cells, mammary cells, and colon cells [35].

In animal studies, oral calcium supplementation decreased colonic epithelial cell hyperproliferation when it was induced by several factors including bile acids and fatty acids, partial enteric resection, dietary fat, and a nutritional stress diet in rodents [35]. A study by Pence et al. [41] used male F344 rats in an AOM-induced colon tumor model to study the single and interactive effects of calcium and aspirin on cholic acid-promoted experimental colon carcinogenesis. The result demonstrated that calcium was a more effective chemopreventive agent in cholic acid-promoted colon carcinogenesis than aspirin. Chemical carcinogenesis in rodents has also been modified by calcium intake [35]. Most studies have shown that calcium intake decreased numbers of tumors induced. On the other hand, several studies failed to show any calcium influence on DMH-induced carcinogenesis [35].

In 18 studies of human subjects, calcium supplementation was effective in decreasing epithelial cell hyperproliferation and correcting abnormal patterns of cell proliferation in colonic mucosa at increased risk for colorectal cancer [35]. In five randomized clinical trials, increased calcium intake resulted in decreased hyperproliferation in four of the five randomized trials [42–45].

The mechanism of chemopreventive action of calcium is not very clear. Calcium and calcium-binding proteins are involved in controlling the cell cycle. Pazianas et al. [46] recently discovered the existence of surface C_a^{2+} receptor on colon cells. Signals from C_a^{2+} receptor on the cell surface trigger a combination of differentiation and apoptosis when external C_a^{2+} concentration reaches their setpoints. Raising the amount of C_a^{2+} in fecal water above a critical level reduces proliferation and thus decreases colorectal carcinogenesis in normal rats and some high-risk humans [47]. Another mechanism of action is attributed to calcium-binding fatty acids and bile acids [48, 49]. Colonic mucosa is easily irritated by fatty acids and free bile acids, resulting in the loss of epithelial cells. A compensatory increase in colonic cellular proliferation provides repair and regeneration. This action may be the basis of the cancer-promoting effect of fat. Calcium inhibits the promoting role of high dietary fat by binding soluble fatty acids and bile acids in the colonic lumen, forming insoluble calcium complexes. This protective effect may occur in the bowel lumen before fat is absorbed across the intestinal brush border. Experiments with bile acids and fatty acids in rodents and in human cells provide evidence to support this hypothesis, showing a reduction in bile-acid and fatty-acid toxicity on colonic mucosa following oral and in vitro calcium supplementation, respectively [35].

The rate of calcium uptake is contingent on adequate vitamin D stimulation of the intestinal mucosa for absorption. 1,25-D_3 enhances the transport of calcium from the lumen across the intestinal wall into the circulatory system. Synergistic interactions between vitamin D_3 and calcium have been reported, with vitamin D_3 playing a permissive role for the expression of a chemopreventive function of calcium. However, the com-

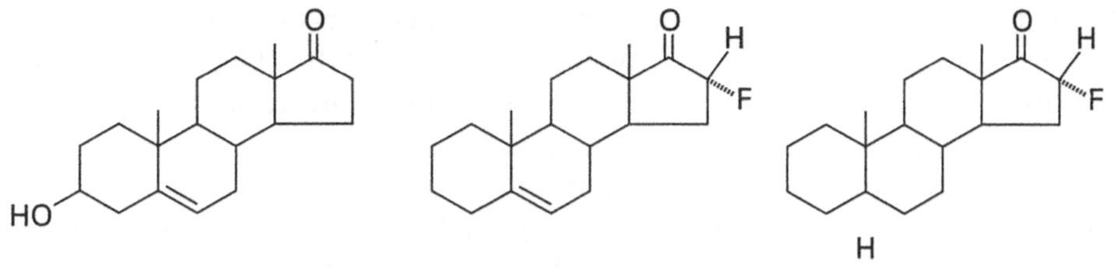

7. DHEA   **8.** 8354   **9.** 8356

Fig. 2
DHEA and its derivatives

bination of both supplemental calcium and vitamin D_3 at very high levels appeared to antagonize the inhibitory effect of each supplement alone on fat-promoted DMH-induced carcinogenesis in rodent colon [50]. Calcium and vitamin D may exert chemopreventive roles through different pathways. Because vitamin D_3 increases calcium absorption, it can inhibit the protective effect of calcium in the colonic lumen. Supplemental calcium, on the other hand, can inhibit the hydroxylation of the inactive form of vitamin D3, thereby decreasing the concentration of the active differentiating dihydroxy form [50]. Apparently, achieving maximum colon cancer chemoprevention requires proper biologically balanced intake of calcium and vitamin D_3, expressed as vitamin-calcium index, large excesses of either one may be counterproductive.

Because of the findings noted above, further clinical trials are currently being planned and are underway to evaluate the possible chemopreventive efficacy of calcium, a promising chemopreventive agent mainly for colorectal cancer [35].

3.3 Dehydroepidandrosterone (DHEA)

DHEA (**7**) (Fig. 2) and its sulfate ester (DHEAS) are major secretory products of the adrenal gland in humans. DHEA is called "the mother of all hormones" by some proponents because it has many functions in the body pertaining to health and longevity; it is also the substance from which other important hormones, such as estrogen, progesterone, and testosterone, are derived. The cancer preventive activities of this group of compounds have been reviewed by Schwartz et al. [51].

Epidemiological studies have shown subnormal plasma levels of DHEA and DHEAS in patients with breast cancer as opposed to controls [51]. Gordon et al. [52] found that DHEA inhibited the differentiation of cultured 3T3 L1 fibroblasts into adipocytes *via* glucose-6-phosphate dehydrogenase (G6PDH) inhibition. Kawai et al. reported that DHEA inhibited B16 mouse melanoma cell growth by induction of differentiation possibly through DHEA receptor mediated protein kinase C (PKC) upregulation [53]. Over the past several years, a number of investigators have demonstrated that DHEA produced broad-spectrum cancer chemopreventive action in animal studies, including inhibition of spontaneous lymphomas [54], mammary cancers [55], and DMBA- and urethane-induced lung ademonas [56], DMBA- and AOM-induced colon tumorigenesis [57,58], dihydroxydi-n-propylnitrosamine-initiated lesions in the thyroid [59], N-nitroso-morpholine-induced hepatocarcinogenesis [60], DMBA-initiated and TPA-promoted skin papillomas [61], and the promotion phase of radiation-induced mammary tumorigenesis [62]. DHEA also inhibited tumor development in the thyroid and small intestine, occurrence of preneoplasias in the urinary bladder and the seminal vesicles in rats [63].

However, significant adverse effects of DHEA have been noted in these animal models. These effects have included weight loss, hepatomegaly, uterine and siminal vesicle enlargement, basophilic loci in the liver and spontaneous ovarian tumor formation [64]. A recent study by Rao et al. [65] indicated that the peroxisome-proliferative property of DHEA made it a hepatocarcinogen.

Considerable evidence indicates that DHEA exerts its tumor preventive activity through suppressing nucleic acid synthesis as a consequence of the inhibition of glucose-6-phosphate dehydrogenase and the pentose phosphate pathway [66].

Two synthetic analogs of DHEA, 16-α-fluoro-5-androstan-17-one (8354) (**8**) and 16-α-fluoro-5-α-androstan-17-one (8356) (**9**) (see Figure 2 for structures), have undergone testing and shown promise as chemopreventive agents. These analogs have been shown to have a greater potency than DHEA without the associated weight loss side effect, and the significant androgenic and estrogenic activity of DHEA [48].

3.4   Coenzyme Q_{10} (CoQ_{10}, Vitamin Q_{10})

CoQ_{10} is a redox component in the respiratory chain. CoQ_{10} is necessary for normal human physiology, and a deficiency of it can lead to ill health and disease. The potential of CoQ_{10} for therapy of human cancer became evident in 1961. The blood levels of CoQ_{10} in a total of 199 American and Swedish cancer patients revealed variable levels of deficiencies of CoQ_{10} and with a deficiency of CoQ_{10} in the cases of both American and Swedish cases of breast cancer being the most statistically significant [67]. The levels of CoQ_{10} in the blood of two groups of subjects ($N = 234$ and $N = 215$) without overt cancer were measured by Folkers et al. [68]. The results revealed that the incidence of low blood CoQ_{10} levels was higher in cancer patients than in the approximately age-matched control subjects. The findings of Shinkai et al. and Okamoto et al. also supported the results [69, 70].

The results of clinical research have been reported by a few groups. Lockwood et al. [71] described the overt, complete regression of breast cancer in two patients during therapy with CoQ_{10}. Accordingly, three additional cases of five breast cancer patients have therapeutically responded to a daily oral dosage of 390 mg of CoQ_{10} [67]. Folkers et al. [72] reported that ten American patients having diverse cancer survived for five to fifteen years, and that six of these patients became free of cancer during therapy with CoQ_{10}. Although clinical regressions of breast cancer can be obtained through conventional treatment by mastectomy, X-ray, and chemotherapy, the apparent complete regression of breast cancer in the five cases has shown the positive effect of CoQ_{10} in cancer treatment. Lockwood et al. [71] observed that a dose level of 90 mg of CoQ_{10} in the treatment of breast cases was ineffective. A minimum effective daily oral dose level of CoQ_{10} appears to be 90–390 mg for the average patient with breast cancer [68].

The regression of tumor in the above cases is biochemically understood to be based upon the immunological activity of CoQ_{10}. Hanioka et al. [73] have shown that the ratio of T_4/T_8 lymphocytes of eleven subjects increased in two months on CoQ_{10}, and the levels of IgG increased in six months. The phagocytic activity in rats was highly enhanced at low dosage of 750 µg/rat 48 hours after an i.v. injection of an emulsion of CoQ_{10} [74]. Oral dosing of CoQ_{10} capsules also increased levels of IgG in three patients with cancer [75].

4   Natural products from foods and vegetables

4.1   Essential oils of vegetables

4.1.1   *Celery seed oil*
In a preliminary screening, celery seed oil, from the ripe fruits of celery *Apium graveolens L.* (Umbelliferae), increased the glutathione-S-transferase (GST) enzyme activity in mouse liver, small intestinal mucosa, and forestomach [76]. This finding led to the isolation of five natural products, including *d*-limonene (**10**), *p*-mentha-2,8-dien-1-ol (**11**), *p*-mentha-

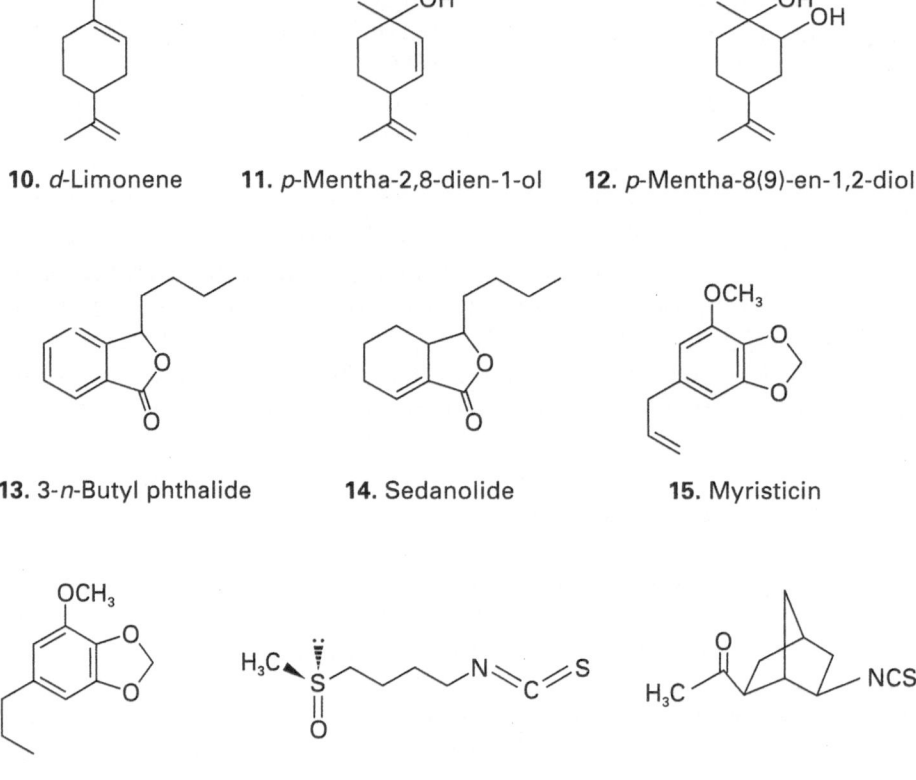

10. *d*-Limonene   **11.** *p*-Mentha-2,8-dien-1-ol   **12.** *p*-Mentha-8(9)-en-1,2-diol

13. 3-*n*-Butyl phthalide   **14.** Sedanolide   **15.** Myristicin

16. Dihydromyristicin   **17.** Sulforaphane   **18.** (+/−)-Exo-2-acetyl-6-
                                                             isothiocyanatonorbornane

Fig. 3
Structures of chemopreventive natural products from foods and vegetables

8(9)-en-1,2-diol (**12**), 3-*n*-butyl phthalide (**13**), and sedanolide (**14**) (see
Fig. 3) [77]. Of these compounds, **11,13,14** exhibited high activities in inducing GST in the target tissues of A/J mice. In B(α)P-induced tumorigenesis in the forestomach of A/J mice, **13** and **14** reduced both tumor incidence and tumor multiplicity, **11** produced only a small or no significant
reduction of tumor formation. Both **13** and **14** have little toxic effect in
mice when given in 20-mg doses.
The five compounds isolated from celery seed oil can be divided into two
groups: limonene-type monoterpenes and butylphthalides. These major
components of the oils appear responsible for the high GST-inducing activity of the oil observed in the preliminary screening. The GST assay data

showed that the phthalide compounds are more active than limonene-type monoterpenes. Among the phthalides found in umbelliferous plants, the five-membered lactone ring appeared to be important for the high enzyme-inducing activity and chemopreventive activity.

4.1.2   Parsley leaf oil

Parsley (*Petroselinum sativum* Hoffm.), a member of edible Umbelliferae plants, is extensively used as a culinary herb for garnishing and seasoning. In the preliminary screening, highly active GST inducers were shown to be present in parsley leaf oil [78]. Myristicin (**15**) (see Fig. 3), a volatile aroma constituent of parsley leaf oil, exhibited high activity as an inducer of GST in the liver and small intestinal mucosa of female A/J mice. Reduction of myristicin yielded dihydromyristicin (**16**) that retained the GST-inducing activity [79]. Both myristicin and dihydromyristicin inhibited B(α)P-induced forestomach cancer in A/J mice. Muristicin reduced the B(α)P-induced lung tumor formation while dihydromyristicin produced insignificant reduction of lung tumor formation in A/J mice [80]. Comparison of the structures and activities indicated that saturation of the isolated double bond in myristicin resulted in a significant decrease in the inhibitory activity against B(α)P-induced tumorigenesis.

Dillweed oil and caraway oil [81], from the plants *Anethum graveolens L.* (Umbelliferae) and *Carum carvi L.* (Umbelliferae), respectively, have been shown to enhance GST activity in several mouse target tissues. Citrus fruit oils and d-limonene, the major constituent of citrus fruit oils, have been shown to have a variety of carcinogen inhibitory effects [82]. Wattenberg [82] found that citrus fruit oils, i.e. orange oil and lemon oil, and d-limonene inhibited NNK-induced neoplasia of the lungs and forestomach of female A/J mice. Citrus fruit oils also inhibited pulmonary adenoma, forestomach and mammary tumor formation after administration of B(α)P or DMBA [83, 84]. These results suggest that consumption of essential oils present in umbelliferous plants and citrus fruits may be effective measures in cancer chemoprevention.

4.2   Sulforaphane

The inhibitory effects of broccoli on mammary tumor formation in female Sprague Dawley rats after an oral dose of DMBA were noted by Wattenberg et al. [85]. Sulforaphane [(-)-1-isothiocyanato-4(R)-(methylsulfinyl)-butane] (**17**) (see Figure 3), recently isolated from broccoli (*Brassica oleracea italica*) [86], is the principal and very potent inducer of detoxication (phase II) enzyme in mouse tissues and murine hepatoma cells in culture.

Barcelo et al. [87] recently found that sulforaphane also inhibited the phase I enzyme cytochrome P450 isoenzyme 2E1. *In vivo*, sulforaphane blocked the formation of DMBA-induced mammary tumors in Sprague-Dawley rats [88].

Zhang et al. [86] synthesized the racemic sulforaphane and several analogs differing in the oxidation state of sulfur and the number of methylene groups: $CH_3-SO_m-(CH_2)_n-NCS$, where m = 0, 1, or 2 and n = 3, 4, or 5. They found that sulforaphane was the most potent inducer of phase II enzyme, the presence of oxygen on sulfur enhanced potency, compounds with 4 or 5 methylene groups in the bridge linking CH_3S- and $N=C=S$ were more potent than those with 3 methylene groups.

Thirty-five structural analogs of sulforaphane have been synthesized by Posner et al. [89]. Among these analogs, the bicyclic ketoisothiocyanate (+/–)-exo-2-acetyl-6-isothiocyanatonorbornane (**18**) was a very potent inducer of quinone reductase in hepatoma cells, and it also induced both quinone reductase and GST in several mouse organs *in vivo*.

4.3   Isoflavonoids and lignans

Several isoflavonoids and lignans are hormone-like diphenolic phytoestrogens. They can be found in soybean products (mainly isoflavonoids but also some lignans), as well as whole grain cereals, seeds, probably berries and nuts (mainly lignans) [90]. Many Chinese medicinal herbs are known to contain isoflavonoids. Das et al. have summarized the structure-activity relationship of phytoestrogenic isoflavonoids [91].

Epidemiological studies indicated that plasma levels and urinary excretion of the lignan and isoflavonoid phytoestrogens correlated negatively with rates of breast and prostate cancer risk [92, 93]. Korpela et al. [94] observed that a high lignan excretion in subjects was associated with a low risk of colon cancer. Epidemiological evidence obtained in Japan pointed to lower colon cancer incidence in areas with high tofu consumption [95]. Diets containing linseed (rich in lignans) seem to protect against colon cancer [96].

Epidemiological studies with regard to the protective role of isoflavonoids and lignans in breast, prostatic and colon cancers have received support from numerous studies. Barnes et al. [97] and Hawrylewicz et al. [98] showed that powdered soybean chips or heated soy decreased mammary tumor formation or inhibited progression of such tumors in rat breast cancer models. Furthermore, linseed containing high amounts of lignans inhibited mammary carcinogenesis in rats [99]. Genistein and biochanin A, the precursor of genistein, inhibited the growth of prostatic cancer cells [100].

Quercetin, a flavonoid with antiestrogenic activity occurring in high amounts in certain plants, inhibited the growth of colon cancer cells in culture [101].

The plant lignan and isoflavonoid glycosides are converted by intestinal bacteria to hormone-like compounds with weak estrogenic and antioxidative activities. They have now been shown to influence not only sex hormone metabolism and biological activity but also intracellular enzymes, protein synthesis, growth factor action, malignant cell proliferation, differentiation and angiogenesis, making them strong candidates as natural cancer chemopreventive compounds [90]. Our group has reported that the estrogenic activities of many isoflavonoids were attributed to their structural similarities with estradiol and diethylstilbestrol [102]. Their diphenolic character also makes them similar to lignans [90]. Isoflavonoids with similar structures have recently been reported by Lien et al. [103].

4.4 Protease inhibitors

Seeds of many plants belonging to the family leguminosae, particularly soybeans and peanuts are rich sources of protease inhibitors. Epidemiological studies demonstrated that consumption of foods which contained protease inhibitors was associated with a decreased incidence of prostate, colon, breast, oral, pharyngeal, pancreas, gastric cancers [104].

In vitro studies have indicated that protease inhibitors are effective suppressors of physical and chemical carcinogenesis. Bowman Birk Inhibitor (BBI) from soybeans significantly reduces the transformation of C3H/10T1/2 cells by X-radiation [105], and by 3-MCA [106].

Experimental studies in vivo have indicated the chemopreventive and anticarcinogenic properties of protease inhibitors from natural food constituents in the diet. Their anticarcinogenic effects are summarized in Table 1. Soybean and soyproducts (usually heat treated) were shown to inhibit skin, breast, liver, colon, bladder, forestomach, stomach/intestine, mammary, leukemias and lymphosarcoma tumor in various animals induced by different chemicals and radiation [107–116]. But contradictory reports also exist. McGuiness et al. [117–119] noted that a diet of raw soya flour (containing trypsin inhibitor) increased the DNA, RNA and protein content and weight of pancreas in rats, and long-term feeding of raw soya flour resulted in further growth in the pancreas, with ultimate development of adenocarcinomas and carcinomas of acinar pancreas. The mechanisms by which raw soya flour stimulates pancreatic growth and neoplastic transformation have not been defined. However, it has been proposed that raw soya flour (containing protease inhibitors) acts on the

Table 1.
Anticarcinogenesis effects of protease inhibitors against chemical- and radiation-induced tumorgenesis in various organs

Organ	Animal	Carcinogen	Anticarcino-genesis effects (%)	Protease inhibitors	Ref.
skin	mice	4-NQO and PMA	+	soybeans	107
breast	Sprague Dawley rats	X-radiation	30–34	soybeans	108
liver	C3H/HeN mice	spontaneous	75–100	soybeans	109
	Swiss mice	nitrite and DBA	+	soybeans	110
colon	CD1 mice	DMH	100	soybean extracts (contain BBI)	111
bladder	Swiss mice	nitrite and DBA	+	soybeans	110
forestomach stomach/	ICR mice	B(α)P	26	soysauce	112
intestine	Fish344 rats	nitrite	+	soysauce	113
mammary mammary–	Sprague Dawley rats	NMU	38	soybean isolate	114
adenocarcinoma	Sprague Dawley rats	DMBA	20	soybean paste	115
lymphosarcoma	C57 B1/6N Crl Br mice	radiation	10–40	soybeans	116

pancreas indirectly by inhibiting trypsin within the lumen of the small intestine [117]. As a consequence of tryptic inhibition by soybean trypsin inhibitor, there is therefore unfettered release of the pancreatic stimulant hormone such as cholecystokinin, which has been shown to stimulate pancreatic hypertrophy and hyperplasia in rats. Continuous release of large amounts of cholecystokinin during feeding of raw soya flour may be responsible for the pancreatic growth. Other factors in raw soya flour may also be involved in raw soya flour-induced pancreatic growth. Undenatured soybean protein can bind trypsin and results in inhibition of trypsin [117]. In addition, free fatty acids can also produce trypsin inhibition [117]. It seems probable that the protease inhibitors contained in the soya proteins are also involved in raw soya flour-induced pancreatic growth by binding pancreatic proteases in the small intestinal lumen [118].

The precise mechanism by which protease inhibitors suppress carcinogenesis is far from clear. Many hypotheses have been proposed and various modes of action have been implicated to account for the role of protease inhibitors [104]. Protease inhibitors may exert their effect through the enzyme system involved in the induction and/or expression of the transformed phenotype. Clark et al. [120] are of the opinion that protease inhibitors appear to inhibit the processing of a growth factor and interfere with the growth regulation of cells at the genetic level. Protease inhibitors have also been considered to be radioprotectors and they appear to

protect animals and tissue culture cells from the damaging effects of ion-
izing radiation which cause neoplastic transformation by interfering with
the oxidation cascade. Furthermore, protease inhibitors might have a role
in the immume mechanism according to a report by Maki et al. [121]. The
data available to date suggest that protease inhibitors are potential chemopreventive agents although their biological role and mechanism of action
are not clearly understood.

5   Natural products from other higher plants

5.1   Polyphenols

5.1.1   Tea polyphenols
Tea, one of the most widely consumed beverages in the world, is grown
in about 30 countries, and is manufactured as either green, black, or oolong
tea [122]. Because green tea is manufactured from fresh tea leaves with
the precaution to avoid excessive oxidation of the polyphenolic compounds which include flavonols, the majority of studies of chemopreventive activities of polyphenolic compounds present in tea have focused on
green tea. Green tea contains 35–52% (measure in weight % of extract
of solids) catechins and flavonols combined. Of the four major catechins
in green tea, (–)-epicatechin (EC) (**19**), (–)-epicatechin-3-gallate (ECG)
(**20**), (–)-epigallocatechin (EGC) (**21**), and (–)-epigallocatechin-3-gallate
(EGCG) (**22**), EGCG is the major component. During the manufactur-
ing process of black tea, the polyphenols undergo oxidative polymerization, resulting in the conversion of catechins to aflavins (**23**) and thearubigins (**24**).
Epidemiological studies, though inconclusive, have shown a protective
effect of tea consumption on human cancer. A case-control study by Kono
et al. [123] has indicated that individuals consuming green tea tend to have
a lower risk for gastric cancer. Studies by Oguni et al. [124] in the Shizu-
oka Prefecture in Japan showed that the stomach cancer death rate in this
tea-producing and -consuming area was lower than the national average.
In recent years, a wide range of studies have demonstrated that a polyphenolic fraction isolated from green tea (GTP), a water extract of green
tea (WEGT), and epicatechin derivatives present in green tea possess
strong anticarcinogenic effects in various tissues, including skin, lung, forestomach, esophagus, duodenum, colon, liver, pancreas, mammary gland.
Studies have also shown that a water extract of black tea (WEBT) has
similar inhibitory effects. Some of the results are summarized in Table 2
[125–130].

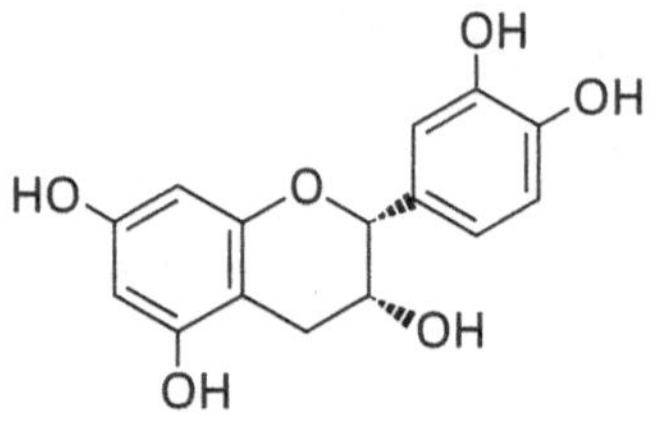

19. EC

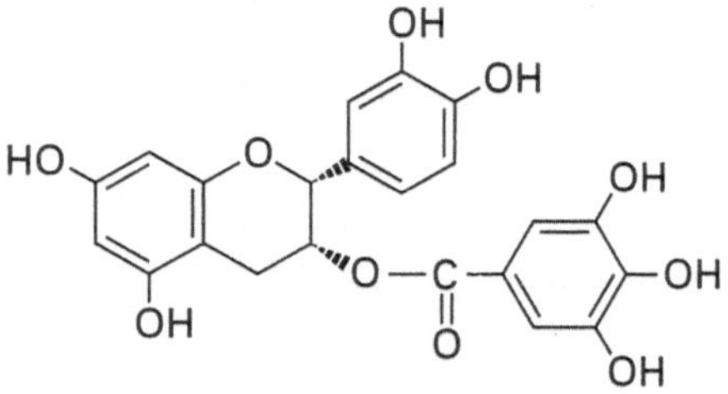

20. ECG

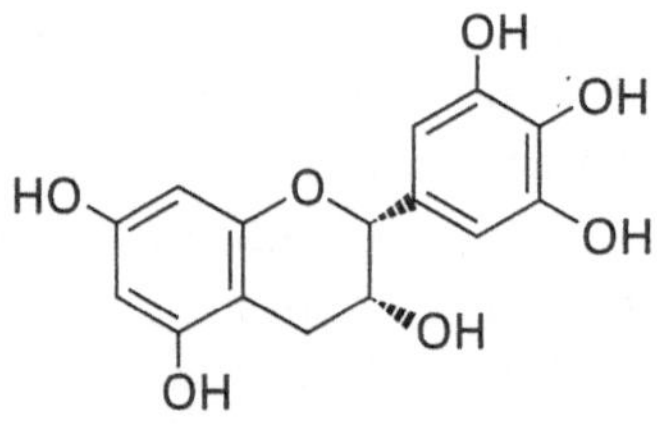

21. EGC

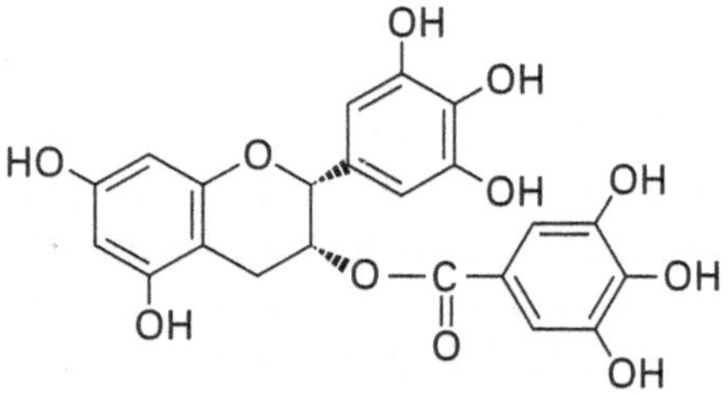

22. EGCG

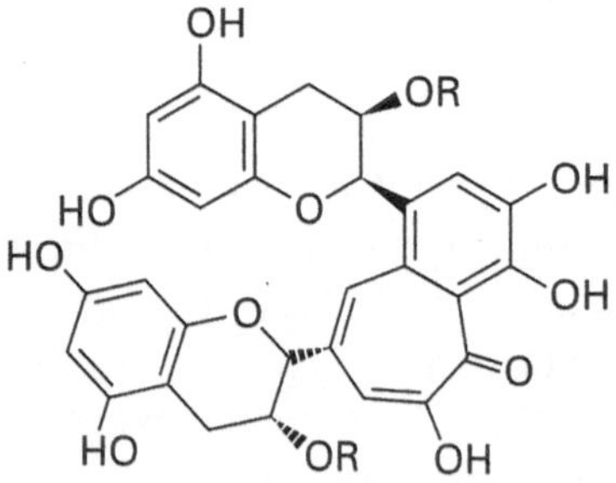

23. Aflavins

R=Galloyl,

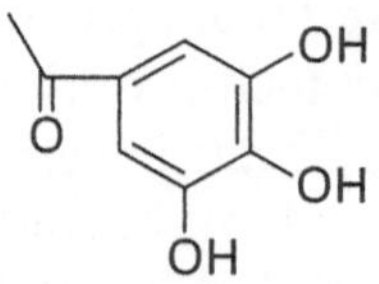

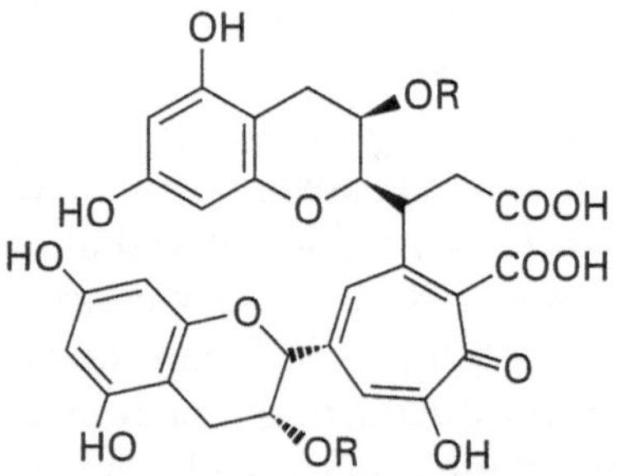

24. Thearubigins

Fig. 4
Polyphenols present in tea

Table 2.
Protective effects of tea polyphenols against chemical carcinogen- and ultraviolet B radiation-induced tumorgenesis in various organs

Organ	Animal	Carcinogen	Polyphenols	% Protection	Ref.
Skin	BALB/c mice	3-MCA	GTP	50	125
	SENCAR mice	DMBA/TPA	GTP	31–84	125
			EGCG	51	125
		BPDE-2/TPA	GTP	38	125
		4-NQO	GTP	43	126
	CD-1 mice	DMBA/TPA	GTP	95	125
				27–50	127
			EGCG	27	125
		UVB/TPA	GTP	11	127
		DMBA/teleocidin	EGCG	95	127
	SKH-1 mice	DMBA/TPA	WEGT	55–84	125
		UVB	GTP	20–41	125
		UVB/TPA	WEGT	64–82	125
		DMBA/UVB	WEGT	88	128
				38–87	125
			WEBT	93	128
Lung	A/J mice	NDEA	WEGT	36–62	125
			GTP	38–43	125
		B(α)P	WEGT	25–56	125
			GTP	25–46	125
		NNK	WEGT	45–85	125
			EGCG	30	125
Forestomach	A/J mice	NDEA	WEGT	59–85	125
			GTP	68–82	125
		B(α)P	WEGT	61–71	125
			GTP	39–66	125
Esophagus	Wistar rats	NMBA	WEGT	40–60	125
	Rats and mice	NS	GTP		129
Duodenum	C57BL/6 mice	ENNG	EGCG	63–75	125
Colon	Fisher rats	AOM	GTP	53–60	125
	F-344 rats	NMU	GTP		129
Liver		Aflatoxin B1	GTP		129
		NDEA	GTP		129
Pancreas	Syrian golden hamsters	NBOPA	GTP		129
Mammary gland	Sprague-Dawley rats	DMBA	WEGT	63	130

Several mechanisms may be responsible for the tumor-inhibitory properties of GTPs, including enhancement of antioxidant (glutathione peroxidase, catalase and quinone reductase) and GST enzyme activities; inhibition of chemically induced lipid peroxidation; inhibition of irradiation-and TPA-induced epidermal ornithine decarboxylase (ODC) and cyclooxygenase activities; inhibition of protein kinase C and cellular proliferation; antiinflammatory activity; and enhancement of gap junction intercellular communication [129].

5.1.2   Curcumin

Turmeric, the powdered rhizome from the root of the plant *Curcuma longa* (Jiang-Huang) Linn. has long been used as a spice in foods and as a naturally occurring medicine for the treatment of inflammatory diseases. Curcumin (diferuloylmethane, 1,7-bis[4-hydroxy-3-methoxyphenyl]-1,6-heptadiene-3,5-dione) (**25**), the yellow pigment in turmeric, has also been used as a coloring agent and spice in foods, as well as in cosmetics and drugs [131]. It is the major phenolic antioxidant and antiinflammatory agent found in *Curcuma longa* and other Chinese herbs like *Curcuma zedoaria, Curcuma aromatica* and *Acorus calamus*. The chemical, biological and pharmacological properties of curcumin have been reviewed by Govindarajan et al., Ammon et al., and Huang et al. [127–129].

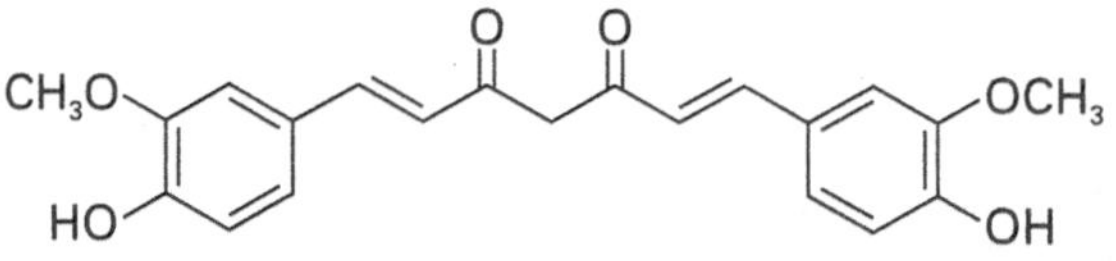

Fig. 5
Structure of curcumin

Recent investigations have demonstrated that curcumin possesses strong anticarcinogenic effects in several tissues. Curcumin inhibited TPA-induced tumor promotion in DMBA-initiated skin tumor [130], and DMBA-induced as well as TPA-promoted skin tumor in CD-1 mice [131]. In addition, curcumin reduced the occurrence of B(α)P-induced forestomach tumors [131], and inhibited the development of precancerous lesion, i.e., DMBA-induced hyperplastic nodules in cultured rat mammary gland tissues [132], azoxymethane-induced crypts in rat colon [133], azoxymethane-induced colon tumor in CF-1 mice, and ENNG-induced duodenal tumors in C57BL/6 mice [134]. In a recent study [135], dietary turmeric was used as a chemopreventive agent in B(α)P induced forestomach tumor in Swiss mice and methyl-(acetoxymethyl)-nitrosamine induced oral mucosal tumors in Syrian golden hamsters. Dietary turmeric significantly inhibited the tumor burden and tumor incidence in both tumor models. Another recent study [136] has shown that administering 5% turmeric in the diet from 2 months of age suppressed mammary tumor virus-related reverse transcriptase activity and preneoplastic changes in the mammary glands, feeding turmeric from 6 months of age resulted in a 100% inhibition of mammary tumors in both of C3H mice and Wistar rats. In the DMBA-induced model of rat mammary tumorigenesis, administration of turmeric resulted in decreased tumor burden and tumor incidence, and a delay in the onset of mammary tumors. Tanaka et al. [141] investigated the modifying effects of curcumin, given during the initiation and post-initiation phase of oral carcinogenesis initiated with 4-NQO in male F344 rats and compared with that of beta-carotene. Feeding of curcumin caused a significant reduction in the frequency of tongue carcinoma, and the chemopreventive efficacy was greater than that of beta-carotene.

Some of the anticarcinogenic effects of curcumin are similar to those of the green tea polyphenols [129]. Curcumin enhances glutathione content and GST activity in liver; and it inhibits lipid peroxidation and arachidonic acid metabolism in mouse skin, protein kinase C activity in TPA-treated NIH 3T3 cells, chemically induced ODC and tyrosine protein kinase activities in rat colon, 8-hydroxyguanosine formation in mouse fibroblasts [129], and xanthine dehydrogenase/oxidase induced by PMA in NIH 3T3 cells [142]. Curcumin suppresses the transcriptional factor c-Jun/AP-1 activation which is believed to play an improtant role in signal transduction of PMA-induced tumor promotion in mouse fibroblast cells [143]. The results of a recent study by Jiang et al. [144] suggest that curcumin induces apoptosis in immortalized NIH 3T3 and malignant cancer cell lines by blocking the cellular signal transduction.

5.2   Polysaccharides from *Acanthopanax* genus

Acanthopanax (A.) chiisanensis Nakai, *A. divaricatus* Seem, *A. giraldii* Harms, *A. hypoleucus* Makino, *A. obovatus*, *A. senticosus* Harms (Ciwujia), *A. sieboldianus*, and *A. spinosus* are traditional Chinese medicinal herbs belonging to the same biological genus but different species. As tonic herbs in Chinese medicine, they are used to treat patients in debilitated conditions due to tumor or chronic diseases. It has been reported [145] that *A. senticosus* as well as its polysaccharides enhanced the phagocytosis of macrophages and inhibited the growth of transplanted tumor in mice.

Polysaccharides (PES) isolated from *A. senticosus* by Shen at al. [146] were found to have a wide spectrum of immunomodulatory activities on experimental animals. PES not only inhibited tumor growth and ameliorated toxicities of cyclophosphamide and thioacetamide in mice but also suppressed human tubercle bacillus propagation in mice and guinea pigs. Recent results of experiments with *A. giradii* polysaccharide (AGP) demonstrated that it inhibited the growth of solid Sarcoma 180 and prolonged the survival time significantly in ICR/SLC mice [147]. In tumor-bearing mice, AGP enhanced the phagocytosis and chemiluminescence of macrophages. *A. obovatus* polysaccharide (AOP) has also been shown to have an enhancing and a modulating activity on immune response [148]. *A. senticosus* Harms extract has been observed to have radioprotective effects on the hemopoiesis of irradiated mice (CBA/olac) when administered before or after irradiation by ^{60}Co [149]. These effects resulted from enhanced stimulation of colony-forming units (CFU-S) not only toward proliferation but also toward CFU-S self-renewal.

The mechanism of antitumor action of these polysaccharides is attributed to the enhancement of immune response [146–148]. In a recent study, Tong et al. [150] reported that antitumor action of *A. senticosus* polysaccharides might be due to the changes of cell membrane and killing the tumor cell directly.

6   Conclusion

A compelling push for the development of chemopreventive strategies has come from diet and cancer epidemiology, with increasing supporting data from laboratory research. A large number of dietary and other natural substances and synthetic compounds have now been identified which can affect the process of carcinogenesis in experimental models. Selected candidates for chemoprevention that appear promising from preliminary evaluations are to be evaluated for possible clinical intervention testing. Vitamin D, calcium, DHEA, CoQ_{10} and their derivatives have been shown to be active in cancer chemoprevention. Consumption of essential oils present in umbelliferous plants, and some vegetables and foods, e.g. broccoli and soybean products, may decrease the risk of cancer. Tea polyphenols and curcumin possess strong anticarcinogenic effects. Polysaccharides from *Acanthopanax* genus inhibited tumor growth in preliminary evaluations and have been shown to be immunomodulators. The data currently available provide the evidence for an optimistic view on the possible use of the above compounds as cancer chemopreventive agents; further preclinical and clinical investigations are clearly warranted. It is the authors' belief that in many cases cancer can be and should be prevented. Early diagnosis is good and necessary, but it is not prevention.

References

1   H. Gao and E. J. Lien: Int. J. Orient. Med. *16* (2), 55–76 (1991).
2   G.G. Schwartz andB.S. Hulka: Anticancer Res. *10*, 1307–1311 (1990).
3   C.F. Garland, G.W. Comstock, F.C. Garland, K.J. Helsing, E.K. Shaw and E.D. Gorham: Lancet *2,* 1176–1178 (1989).
4   C.F. Garland, F.C. Garland and E.D Gorham: Am. J. Clin. Nutr. *54* (suppl. 1), 193 S–201S (1991).
5   E.H. Corder, H.A. Guess, B.S. Hulka, G.D. Friedman, M. Sadler, R.T. Vollmer, B. Lobaugh, M.K. Drezner, J.H. Vogelman and N. Orentreich: Cancer Epidemiology, Biomarkers & Prevention *2,* 467–472 (1993).
6   M.M. Braun, K.J. Helzlsouer, B.W. Hollis and G.W. Comstock: Cancer Causes and Control *6* (3), 235–239 (1995).
7   M.M. Braun, K.J. Helzlsouer, B.W. Hollis and G.W. Comstock: Am. J. Epidemiology *142* (6), 608–611 (1995).
8   E.S. Lefkowitz, C.F. Garland: Inter. J. Epidem. *23* (6), 1133–1136 (1994).
9   A.W. Norman, J. Roth and L. Orci: Endocr. Rev. *3*, 331 (1982).
10   J.W. Pike: Ann. Rev. Nutr. *11*, 189–216 (1991).
11   A.W. Norman: J. Cell. Biochem. *22*, 218–225 (1995 suppl.).
12   E. Abe, C. Miyayra, H. Sakagami, M. Takeda, K. Konno, T. Yamazaki, S. Yoshiki and T. Suda: Proc. Natl. Acad. Sci. USA *78*, 4990–4994 (1981).
13   K.W. Colston, U. Berger and R.C. Coombes: Lancet *1*, 188–191 (1989).
14   J.A. Eisman, D.H. Barkla and P.J. Tutton: Cancer Res. *47*, 21–25 (1987).
15   K. Colston, J.M. Colston and D. Feldman: Endocrinology *108*, 1083–1086 (1981).
16   M.G. Thomas, S. Tebutt, R.C. Williamson: Gut *33*, 1660–1663 (1992).
17   K.D. Harper, R.V. Iozzo and J.G. Haddad: Metabolism *38*, 1062–1069 (1989).
18   X. Zhao and D. Feldman: Endocrinology *132*, 1808–1814 (1993).
19   D. Feldman, R.J. Skowronski and D.M. Peehl: Advan. Exper. Med. Biology *375*, 53–63 (1995).
20. H.A.P. Pols, J.C. Birkenhager, J.A. Foekens and J.P.T.M. Van Leeuwen: J. Steroid Biochem. *37*, 873–876 (1990).
21   T.A. Owen, M.S. Aronow, L.M. Barone, B. Bettencourt, G.S. Stein and J.B. Lian: Endocrinology *128*, 1496–1504 (1991).
22   E.M. Costa, H.M. Blau and D. Feldman: Endocrinology *119*, 2214–2220 (1986).
23   S. Pillai, D.D. Bikle and P.M. Elias: J. Biol. Chem. *263*, 5396–5401 (1988).
24   T. Suda, T. Shinki and N. Takahashi: Ann. Rev. Nutr. *10*, 195–211 (1990).
25   C.F. Garland and F.C. Garland: Int. J. Epidemiol. *9*, 227–231 (1980).
26   D.D. Bikle: Endocrine Rev. *13*, 765–784 (1992).
27   A.W. Norman, J.Y. Zhou, H.L. Henry, M.R. Uskokovic and H.P. Koeffler: Cancer Res. *50*, 6857–6864 (1990).
28   K.W. Colston, A.G. Mackay, S.Y. James, L. Binderup, S. Chander and R.C. Coombes: Biochem. Pharm. *44* (12), 2273–2280 (1992).

29   K.W. Colston, A.G. Mackay, S.Y. James, L. Binderup and R.C. Coombes: Vitamin D, Gene Regulation. Structure–Function Analysis and Clinical Application. Proceedings of the Eighth Workshop on Vitamin D, Berlin, de Gruyter, pp. 465 (1991).

30   I.S. Mathiasen, K.W. Colston and L. Binderup: J. Steroid Biochem. Molec. Biol. *46*, 365–371 (1993).

31   M.A. Anzano, J.M. Smith and M.R. Uskokovic: Cancer Res. *54*, 1653–1656 (1994).

32   M.S. Lucia, M.A. Anzano, M.V. Slayter, M.R. Anver, D.M. Green, M.W. Shrader, D.L. Logsdon, C.L. Driver, C.C. Brown and C.W. Peer: Cancer Res. *55*, 5621–5627 (1995).

33   J.Y. Zhou, A.W. Norman, M. Lubbert, E.D. Collins, M.R. Uskokovic and H.P. Koeffler: Blood *74*, 82–93 (1989).

34   J. Abe-Hashinoto, T. Kikuchi, T. Matsumoto, Y. Nishii, E. Ogata and K. Ikeda: Cancer Res. *53*, 2534–2537 (1993).

35   M. Lipkin and H. Newmark: J. Cell Biochem. *22*, 65–73 (1995).

36   C. Garland, R.B. Shekelle, E. Barrett-Connor, M.H. Criqui, A.H. Rossof and O. Paul: Lancet *1*, 307–309 (1985).

37   M.L. Slattery, A.W. Sorenson and M.H. Ford: Am. J. Epidemiol. *128*, 504–514 (1988)

38   C. Garland and F.C. Garland: Int. J. Epidemiol. *27*, 155 (1979).

39   E. Kampman, E. Giovannucci, P.V.T. Veer and E. Rimm: Am. J. Epidemiol. *139* (1), 16–29 (1994).

40   J.H. Kleibeuker, R. van-der-Meer and E. G. de-Vries: European J. Cancer *31*A(7–8), 1081–1084 (1995).

41   B.C. Pence, D.M. Dunn, C. Zhao, M. Landers and M.J. Wargovich: Carcinogenesis, *16* (4), 757–765 (1995).

42   M.J. Wargovich, G. Isbell, M. Shabot, R. Winn, F. Lanza, L. Hochman, E. Larson, P. Lynch, L. Roubein and B. Levin: Gastroenterology *103*, 92–97 (1992).

43   K.R. O'Sullivan, P.M. Mathias, S. Beattie and C. O'Morain: Eur. J. Gastroenterol. Hepatol. *5*, 85–89 (1993).

44   G.H. Barsoum, C. Hendrickse, M.C. Winslet, D. Youngs, I.A. Donovan, J.P. Neoptolemos and M.R.B. Keighley: Br. J. Surg. *79*, 581–583 (1992).

45   R.M. Bostick, J.D. Potter, L. Fosdick, P. Grambsch, J.W. Lampe, J.R. Wood, T.A. Louis, R. Ganz and G. Grandits: J. Natl. Cancer Inst. *85*, 132–141 (1993).

46   M. Pazianas, J.D. Maxwell, V.S. Shankar, O.A. Adebanjo, F.A. Lai, A. Ventikoraman, V. C.-L. Huang, K.W. Colston, E.M. Brown and M. Zaidi: J. Bone Miner. Res. *S220* (1994).

47   F.J. Whitfield, R.P. Bird, B.R. Chakravarthy, R.J. Isaacs and P. Morley: J. Cell Biochem. Suppl. *22*, 74–91 (1995).

48   C.E. Szarka, G. Grana and P.F. Engstrom: Curr. Probl. Cancer, pp.6–79 (1994).

49   H.L. Newmark, M.J. Wargovich and W.R. Bruce: J. Natl. Cancer Inst. *72*, 1324–1325 (1984).

50   B.C. Pence and F. Buddingh: Carcinogenesis *9*, 187–190 (1988).

51   A.G. Schwartz, J.M. Whitcomb and J.W. Nyce: Adv. Cancer Res. *51*, 391–424 (1988).

52   R. Raineri and H.R. Levy: Biochem. *9*, 2233–2243 (1970).

53   S. Kawai, N. Yahata, S. Nishida, K. Nagai and Y. Mizushirna: Anticancer Res. *15*, 427–431 (1995).

54   S.D. Hursting, S.N. Perkins, D.C. Haines, J.M. Ward and J.M. Phang: Cancer Res. *55*, 3949–3953 (1995).

55   A.G. Schwartz: Cancer Res. *39*, 1129–1132 (1979).

56   A.G. Schwartz and R.H. Tannen: Carcinogenesis *2*, 1335–37 (1981).

57   J.W. Nyce, P.N. Magee, G.C. Hard and A.G. Schwartz, Carcinogenesis 5, 57–62 (1984).

58   M.A. Pereira and M.D. Khoury: Cancer Lett. 61, 27–33 (1991).

59   M.A. Moore, W. Thamavit, H. Tsuda, K. Sato, A. Ichibara and N. Ito: Carcinogenesis 7, 311–316 (1986).

60   E. Weber, M.A. Moore and P. Bannasch: Carcinogenesis 9, 1191–1195 (1988).

61   L.L. Pashko, R.J. Rovito, J.R. Williams, E.L. Sobel and A.G. Schwartz: Carcinogenesis 5, 463–466 (1984).

62   H. Inano, O.H. Ishii, K. Suzuki, H. Yamanouchi and M. Onoda: J. Steroid Biochem. Mole. Biol. 54, 47–53 (1995).

63   M. Shbata, R. Hasegawa, K. Imaida, A. Hagiwara and K. Ogawa: Cancer Res. 55, 4870–4874 (1995).

64   G.J Kelloff, W.F. Maline and C.W. Boone: Semin. Oncol. 17, 438–455 (1990).

65   M.S. Rao, V. Subbarao, A.V. Yeldandi and J.K. Reddu: Cancer Res. 52, 2977–2979 (1992).

66   A.G. Schwartz and L.L. Pashko: J. Cell Biochem. 17G, 73–79 (1993).

67   K. Lockwood, S. Moesgaard, T. Yamamoto and K. Folkers: Biochem. Biophys. Res. Comm. 212, 172–177 (1995).

68   K. Flokers, J. Ellis, O. Yang, H. Tamagawa, Y. Nara, K. Nara, C. Ye and Z. Shen: Vitamins and Cancer Prevention, Chapter 8, pp. 103– 110.

69   T. Shinkai, K. Tominaga, Z. Shimabukuro, E. Shimizu, K. Eguchi, N. Saijo, K. Iwashita and H. Niitani: Jap. J. Cancer Chemother. 11, 87–96 (1984).

70   T. Okamoto, K. Fukui, M. Nakamoto, T. Kishi, N. Kanamori, K. Kataoka, S. Nishii, H. Kishi, E. Hiraoka and A. Okada: J. Nutri. Sci. Vitamino. 32, 1–12 (1986).

71   K. Lockwood, S. Moesgaard, and K. Folkers: Biochem. Biophys. Res. Comm. 199, 1504–1508 (1994).

72   K. Folkers, R. Brown, W. Judy and M. Morita: Biochem. Biophys. Res. Comm. 192, 241–245 (1993).

73   T. Hanioka, J. Mcree, L. Xia, S. Shizukuishi and K. Folkers: J. Dental Health 43, 5 (1993).

74   E.G. Bliznakov, A.C. Casey and E. Premuzic: Experientia 26, 953–954 (1970).

75   K. Folkers, S. Shizukuishi, K. Tademura, J. Drzewoski, P. Richardson, J. Ellis and W.C. Kuzell: Res. Commun. Chem. Path. Pharm. 38, 335–338 (1982).

76   L.K.T. Lam and B.L. Zheng: J. Agric. Food Chem. 39, 660–662 (1991).

77   G. Zheng, P.M. Kenney, J. Zhang and L.K.T. Lam: Nutr. Cancer 19, 77–86 (1993).

78   L.K.T. Lam and B.L. Zheng: J. Agric. Food Chem. 39, 660–662 (1991).

79   G. Zheng, P.M. Kenney and L.K.T. Lam: J. Agric. Food Chem. 40, 107–110 (1992).

80   G. Zheng, P.M. Kenney, J. Zhang and L.K.T. Lam: Carcinogenesis 13, 1921–1923 (1992).

81   G. Zheng, P.M. Kenney and L.K.T. Lam: Planta Medica 58, 338–341 (1992).

82   L.W. Wattenberg and J. Coccia: Carcinogenesis (Lond.) 12, 115–117 (1991).

83   L.W. Wattenberg, A.B. Hanley, G. Barany, V.L. Sparnins, L.K.T. Lam and G.R. Fenwick: in U. Hayashi et al. (eds): Diet, Nutrition and Cancer, Japan Scientific Societies Press, Tokyo, pp. 193–203 (1985).

84   L.W. Wattenberg: Cancer Res. 43 (suppl.), 2448s–2453s (1983).

85   L.W. Wattenberg, H.W. Shafer, L. Waters and D.W. Davis: Proc. Am. Asso. Cancer Res. 30, 181 (1989).

86   Y. Zhang, P. Talalay, C.G. Cho and G.H. Posner: Proc. Natl. Acad. Sci. USA 89, 2399–2403 (1992).

87   S. Barcelo, J.M. Gardiner, A. Gescher and J.K. Chipman: Carcinogenesis 17, 277–282 (1996).

88   Y. Zhang, T.W. Kensler, C.G. Cho, G.H. Posner and P. Talalay: Proc. Natl. Acad. Sci. USA *91*, 3147–3150 (1994).
89   G.H. Posner, C.G. Cho, J.V. Green, Y. Zhang and P. Talalay: J. Med. Chem. *37*, 170–176 (1994).
90   C. Herman and T. Adlercreutz: J. Nutr. *125*, 757s–770s (1995).
91   A. Das and E.J. Lien: Pharm. Res. *11*, S118 (1994).
92   H. Adlercreutz, T. Fotsis, J. Lampe, K. Wahala, T. Makela, G. Brunow and T. Hase: Scand. J. Clin. Lab. Invest. *53* (suppl. 215), 5–18 (1993).
93   H. Adlercreutz, T. Fotsis, C. Bannwart, K, Wahala, T. Makela, G. Brunow and T. Hase: J. Steroid Biochem. *25*, 791–797 (1986).
94   J.T. Korpela, R. Korpela and H. Adlercreutz: Gastroenterology *103*, 1246–53 (1992).
95   S. Watanabe and S. Koessel: J. Epidemiol. *3*, 47–61 (1993).
96   M. Serraino and L.U. Thompson: Cancer Lett. *63*, 159–165 (1992).
97   S. Barnes, C. Grubbs, K.D.R. Setchell and J. Carlson: in M.W. Pariza, H.U. Aeschbacher, J.S. Eton and S. Sato (eds.): Mutagens and carcinogens in the diet. progress in clinical and biological research, vol. 347, pp 239–253. Wiley-Liss, Inc. New York 1990.
98   E.J. Hawrylewicz, H.H. Huang and W.H. Blair: J. Nutr. *121*, 1693–1698 (1991).
99   M. Serraino and L.U. Thompson: Nutr. Cancer *17*, 153–159 (1992).
100 G. Peterson and S. Barnes: Prostate *22*, 335–345 (1993).
101 F.O. Ranelletti, R. Ricci, L.M. Larocca, N. Maggiano, A. Capelli, G. Scambia, P. Benedettipanici, S. Mancuso, S. Rumi and M. Piantelli: Int. J. Cancer *50*, 486–492 (1992).
102 A. Das, J.H. Wang and E.J. Lien: Prog. Drug Res. *42*, 133–166 (1994).
103 E.J. Lien, A. Das and L.L. Lien: Prog. Drug Res. *46*, 263–280 (1996).
104 S. Das and P. Mukhopadhyay: Acta Oncol. *33*, 859–865 (1994).
105 J. Yavelow, T.H. Finlay, A.R. Kennedy and W. Troll: Cancer Res. *43* (Suppl.), 2454–2459s (1983).
106 W.H. St Clair: Carcinogenesis *12*, 935–937 (1991).
107 B. Zemplen, I. Tulok and I. Palasti: Orv. Hetil. *132*, 2139–2142 (1991).
108 W. Troll, R. Weisner, C.J. Shellabarger, S. Holtzman and J.P. Stone: Carcinogenesis *1*, 469–472 (1980).
109 F.F. Becker: Carcinogenesis *2*, 1213–1214 (1981).
110 N.M. Mokhtar, A.A. EL-Aaser and M.N. EL-Bolkainy: Eur. J. Cancer Clin. Oncol. *24*, 403–11 (1988).
111 H. Weed, R.B. Mc Gandy and A.R. Kennedy: Carcinogenesis *6*, 1239–1241 (1985).
112 H. Benjamin, J. Storkson, A. Nagahara and M. W. Pariza: Cancer Res. *51*, 2940–2942 (1991).
113 M. Nagao, K. Wakabayashi and Y. Fujita: Int. Symp. Princess Takamatsu Cancer Res. Fund *16*, 77–86 (1985).
114 E.J. Hawrylewiez, H.H. Huang and W.H. Blair: J. Nutr. *121*, 1693–1698 (1991).
115 J.E. Baggott, T. Ha, W.H. Vaughn, M.M. Julliana, J.M. Hardin and C.J. Grubbs: Nutr. Cancer *14*, 103–109 (1990).
116 S.M. Evans, T. Van Winkle, B. Szuhaj, K.E. Michel and A.R. Kennedy: Radiat. Res. *132*, 259–262 (1992).
117 E.E. McGuinness, R.G. Morgan and K.G. Worrnsley: Environ. Health Persp. *56*, 205–212 (1984).
118 E.E. McGuinness, R.G. Morgan and K.G. Wormsley: Scand. J. Gastroenterol. *112* (suppl.), 64–67 (1985).
119 E.E. McGuinness, R.G. Morgan and K.G. Wormsley: Gut *28* (suppl.), 207–212 (1987).

120 U.A. Clark, R. Uay, N. Seldan, I.W. Moody, T. Cuttitta and I.P. Davis: Peptides *14*, 1021–1028 (1993).

121 P.A. Maki and A.R. Kennedy: J. Nutr. Cancer *18*, 165–173 (1992).

122 H. Mukhtar, S.K. Katiyar and R. Agarwal: J. Invest. Dermatol. *102*, 3–7 (1994).

123 S. Kono, M. Lkeda, S. Tokudome and M. Kuratsune: Jpn. J. Cancer Res. *79*, 1067–1074 (1988).

124 I. Oguni, K. Nasu, S. Yammamoto and T. Nomura: Agric. Biol. Chem. *52*, 1879 (1988).

125 H. Mukhtar, S.K. Katiyar and R. Agarwal: Diet Cancer, Markers, Prevention, and Treatment, 123–134 (1994).

126 S.K. Katiyar, R. Agarwal and H. Mukhtar: Cancer Res. *53*, 5409–5412 (1993).

127 Z.Y. Wang, M.T. Huang, C.T. Ho, R. Chang, W. Ma, T. Ferraro, K.R. Reuhl, C.S. Yang and A.H. Conney: Cancer Res. *52*, 6657–6665 (1992).

128 Z.Y. Wang, M.T. Huang, Y.R. Lou, J.R. Xie, K.R. Reuhl, H.L. Newmark, C.T. Ho, C.S. Yang and A.H. Conney: Cancer Res. *54*, 3428–3435 (1994).

129 G.D. Stoner and H. Mukhtar: J. Cell Biochem. (Suppl.) *22*, 169–180 (1995).

130 M. Hirose, T. Hoshiya, K. Akagi, M. Futakuchi and N. Ito: Cancer Lett. *83*, 149–156 (1994).

131 V.S. Govindarajan: CRC Rev. Food Sci. Nutr. *12*, 199–301 (1980).

132 H.P T Ammon and M.A. Wahl: Planta Med. *57*, 1–7 (1990).

133 M.T. Huang, F.M. Robertson, T. Lysz, T. Ferraro, Z.Y. Wang, C.A. Georgiadis, J.D. Laskin and A.H. Conney: in M.T. Huang, C.T. Ho, C.Y. Leed (eds.): Phenolic compounds in food and their effects on health II, Antioxidants and cancer prevention, p. 339–349. American Chemical Society, Washington, DC 1992.

134 M.T. Huang, R.C. Smart, C.Q. Wong and A.H. Conney: Cancer Res. *48*, 5941–5946 (1988).

135 M. Nagabhushan and S.V. Bhide: J. Am. Coll. Nutr. *11*, 192–198 (1992).

136 R.G. Mehta, and R.C. Moon: Anticancer Res. *11*, 593–596 (1991).

137 C.V. Rao, B. Simi and B.S. Reddy: Carcinogenesis *14*, 2219–2225 (1993).

138 M.T. Huang, Y.R. Lou, W. Ma, H.L. Newmark, K.R. Reuhl and A.H. Conney: Cancer Res. *54*, 5841–5847 (1994).

139 M.A. Azuine and S.V. Bhide: J. Ethnopharm. *44* (3), 211–217 (1994).

140 S.V. Bhide, M.A. Azuine, M. Lahiri and N.T. Telang: Breast Cancer Res. Treat. *30* (3), 233–242 (1994).

141 T. Tanaka, H. Makita, M. Ohnishi, Y. Hirose, A. Wang, H. Mori, K. Satoh, A. Hara and H. Ogawa: Cancer Res. *54* (17), 4653–4659 (1994).

142 J.K. Lin and C.A. Shih: Carcinogenesis *15*, 1717–1721 (1994).

143 T.S. Huand, S.C. Lee and J.K. Lin: Proc. Natl. Acad. Sci. USA *88*, 5292–5296 (1991).

144 M.C. Jiang, H.F. Yang-Yen, J.J.Y. Yen and J.K. Lin: Nutr. Cancer *26*, 111–120 (1996).

145 J.N. Fang, A. Proksch and H. Wagner: Phytochemistry *24*, 2619–2622 (1985).

146 M.L. Shen, S.K. Zhai, H.L. Chen, Y.D. Luo, G.R. Tu and D.W. Ou: Int. J. Immunopharm. *13*, 549–554 (1991).

147 J.Z. Wang, H. Tsumura, K. Shimura and H. Ito: Cancer Letters *65*, 79–84 (1992).

148 J.Z. Wang, X.J. Mao, H. Ito and K. Shimura: Planta Medica *57*, 335–336 (1991).

149 T. Miyanomae and E. Frindel: Experimental Hematology *16*, 801–806 (1988).

150 L. Tong, T.Y. Huang and J.L. Li: Chung-kuo Chung Hsi I Chieh Ho Tsa Chih *14*, 482–484 (1994).

Progress in Drug Research, Vol. 48 (E. Jucker, Ed.)
© 1997 Birkhäuser Verlag, Basel (Switzerland)

Dopamine receptor diversity:
Molecular and pharmacological perspectives

By Deborah S. Hartman[1] and Olivier Civelli[2]

[1]Pharmaceutical Research, Preclinical Neurosciences, Hoffmann-La Roche AG, CH-4070 Basel, Switzerland, and [2]Department of Pharmacology, College of Medicine, University of California at Irvine, Irvine, CA 92717, USA

1   Introduction

Five distinct dopamine (DA) receptors, named D1–D5, have now been identified. All five DA receptors are expressed in the central nervous system where they control motor function, emotional states, and endocrine physiology, and all receptor subtypes are also found in peripheral tissues where they regulate transmembrane ion transport, catecholamine secretion, and cardiovascular function. Significant advances have been made following the cloning and heterologous expression of individual DA receptor subtypes, which has allowed the production of specific cDNA probes, receptor subtype-specific antibodies, and most recently the development of receptor-specific ligands. In this review we will discuss both molecular and pharmacological aspects of DA receptor diversity ranging from nucleotide sequences to behavioral aspects of DA receptor knockout mice.

In 1979 dopamine receptors were classified as 'D1' and 'D2' receptors based on pharmacological differences observed in brain tissue [1], and it was shown that the antipsychotic action of neuroleptics, which are used to treat psychosis, was correlated with their ability to block the 'D2' receptors [2,3]. This was consistent with an earlier hypothesis implicating overactivity of the central dopaminergic system in schizophrenia [4]. Fifteen years later molecular cloning efforts revealed that the D2-like receptors observed in brain actually included three distinct receptor subtypes (D2, D3, and D4) and that the D1-like receptors included both D1 and D5 receptors.

Schizophrenia is a chronic, debilitating mental disorder that involves injury to a vast array of emotional and cognitive systems. It is believed to be connected to an imbalance of the dopaminergic system resulting from or consequently affecting glutaminergic and serotonergic pathway transmission. Although dopaminergic antagonists show therapeutic efficacy in psychosis, it should be emphasized that it is not known whether alterations in dopaminergic systems in the brain play a role in causing schizophrenia, or whether they represent secondary consequences of an unidentified primary insult.

DA is highly related to two other catecholamine neurotransmitters, norepinephrine (NE) and epinephrine (EP), which also have powerful activities in the central nervous system and periphery. EP and NE activate a large family of adrenergic receptors including $\alpha 1$ subtypes ($\alpha 1a/b/c$), $\alpha 2$ subtypes ($\alpha 2a/b/c$-1/c-2), and the β-receptors ($\beta 1$, $\beta 2$, $\beta 3$). Noradrenergic pathways in the central nervous system play key roles in learning and memory [5], attention and vigilance, as well as depression and anxiety [6], and in the periphery regulate the cardiovascular system. There is close interaction between dopaminergic and adrenergic pathways in the brain involving crosstalk between signal transduction pathways activated by DA and noradrenergic receptors in the same cell, but interaction also occurs upstream of receptor activation, i.e. adrenergic innervation of the DA neurons in the hypothalamus [7]. We have recently obtained evidence that the human D4R may be activated by DA, EP and NE, and discuss here implications of this data, i.e. that the D4R may play a key role in coordinating signaling between different neurotransmitter systems.

The discovery of multiple subtypes of dopamine receptors has opened up the possibility that improved antipsychotic drugs may be obtained by developing more selective compounds, and this has led to a flurry of activity in the pharmaceutical industry. In discussing receptor pharmacology, we present a number of recently reported D4 specific ligands currently under development as potential new treatment for schizophrenia. Importantly, even if these compounds fail as drugs, they hold great promise as tools for dissecting the function of this receptor *in vivo*. This review provides only a snapshot of a rapidly expanding area of research which has important implications for human behaviors including motivation and cognition, and for human diseases including Parkinson's and schizophrenia.

2   Structural features of dopamine receptor subtypes

The deduced amino acid sequences of all DA receptors exhibit seven highly hydrophobic stretches of approximately 24 amino acids which are believed to represent membrane-spanning domains. The proposed transmembrane topology predicts an extracellular amino-terminus and an intracellular carboxy-terminus, with alternating intra- and extracellular loops connecting the transmembrane regions.

The D2R was the first of the DA receptors to be cloned, and was identified by using low stringency hybridization with the related β-adrenergic receptor sequence [8]. Additional DA receptor subtypes were subsequently identified by sequence homology. The binding domain for both agonists and antagonists is believed to occur within the transmembrane domains, particularly the 3rd and 5th transmembrane domains for agonist binding, and including the 7th transmembrane domain for antagonist binding (see [9] for review). These regions are highly conserved among the D1-like and D2-like receptors, leading to similar pharmacological profiles between closely related receptor subtypes.

2.1   Sequence characteristics

The original D2 receptor cDNA contained an open reading frame encoding 415 amino acids with 7 hydrophobic stretches. This sequence has 3 potential N-linked glycosylation sites in the putative extracellular N-terminal tail, and exhibits a relatively long third cytoplasmic loop and a short cytoplasmic C-terminal tail. Transfection of this clone into mouse fibroblasts resulted in the expression of high affinity, saturable binding of the D2 antagonist [3H]-spiroperidol [8], which showed a pharmacological profile indicative of binding to a D2 dopamine receptor based on data obtained with rat striatum membranes.

At the level of amino acid sequence, the D3R is most homologous to the D2 receptor, exhibiting 75% homology in the transmembrane domains [10]. In addition, other structural features, such as a long third cytoplasmic loop and a short C-terminal domain, reinforce the similarity to the previously cloned D2 receptor and dissimilarity to D1 and D5 receptors. The deduced amino acid sequence of the D4R, based on combined genomic and cDNA sequences, results in a 387 amino acid open reading frame containing 7 hydrophobic regions corresponding to the putative transmembrane regions found in the D2 and D3 receptors [11]. The human genomic clone contained sequences corresponding to the N-terminus through the fourth transmembrane region, as well as several introns which interrupted the coding sequence in transmembrane regions 1, 3, 6 and the third cytoplasmic loop. These introns are in positions analogous to the introns found in both the D2 and D3 receptors [10–16]. Overall, the homology with the D2 and D3 receptors is 41% and 39% respectively, and about 56% for both receptors within the transmembrane regions.

The deduced amino acid sequences of the D1R and D5R, respectively, are approximately 41% and 44% homologous to that of the D2R. The D1-like receptors, D1 and D5, show higher homology with each other than with the D2-like receptors, and have shorter third intracellular loops and longer carboxy-terminal cytoplasmic tails. D1 and D5 receptors are encoded by genes lacking introns, and in humans these genes encode 446 and 477 amino acids, respectively. The D1R gene is located on human chromosome 5, the D5R on chromosome 4, and the D3R on chromosome 3, while D2R and D4R genes are found on chromosome 11.

2.2   Receptor isoforms

Multiple receptor isoforms have been identified for all D2-like DA receptors resulting either from differential splicing or allelic variation. These

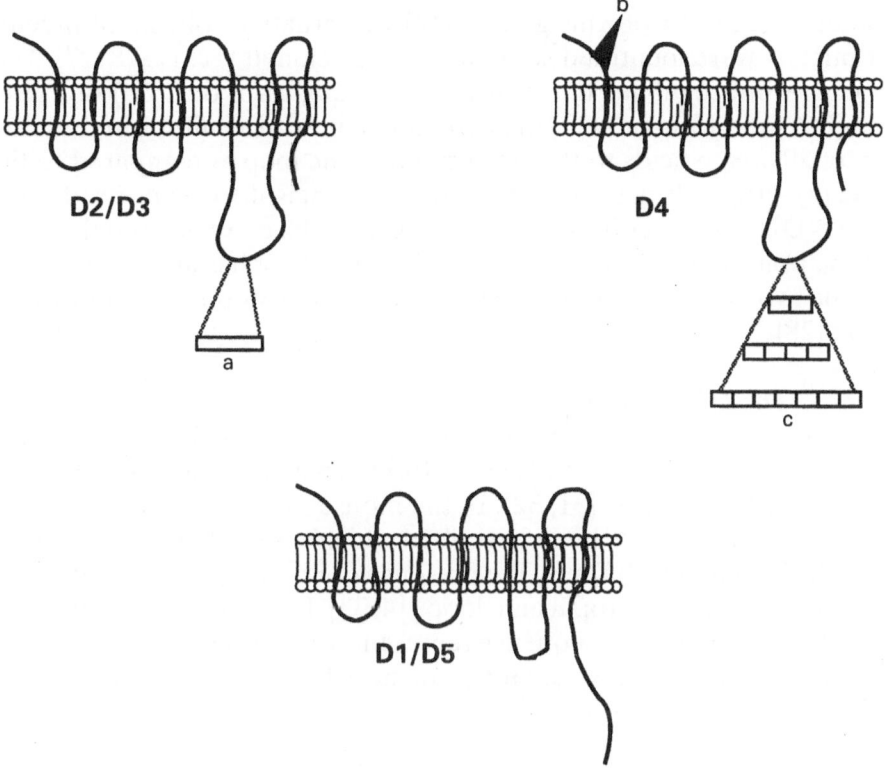

Figure 1
Schematic representation of the predicted secondary structure of dopamine receptors and receptor isoforms. D2 and D3 receptor isoforms are generated by alternative splicing which results
in the addition of 29 and 21 amino acids, respectively, to the predicted third cytoplasmic loop
(a). Two major polymorphisms in the D4R gene locus have been described including a 12 base
pair deletion in first exon (b) and variation in the number of 16 amino acid proline-rich repeats
in the putative third cytoplasmic loop (c). The D1-like receptors, including D1 and D5, have
shorter third intracellular loops and longer carboxy-terminal cytoplasmic tails.

are described in greater detail in the following section, and are drawn sche-
matically in Figure 1. There are no splice variants for the D1 or D5 receptor sequences since they contain no introns, however a polymorphism in
the human D5 gene promoter has recently been reported. This polymorphism consists of a TC dinucleotide repeat within the major trans-
activation domain located 119-182 base pairs upstream of the transcriptional start site [17]. Although no differences between D5R polymorphic
variants were detected in an *in vitro* reporter gene assay, this variation
may prove useful for genetic linkage studies.

2.2.1   The D2 receptor

Two distinct D2R isoforms generated by alternative splicing of precursor mRNA were identified soon after it was cloned [12, 13, 18–27]. This splicing event regulates the inclusion (D2-long form or D2L) or exclusion (D2-short form or D2S) of an 87 base pair exon, resulting in the addition of 29 amino acids to the third cytoplasmic loop as compared to the sequence originally described. The predominant isoform expressed in the brain is D2L, however both isoforms appear to be co-expressed throughout the brain [12, 13, 15, 19, 21, 22, 24, 26, 28–30]. It has also been shown that the two isoforms do not represent pre-synaptic vs. post-synaptic forms of D2 [28].

2.2.2   The D3 receptor

Characterization of the gene for the D3R has revealed alternate splicing events which give rise to D3R isoforms, some of which encode truncated receptor proteins [31, 32]. In the mouse, two alternatively spliced forms of the D3R have been described which resemble the isoforms of the D2R in that they differ by the presence or absence of a 21 amino acid segment in the third cytoplasmic loop [14, 33]. It is not clear whether the published human cDNA sequence represents a short, alternatively spliced isoform, or whether these exonic sequences have been lost during evolution.

2.2.3   The D4 receptor

Although no splice variants of the D4R have been identified, the existence of multiple D4R proteins is predicted in humans and primates by the highly polymorphic nature of the D4R gene locus (DRD4). The most striking polymorphism involves a 48 base pair sequence which encodes an imperfect 16 amino acid repeat in the putative third cytoplasmic loop of the protein [34]. DRD4 alleles differ not only in the number of these repeat units, which can vary from 2 to 10 (4 is most common, and no alleles with 9 repeats have been found), but they also vary in nucleotide sequence and in the order in which they are arranged [35]. In one study, eighteen distinct D4R protein sequences were identified among 178 human alleles [35], and although this repeat structure is not apparent in rat or mouse D4R sequences, similar repeat units have been identified in primates [36]. These repeats are proline-rich, and appear to consist of tandem copies of consensus SH3 binding domains suggesting that the D4R may be capable of direct interaction with proteins containing SH3-domains (i.e. cytoskeletal proteins, serine/threonine and tyrosine kinases) [37] in addition to the heterotrimeric G-proteins. Although the functional significance of D4 repeat sequence variation is not clear, one report indicated differential effects of sodium on antagonist binding depending on the number of repeat sequences [34].

A second D4R polymorphism involves a 12 base pair (bp) repeat within the first exon, bordering the first putative transmembrane domain [38]. The more common allele (A1) contains two 12 bp repeats, while the less common allele (A2) contains only one copy of the repeat.

2.2.4   Gene linkage studies

The discovery of extensive genetic polymorphism at the DRD4 locus has led to studies investigating whether specific variants of the D4R might be associated with schizophrenic pathology. Numerous groups have conducted linkage studies examining D4R variants in schizophrenic patients, but so far no linkage of D4R isoforms to genetic susceptibility for schizophrenia has been observed in the populations studied [39–44]. On the other hand, a different polymorphism involving the presence (A1) or absence (A2) of the 12 base pair repeat within the first exon has been shown to be associated with a form of psychosis called delusional disorder [38]. Interestingly, patients with the A2 allele respond poorly to neuroleptics, so that the effect of this sequence difference on functional properties of the corresponding D4R proteins will be of great interest.

Genetic linkage studies have found no correlation between the number of D4R 16-amino acids repeats and incidence of schizophrenia [45], however the significance of individual repeat sequences or combinations of repeats is not yet clear. Two recent studies suggest that the presence of the D4.7 allele (containing seven 16-amino acids repeats) correlates with a higher level of 'novelty seeking' behavior than that found in persons with the shorter D4.4 allele [46, 47]. These results would suggest that the D4R can contribute to variation in a human personality trait, however it is clear that such complex behavior is also influenced by other genetic elements, as well as environmental factors.

A natural D4R null mutation has also been found in humans with a frequency of about 2% in the general population, but no correlation has been found between the presence of heterozygosity for this mutation and either schizophrenia, bipolar disorder or Tourette's syndrome [48]. A single individual homozygous for the null mutation at the D4 locus has been identified, and this person suffers from acoustic neuroma, obesity, and some disturbances of the autonomic nervous system, but does not show signs of major psychiatric illness [48]. Identification of additional homozygous individuals (predicted frequency of 4/10000) will be required to establish a causal relationship between the D4R and these symptoms.

A restriction fragment length polymorphism observed for the D3R gene has been identified, but in several studies this showed no association with schizophrenia [49–60]. Interestingly, loss of D3R mRNA from parietal and motor cortex in postmortem brain samples from schizophrenic patients has been reported [61], however it will be necessary for such a finding to be replicated in a larger patient sample to control for medication history and other possible confounding variables.

2.3 Expression patterns

Two major dopaminergic pathways are found in the brain, the nigrostriatal pathway which controls motor function, and the mesolimbic pathway which mediates affective/emotional behavior. Overall, the D1 and D2 are the most abundant DA receptor subtypes in the brain, with particularly high expression in the nigrostriatal pathway, especially in striatum and nucleus accumbens with lower levels in the olfactory tubercle [62]. In human prefrontal cortex, both D1 and D2 receptor mRNA are also detected at significantly higher levels than D3, D4, or D5 transcripts [63]. The D2R is the most prominent receptor in the substantia nigra, a region where the D1R is absent. The levels of D3, D4, and D5 receptors in the brain are approximately 10–100 fold lower overall as compared to D1 and D2 receptor levels.

The expression of D3R mRNA in the rat brain is localized to limbic areas including the nucleus accumbens, islands of Calleja, olfactory tubercle, hippocampus, mammary nuclei and hypothalamus [10]. Low levels of D3R mRNA have also been found in the striatum and certain regions of the cerebral cortex, as well as in dopaminergic cells of the substantia nigra, where the D3R may also function as a presynaptic autoreceptor. Overall, the pattern of D3 receptor expression suggests that this dopamine receptor subtype may be well positioned to mediate the effects of dopamine on cognitive and emotional functions, and thus could prove to be a relevant target for anti-psychotic drug therapy.

The D4R is particularly interesting because of its localization in limbic and cortical areas of the brain which are involved in emotional/affective behavior and cognition [64]. D4R mRNA expression has been found in human tissue from frontal cortex, amygdala, thalamus, hypothalamus, cerebellum, and pituitary, with lower levels in hippocampus [65]. *In situ* hybrization in human temporal lobe has shown D4R mRNA expression in the dentate gyrus and CA2 regions of the hippocampus, as well as in entorhinal cortex [64]. In mouse retina, D4R mRNA has been localized in the photoreceptor cells, the inner nuclear layer, and the ganglion cell layer [66]. High levels of D4R mRNA were found in rat heart [67], however this was not confirmed in human tissue [65]. A D4R-specific antisera has recently been reported which labeled GABAergic neurons in cerebral cortex, hippocampus, thalamic reticular nucleus, globus pallidus, and substantia nigra [68], providing the first look at D4R protein distribution in the brain.

D5R mRNA expression is restricted to the parafascicular nucleus of the thalamus, the hippocampus and the hypothalamus [62]. D5R-specific antibodies have been reported which recognize polypeptides ranging in size from 50 to 200 kDa in primate hippocampus, caudate, and substantia nigra, and label pyramidal neurons in the prefrontal cortex [69].

2.4 Signal transduction and second messenger systems

When dopamine receptor subtypes are expressed at high levels in heterologous cells, the primary signaling pathway activated by both the D1R and D5R is stimulation of adenylyl cyclase (AC), while D2R, D3R, and D4R inhibit AC activity. However, the signalling potential of each of these receptors is much broader. For example, D2L and D2S inhibit AC activity in some heterologous expression systems [70, 71], as well as stimulate PLC activation [71], mobilize intracellular calcium [72] and activate Na^+/H^+ exchange [73]. Interestingly, phosphorylation of D2R isoforms by protein kinase C can direct preferential coupling away from inhibition of AC activity and toward potentiation of arachidonic acid release (reviewed in [74]). D2, D4, and to a lesser extent D3 receptors expressed in Xenopus oocytes have also been shown to activate inward currents when coexpressed with a G-protein regulated potassium channel (GIRK1) [75].

Although the demonstration of second messenger responses to D3R stimulation has been difficult, at least one group has been able to demonstrate inhibition of AC activity and stimulation of extracellular acidification through D3 receptors expressed in a Chinese Hamster Ovary (CHO) cell line, but this appears to require relatively high levels of expression [76]. In addition, the D3R has been shown to mediate inhibition of calcium currents [77]; to activate c-*fos* expression and stimulate [3H]-thymidine incorporation in undifferentiated NG108-15 cells [78]; and to inhibit dopamine release in a mesencephalic cell line [79].

Heterologous expression of the D4 receptor has shown that this receptor couples to inhibition of AC activity [80, 81], but also to stimulation of Na^+/H^+ exchange [80], and potentiation of stimulated arachidonic acid release [80]. In cultured cerebral granule cells, D4R activation inhibits an L-type calcium current via a G_i/G_o protein, but independent of AC inhibition [82]. D4R activation may also regulate the light sensitive pool of cAMP in retina [66], mediate DA-induced contraction and elongation of cone photoreceptor cells [83], and regulate serotonin N-acetyltransferase activity, which controls melatonin synthesis [84].

The D1R and D5R stimulate AC through $G\alpha_s$ [62] but can also mediate phosphoinositol turnover through the promiscuous G proteins, $G\alpha_{15}$ and $G\alpha_{16}$ [85]. Activation of the D1R was shown to induce long-lasting long-term synaptic potentiation (L-LTP) in a synaptic model of memory formation [86], and was required for induction of long-term synaptic depression (LTD) in mammalian brain [87].

2.5   Physiology of knockout mice

Targeted mutation of D1, D2 and D3 receptors in mice has recently been reported. D1 knockout mice failed to show the increased locomotor activity normally observed after cocaine administration in the wildtype mice, however no change in the rewarding and reinforcing effects of the drug were seen in the knockout mice [88]. Parkinsonian-like locomotor impairment was observed in D2R deficient mice with significant reduction in spontaneous movements, and both akinetic and bradykinetic behavior [89]. In contrast, D3R knockout mice showed hyperactivity with increased locomotor activity and rearing behavior in an exploratory test [90]. These animals provide evidence for distinct roles of each of these receptors in dopaminergic signaling in the brain.

3   Dopamine receptor pharmacology

The behavioral and neurophysiological effects of antipsychotic drugs have been shown to be mediated in part via D2-like receptor blockade. Two classical neuroleptics, chlorpromazine and haloperidol, show high affinity binding to D2, D3, and D4 receptors and display efficacy in alleviating acute 'positive' psychotic symptoms (i.e. hallucinations and paranoia) and reducing the number or frequency of psychotic episodes [91–93]. However, these drugs are associated with a high incidence of side effects [91, 94], with up to 40% of patients experiencing neuroleptic-induced parkinsonism severe enough to require additional drug therapy, or complete withdrawal of treatment.

New hopes for better antipsychotic drugs have been raised with the discovery that the D4 and D3 receptor subtypes are expressed primarily outside the nigrostriatal pathway, suggesting that compounds specific for these

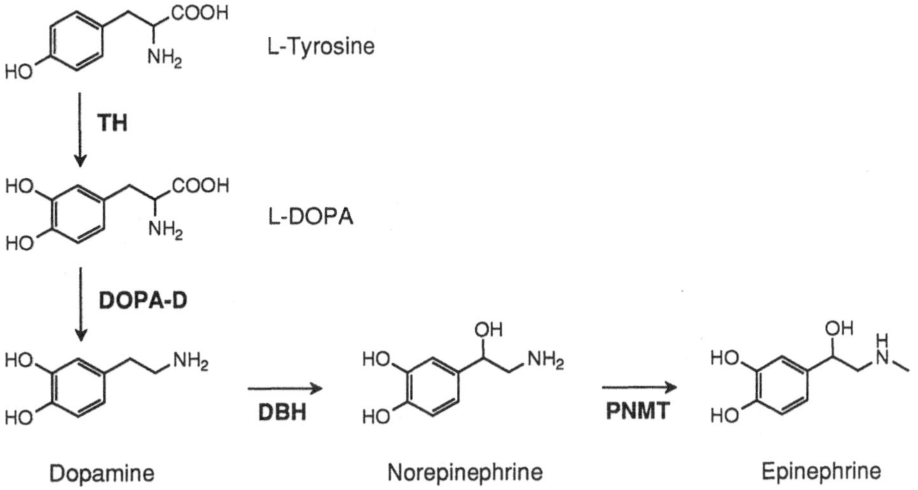

Figure 2
DA, EP, and NE which are synthesized in a single biosynthetic pathway originating with the amino acid, L-tyrosine. TH, tyrosine hydroxylase; DOPA-D, dopamine decarboxylase; DBH, dopamine β-hydroxylase; PNMT, phenylethanolamine N-methyltransferase.

receptor subtypes may have a reduced liability for motor side effects. In addition, recent evidence has suggested a unique role for the D4R in integration and coordination of DA, EP and NE signaling.

3.1   Interaction of catecholamines with the D4R

DA belongs to the family of catecholamine neurotransmitters including EP and NE which are synthesized in a single biosynthetic pathway originating with the amino acid, L-tyrosine (Figure 2). DA interacts with the D1 and D2 receptors with two different affinity states displaying micromolar and nanomolar binding constants, respectively. The D3, D4, and D5 receptors bind DA with nanomolar affinity, however some low affinity binding sites have been reported in heterologous expression systems. The D5 receptor shows a 10-fold higher affinity for dopamine than the D1 receptor [95–99].

DA, Ep and NE have been shown to stimulate distinct receptor superfamilies, activating different neuronal pathways in the brain. Surprisingly, we have recently discovered that all three catecholamines bind with high affinity to the recombinant human D4R heterologously expressed in CHO cells [100], and that each acts as a potent, full agonist at the D4R in stimulating ^{35}S-GTPγS binding and in decreasing forskolin-induced cAMP accu-

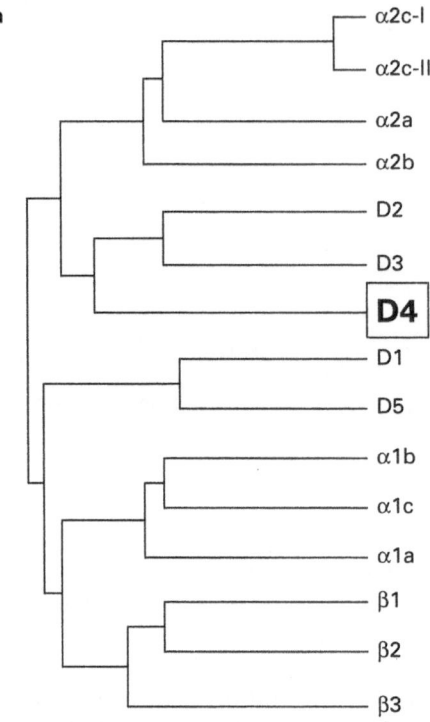

b Amino acid identities between the D4R vs. DA and adrenergic receptors

D4R	100%
D2R	43%
D3R	41%
α2C-1	41%
α2C-2	41%
α2A	37%
α2B	38%

Figure 3
a) Dendritic tree diagram comparing amino acid homologies between human DA and adrenergic receptors (generated by Wisconsin GCG software). b) Amino acid identities between the human D4R vs. other D2-like DA receptors and α2 adrenergic receptors.

mulation in intact CHO-D4.4 cells. Three D4R isoforms, D4.2, D4.4, and D4.7, showed identical pharmacological profiles in both receptor binding and receptor activation assays. These results demonstrate direct activation of the D4R by three distinct neurotransmitters, providing a novel mechanism for interaction between the dopaminergic and adrenergic neuronal pathways. In addition, it suggests that the D4R should be classified as both a dopaminergic and an adrenergic receptor.

Why do EP and NE bind with much higher affinity to the D4R than the D1R and D2R? Comparison of deduced amino acid sequences reveals a high degree of homology between the D4R and the adrenergic α2 receptor subfamily (Figure 3). In fact, the D4R is as similar to the adrenergic α2c receptor as it is to D2 and D3 receptors, with overall amino acid identities of 41%, 43% and 41%, respectively. In contrast, the human D2R shows 57% identity with the D3R, and only 33% identity with the α2C receptor. Molecular modeling of the β-adrenergic receptor and site-directed mutagenesis studies of the D2R have implicated a conserved aspartic acid residue in putative transmembrane domain 3 (TM3) and three serine residues in TM5 in catecholamine binding interactions [101–104]. In TM3, divergence between D4 and D2 is clustered near the critical aspartic acid residue, Asp115 (D4R numbering) (Figure 4A), close to the extracellular surface (Figure 4B). Amino acid changes in this region could theoretically affect receptor binding specificity by altering ligand orientation within the receptor binding pocket, or by restriction or facilitation of ligand access to the binding pocket. The D4R sequence in this region also differs from the adrenergic receptors, however only two amino acids differ between the human and rat TM3 sequences.

At the extracellular surface of TM5, the D4R contains one positively charged and three negatively charged residues, similar to α2 receptors which contain one or two negatively charged residues in this region. In contrast, the D2R and D3R residues are uncharged, and the D1R and D5R contain a single positive charge. Divergence between D4 and D2 is also observed downstream of the critical serines (Cys205-Met208), where the D4 sequence strongly resembles that of the α2 receptors. In addition, a cysteine residue (Cys199 in the D4R) located between two critical serine residues (Ser197 and Ser200 in D4) does not occur in any other DA receptor, but is observed in α2a and α2c receptors, and Phe202 in D4 is conserved in all α2 receptors but corresponds to a tyrosine residue in other DA receptors. TM5 sequences are highly conserved between the human and rat D4R, with only a single conservative amino acid change (Val198 in human to Ile198 in rat), again suggesting that the human and rat D4R may show similar pharmacological profiles.

▼

```
TM3  CEIYLALDVLFCTSSIVHLCAISLDRY    α2a
     CEVYLALDVLFCTSSIVHLCAISLDRY    α2b
     CGVYLALDVLFCTSSIVHLCAISLDRY    α2c-1
     CGVYLALDVLFCTSSIVHLCAISLDRY    α2c-2
     CDALMAMDVMLCTASIFNLCAISVDRF    D4
     CDIFVTLDVMMCTASILNLCAISIDRY    D2
     CDVFVTLDVMMCTASILNLCAISIDRY    D3
     CNIWVAFDIMCSTASILNLCVISVDRY    D1
     CDVWVAFDIMCSTASILNLCVISVDRY    D5
```

```
TM5  DQKWYVISSCIGSFFAPCLIMILVYLR    α2a
     QEAWYILASSIGSFFAPCLIMILVYLR    α2b
     DETWYILSSCIGSFFAPCLIMGLVYAR    α2c-1
     DETWYILSSCIGSFFAPCLIMGLVYAR    α2c-2
     EDRDYVVYSSVCSFFLPCPLMLLLYWA    D4
     ANPAFVVYSSIVSFYVPFIVTLLVYIK    D2
     SNPDFVIYSSVVSFYLPFGVTVLVYAR    D3
     LSRTYAISSSVISFYIPVAIMVTYTR     D1
     LNRTYAISSSLISFYIPVAIMIVTYTR    D5
```

▲   ▲

A

Figure 4

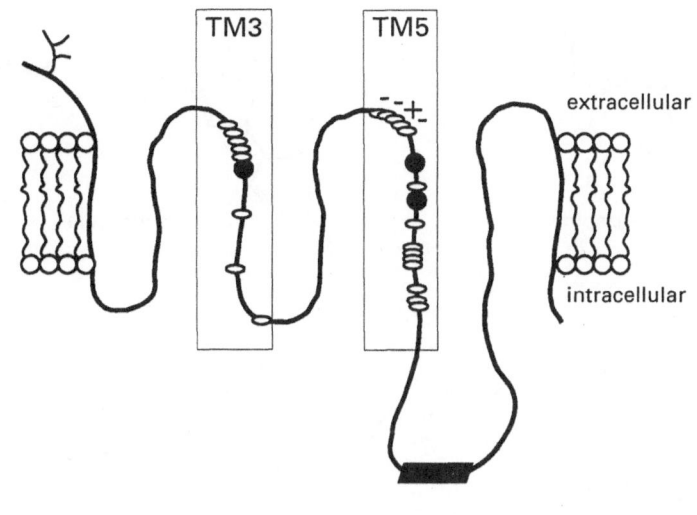

B

○   residues not conserved between D4 and D2
●   residues implicated in ligand binding
▰   16 amino acid repeat units in D4.4

Figure 4
A) Line-up of amino acid sequences from putative transmembrane domains (TM) 3 and 5 from human DA and alpha2 adrenergic receptors. The D4R sequence and conserved residues in other sequences are shown in bold. Arrows indicate conserved aspartate (D) and serine (S) residues implicated in ligand binding.
B) Schematic representation of amino acid residue divergence between D4 and D2 receptors. Open circles indicate residues in the D4R sequence that are not conserved in the D2R which may contribute to the selective activation of the D4R by EP and NE.

Divergence between receptor subtypes may provide a possible structural basis for future site-directed mutagenesis studies aimed at elucidating key receptor-ligand interactions.

3.2   New antipsychotic drugs

The binding of known antipsychotic drugs and related compounds to heterologously expressed recombinant DA receptors has been extensively reviewed in [105]. Many small molecules have been identified which interact with the DA receptors with some degree of selectivity and serve as useful tools for the study of these receptors.
In general, very similar pharmacological profiles are seen among the D2-like receptors and among the D1-like receptors, as expected from the high

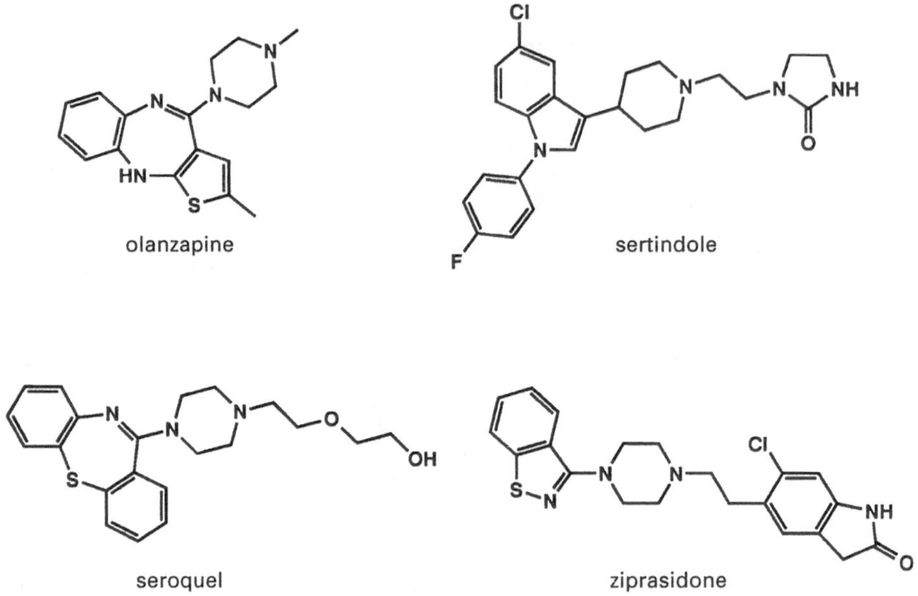

Figure 5
Chemical structures of four new atypical antipsychotic drugs about to enter the market: olanzapine (Lilly), sertindole (Abbott), seroquel (Zeneca), and ziprasidone (Pfizer).

degree of sequence conservation within these groups. For example, the neuroleptic haloperidol shows strongest affinity for D2 receptors, but it also binds to D3, D4, D1 and D5 receptors with affinities in the nanomolar range. In contrast to the classical neuroleptics, the dibenzazepine clozapine has been found to alleviate psychiatric symptoms of schizophrenia without producing adverse extrapyramidal and motor side effects. Interestingly, clozapine, which has been termed an 'atypical' antipsychotic drug, binds to a broad spectrum of receptor sites including the DA receptors. A large number of new antipsychotic drugs, shown in Figure 5, are entering or predicted to enter the market this year including olanzapine (Lilly), ziprasidone (Pfizer), sertindole (Abbott) and seroquel (Zeneca). Ziprasidone is a combined serotonin and dopaminergic receptor antagonist which is particularly potent at 5HT2A, D2, 5HT1A, 5HT 1D, and 5HT2C receptors. This compound showed very good tolerability in phase II clinical trials [106] and is now in phase III. Seroquel is a mixed serotonin and dopaminergic antagonist which has shown good tolerability and lack of significant extrapyramidal side effects in phase III clinical trials [107]. Sertindole has high affinity for D2, 5HT2A, and alpha1 adrenergic receptors. It was demonstrated to be effective, well tolerated, and not associated with significant motor side effects in phase III trials for schizophrenia [108]. Olanzapine shows a broad pharmacological profile similar to clozapine, with high affinity binding to 5HT2A, 5HT2C, D1, D2, muscarinic M1, alpha 1 adrenergic, and histamine H1 receptors. New Drug Applications (NDA) have been filed in the U.S. for both olanzapine and sertindole.

3.3   New D4R selective ligands

Particular attention has been devoted to the development of D4R-specific ligands as potential treatment for schizophrenia for two main reasons, i) an early report showing that clozapine had up to 10-fold higher affinity for the D4R vs. the D2R [11], and ii) reports claiming elevated densities of D4R in striatal homogenates from schizophrenic vs. control subjects [109–111]. Subsequent D4R expression and binding studies have shown that clozapine binding to the D4R may be only about 3-fold higher affinity than to the D2R [80, 81, 112, 113]. With respect to ligand-binding studies in post-mortem tissue, lack of a D4R-specific radioligand led to use of an indirect method to measure D4R density by subtraction of 3H-raclopride binding sites (labels D2R + D3R) from 3H-emonapride sites (labels D2R + D3R + D4R). The results of these studies await confirmation with D4R-selective radioligands or antibodies.

Nevertheless, the pharmaceutical industry has devoted a major effort to the development of D4R specific compounds over the past three years. The earliest reports came from companies such as Neurogen [114], Merck, Sharp & Dohme [115, 116], and Pharmacia & Upjohn [117]. At the Society for Neuroscience meeting held in Washington, D.C. in November, 1996, at least eight different pharmaceutical companies reported identification and characterization of D4R selective compounds. A selection of these compounds is shown in Figure 6.

An alternate approach to treatment of schizophrenia might include development of dopaminergic agonists. Several studies have shown that depletion of DA levels in the prefrontal cortex of aged monkey brain has been found to correlate with cognitive deficits [118, 119] which can be reduced by quinpirole, an agonist at the D2R, D3R, and D4R, suggesting a possible role for these receptors as well in DA-mediated cognitive functions [120]. Schizophrenic patients are known to suffer from cognitive deficits including reductions in working and semantic memory, attention, verbal fluency, and executive function which may in fact be a consequence of reduced DA activity in the frontal cortex [121]. The results obtained in primates suggest that DA receptor agonists may be able to partially alleviate these deficits.

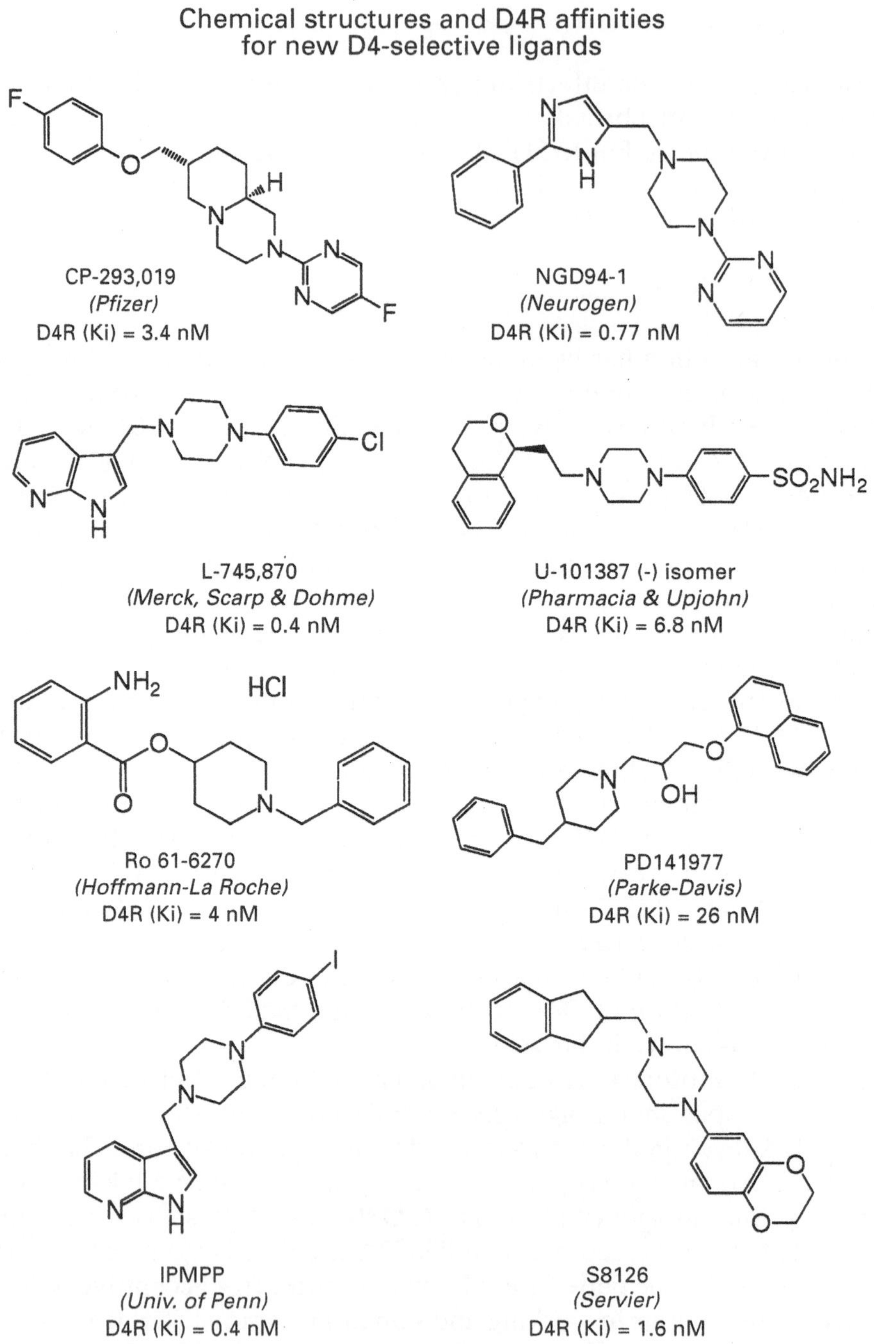

Chemical structures and D4R affinities
for new D4-selective ligands

CP-293,019
(Pfizer)
D4R (Ki) = 3.4 nM

NGD94-1
(Neurogen)
D4R (Ki) = 0.77 nM

L-745,870
(Merck, Scarp & Dohme)
D4R (Ki) = 0.4 nM

U-101387 (-) isomer
(Pharmacia & Upjohn)
D4R (Ki) = 6.8 nM

Ro 61-6270
(Hoffmann-La Roche)
D4R (Ki) = 4 nM

PD141977
(Parke-Davis)
D4R (Ki) = 26 nM

IPMPP
(Univ. of Penn)
D4R (Ki) = 0.4 nM

S8126
(Servier)
D4R (Ki) = 1.6 nM

Figure 6
Chemical structures and D4R affinities of new D4R selective compounds reported at the American Society for Neuroscience Meeting held in Washington, D.C. from November 16–21, 1996.

4 Conclusions

Although no genetic linkage has been established between schizophrenia and any of the DA receptor genes, DA clearly plays a central role in the pathophysiology of this disease. A putative susceptibility locus for schizophrenia has been identified on chromosome 6p by several independent groups [122–125], which may provide new clues to the genetic factors involved in schizophrenia. Other important developments in the area of dopaminergic signaling include production of a dopamine transporter knockout mouse which provides new insight into the physiological role of the dopaminergic system in behavior [126].

The expression patterns of the D3 and D4 receptors suggest that these receptor subtypes may be appropriately positioned to mediate the effects of DA on affective, emotional, and cognitive functions, and thus may represent relevant targets for antipsychotic drug development. The discovery of multiple DA receptor subtypes with distinct pharmacological profiles and localization patterns, and the explosion of compounds specific for these receptor subtypes, provides a means for better understanding of this complex and essential system.

References

1   Kebabian, J.W. and Calne, D.B.: Nature 277, 93–96 (1979).
2   Seeman, P., Lee, T., Chan-Wong, M. and Wong, K.: Nature 261, 717–719 (1976).
3   Creese, I., Burt, D.R. and Snyder, S.H.: Science 192, 481–483 (1976).
4   Carlsson, A.: Neuropsychopharm 1, 179–186 (1988).
5   Cahill, L., Prins, B., Weber, M. and McGaugh, J.L.: Nature 371, 702–704 (1994).
6   Pacak, K., Palkovits, M., Kopin, I.J. and Goldstein, D.S.: Front. Neuroendocrinol. 16, 89–150 (1995).
7   Hrabovsky, E. and Liposits, Z.: Neurosci. Lett. 182, 143–146 (1994).
8   Bunzow, J.R., et al.: Nature 336, 783–7 (1988).
9   Savarese, T.M. and Fraser, C.M.: Biochemical Journal 283, 1–19 (1992).
10   Sokoloff, P., Giros, B., Martres, M.-P., Bouthenet, M.-L. and Schwartz, J.-C.: Nature 347, 146–151 (1990).
11   Van Tol, H.H.M., et al.: Nature 350, 610–614 (1991).
12   Grandy, D.K., et al.: Proc. Natl. Acad. Sci. USA 86, 9762–9766 (1989).
13   O'Malley, K.L., Mack, K.J., Gandelman, K.Y. and Todd, R.D.: Biochemistry 29, 1367–71 (1990).
14   Park, B.-H., Fishburn, S., Carmon, S., Accili, D. and Fuchs, S.: Journal of Neurochemistry 64, 482–486 (1995).
15   Mack, K.J., Todd, R.D. and O'Malley, K.L.: J. Neurochem. 57, 795–801 (1991).
16   Giros, B., Martres, M.P., Sokoloff, P. and Schwartz, J.C.: C. R. Acad. Sci. Iii. 311, 501–8 (1990).
17   Beischlag, T.V., Nam, D., Ulpian, C., Seeman, P. and Niznick, H.B.: Neurosci. Lett.

205, 173–176 (1996).

18   Chio, C.L., Hess, G.F., Graham, R.S. and Huff, R.M.: Nature *343*, 266–9 (1990).
19   Dal Toso, R., et al.: Embo. J. *8*, 4025–34 (1989).
20   Eidne, K.A., Taylor, P.L., Zabavnik, J., Saunders, P.T. and Inglis, J.D.: Nature *342* (1989).
21   Gandelman, K.Y., Harmon, S., Todd, R.D. and O'Malley, K.L.: J. Neurochem. *56*, 1024–9 (1991).
22   Giros, B., et al.: Nature *342*, 923–6 (1989).
23   Miller, J.C., Wang, Y. and Filer, D.: Biochem. Biophys. Res. Commun. *166*, 109–12 (1990).
24   Monsma, F.J., Jr., McVittie, L.D., Gerfen, C.R., Mahan, L.C. and Sibley, D.R.: Nature *342*, 926–9 (1989).
25   Montmayeur, J.P. and Borrelli, E.: Proc. Natl. Acad. Sci. USA *88*, 3135–9 (1991).
26   Mack, K.J., O'Malley, K.L. and Todd, R.D.: Brain Res. Dev. Brain Res. *59*, 249–51 (1991).
27   O'Dowd, B.F., et al.: Febs Lett. *262*, 8–12 (1990).
28   Le Moine, C. and Bloch, B.: Brain Res. Mol. Brain Res. *10*, 283–9 (1991).
29   Neve, K.A., Neve, R.L., Fidel, S., Janowsky, A. and Higgins, G.A.: Proc. Natl. Acad. Sci. USA *88*, 2802–6 (1991).
30   Snyder, L.A., Roberts, J.L. and Sealfon, S.C.: Neurosci. Lett. *122*, 37–40 (1991).
31   Giros, B., Martres, M.P., Pilon, C., Sokoloff, P. and Schwartz, J.C.: Biochem. Biophys. Res. Commun. *176*, 1584–92 (1991).
32   Snyder, L.A., Roberts, J.L. and Sealfon, S.C.: Biochem. Biophys. Res. Commun. *180*, 1031–5 (1991).
33   Fishburn, C.S., Belleli, D., David, C., Carmon, S. and Fuchs, S.: J. Biol. Chem. *268*, 5872–8 (1993).
34   Van Tol, H.H.M., et al.: Nature *358*, 149–152 (1992).
35   Lichter, J.B., et al.: Hum. Mol. Genet. *2*, 767–73 (1993).
36   Livak, K.J., Rogers, J. and Lichter, J.B.: Proc. Natl. Acad. Sci. USA *92*, 427–431 (1995).
37   Hartman, D.S. and Civelli, O.: Ann. Med. *28*, 211–219 (1996).
38   Catalano, M., Nobile, M., Novelli, E., Nothen, M.M. and Smeraldi, E.: Biol. Psychiatry *34*, 459–64 (1993).
39   Barr, C.L., et al.: Am. J. Med. Genet. *48*, 218–22 (1993).
40   Campion, D., et al.: Psychiatry Res. *51*, 215–30 (1994).
41   Coon, H., et al.: Am. J. Hum. Genet. *52*, 327–34 (1993).
42   Macciardi, F., et al.: Arch. Gen. Psychiatry *51*, 288–93 (1994).
43   Shaikh, S., et al.: Am. J. Med. Genet. *54*, 8–11 (1994).
44   Sommer, S.S., Lind, T.J., Heston, L.L. and Sobell, J.L.: Am. J. Med. Genet. *48*, 90–3 (1993).
45   Nanko, S., et al.: Lancet *341*, 689–90 (1993).
46   Benjamin, J., et al.: Nature Genetics *12*, 81–84 (1996).
47   Ebstein, R.P., et al.: Nature Genetics *12*, 78–80 (1996).
48   Nothen, M.M., et al.: Hum. Mol. Genet. *3*, 2207–2212 (1994).
49   Di Bella, D., et al.: Psychiatr. Genet. *4*, 39–42 (1994).
50   Laurent, C., et al.: J. Med. Genet. *31* (1994).
51   Mant, R., et al.: Am. J. Med. Genet. *54*, 21–6 (1994).
52   Nimgaonkar, V.L., Zhang, X.R., Caldwell, J.G., Ganguli, R. and Chakravarti, A.: Am. J. Med. Genet. *48*, 214–7 (1993).
53   Nanko, S., Hattori, M., Ueki, A. and Ikeda, K.: Lancet *342* (1993).
54   Nothen, M.M., et al.: J. Med. Genet. *30*, 708–9 (1993).

55 Sabate, O., et al.: Am. J. Psychiatry *151*, 107–11 (1994).
56 Morel, R.T.: J. Med. Genet. *30*, 708–9 (1993).
57 Yang, L., et al.: Am. J. Med. Genet. *48*, 83–6 (1993).
58 Wiese, C., et al.: Psychiatry Res. *46*, 69–78 (1993).
59 Jonsson, E., Lannfelt, L., Sokoloff, P., Schwartz, J.C. and Sedvall, G.: Acta Psychiatr. Scand. *87*, 345–9 (1993).
60 Crocq, M.A., et al.: J. Med. Genet. *29*, 858–60 (1992).
61 Schmauss, C., Haroutunian, V., Davis, K.L. and Davidson, M.: Proc. Natl. Acad. Sci. USA *90*, 8942–6 (1993).
62 Civelli, O., Bunzow, J.R. and Grandy, D.K.: Ann. Rev. Pharmacol. Toxicol. *32*, 281–307 (1993).
63 Meadorwoodruff, J.H., et al.: Neuropsychopharmacol. *15*, 17–29 (1996).
64 Meador–Woodruff, J.H., et al.: Neuropsychopharm. *10*, 239–248 (1994).
65 Matsumoto, M., Hidaka, K., Tada, S., Tasaki, Y. and Yamaguchi, T.: Mol. Brain Res. *29*, 157–162 (1995).
66 Cohen, A.I., Todd, R.D., Harmon, S. and O'Malley, K.L.: Proc. Natl. Acad. Sci. USA *89*, 12093–7 (1992).
67 O'Malley, K.L., Harmon, S., Tang, L. and Todd, R.D.: New Biol. *4*, 137–46 (1992).
68 Mrzljak, L., et al.: Nature *381*, 245–248 (1996).
69 Bergson, C., Mrzljak, L., Lidow, M.S., Goldman-Rakic, P.S. and Levenson, R.: Proc. Natl. Acad. Sci. USA *92*, 3468–3472 (1995).
70 Senogles, S.E.: The Journal of Biological Chemistry *269*, 23120–23127 (1994).
71 Liu, Y.F., Civelli, O., Grandy, D.K. and Albert, P.R.: Journal of Neurochemistry *59*, 2311–2317 (1992).
72 Hayes, G., Biden, T.J., Selbie, L.A. and Shine, J.: Mol. Endocrinol. *6*, 920–6 (1992).
73 Neve, K.A., Kozlowski, M.R. and Rosser, M.P.: The Journal of Biological Chemistry *267*, 25748–25753 (1992).
74 Jackson, D.M. and Westlind-Danielsson, A.: Pharmac. Ther. *64*, 291–369 (1994).
75 Werner, P., Hussy, N., Buell, G., Jones, K.A. and North, R.A.: Mol. Pharmacol. *49*, 656–61 (1996).
76 Chio, C.L., Lajiness, M.E. and Huff, R.M.: Molecular Pharmacology *45*, 51–60 (1994).
77 Seabrook, G.R., et al.: British Journal of Pharmacology *111*, 391–393 (1994).
78 Pilon, C., et al.: European Journal of Pharmacology – Molecular Pharmacology Section *268*, 129–139 (1994).
79 Tang, L., Todd, R.D., Heller, A. and O'Malley, K.L.: J. Pharmacol. Exp. Ther. *268*, 495–502 (1994).
80 Chio, C.L., et al.: J. Biol. Chem. *269*, 11813–9 (1994).
81 McHale, M., et al.: Febs Lett. *345*, 147–50 (1994).
82 Mei, Y.A., et al.: Neurosci. *68*, 107–116 (1995).
83 Hillman, D.W., Lin, D. and Burnside, B.: J. Neurochem. *64*, 1326–1335 (1995).
84 Zawilska, J.B. and Nowak, J.Z.: Neurochem. Int. *24*, 275–80 (1994).
85 Offermanns, S. and Simon, M.I.: J. Biol. Chem. *270*, 15175–15180 (1995).
86 Frey, U., Huang, Y.-Y. and Kandel, E.R.: Science *260*, 1661–1664 (1993).
87 Surmeier, D.J., Bargas, J., Hemmings, J.H.C., Nairn, A.C. and Greengard, P.: Neuron *14*, 385–397 (1995).
88 Miner, L.L., Drago, J., Chamberlain, P.M., Donovan, D. and Uhl, G.R.: Neuroreport *6*, 2314–6 (1995).
89 Baik, J.H., et al.: Nature *377*, 424–8 (1995).
90 Accili, D., et al.: Proc. Natl. Acad. Sci. USA *93*, 1945–9 (1996).

91   Kane, J.M.: Journal of Clinical Psychiatry *50*, 322–328 (1989).
92   Cole, J.O., Goldberg, S.C. and Klerman, G.L.: Archives of General Psychiatry *10*, 246–261 (1966).
93   Davis, J.M., Schaffer, C.B., Killian, G.A. et al.: Schizophrenia Bulletin *6*, 70–87 (1980).
94   Ayd, F.R., Jr.: J. Amer. Med. Assoc. *175*, 1054–1060 (1961).
95   Jarvie, K.R., Tiberi, M., Silvia, C., Gingrich, J.A. and Caron, M.G.: Journal of Receptor Research *13*, 573–590 (1993).
96   Grandy, D.K., et al.: Proc. Natl. Acad. Sci. USA *88*, 9175–9179 (1991).
97   Sunahara, R.K., et al.: Nature *350*, 614–619 (1991).
98   Tiberi, M., et al.: Proc. Natl. Acad. Sci. USA *88*, 7491–7495 (1991).
99   Weinshank, R.L., et al.: The Journal of Biological Chemistry *266*, 22427–22435 (1991).
100   Lanau, F., Zenner, M.-T., Civelli, O. and Hartman, D.S.: J. Neurochem. *68*, 804–812 (1997).
101   Neve, K.A., Cox, B.A., Henningsen, R.A., Spanoyannis, A. and Neve, R.L.: Mol. Pharmacol. *39*, 733–9 (1991).
102   Mansour, A., et al.: Eur. J. Pharmacol. *227*, 205–214 (1992).
103   Fong, T.M. and Strader, C.D.: Med. Res. Rev. *14*, 387–399 (1994).
104   Woodward, R., Coley, C., Daniell, S., Naylor, L.H. and P.G., S.: J. Neurochem. *66*, 394–402 (1996).
105   Hartman, D.S., Monsma, F. and Civelli, O.: in: Handbook of Experimental Pharmacology (ed. Csernansky, J.G.) 43–75, Springer-Verlag, New York 1996.
106   Seeger, T.F., et al.: J. Pharmacol. Exp. Ther. *275*, 101–113 (1995).
107   Borison, R.L., Arvanitis, L.A., Miller, B.G. and Group, U.S.S.S.: J. Clin. Psychopharmacol. *16*, 158–169 (1995).
108   van Kammen, D.P., et al.: Psychopharmacol. *124*, 168–175 (1996).
109   Murray, A.M., et al.: J. Neurosci. *15*, 2186–2191 (1995).
110   Seeman, P., Guan, H.C. and Van Tol, H.: Nature *365*, 441–5 (1993).
111   Sumiyoshi, T., Stockmeier, C.A., Overholser, J.C., Thompson, P.A. and Meltzer, H.Y.: Brain Research *681*, 109–116 (1995).
112   Mills, A., et al.: FEBS *320*, 130–134 (1993).
113   Lahti, R.A., Evans, D.L., Stratman, N.C. and Figur, L.M.: Eur. J Pharm. *236*, 483–486 (1993).
114   Thurkauf, A., et al.: J. Med. Chem. *38*, 4950–2 (1995).
115   Kulagowski, I.J., et al.: J. Med. Chem. *39*, 1941–2 (1996).
116   Rowley, M., et al.: J. Med. Chem. *39*, 1943–5 (1996).
117   TenBrink, R.E., et al.: J. Med. Chem. *39*, 2435–7 (1996).
118   Wenk, G.L., Pierce, D.J., Struble, R.G., Price, D.L. and Cork, L.C.: Neurobiol. Aging *10*, 11–19 (1989).
119   Goldman-Rakic, P.S. and Brown, R.M.: Neurosci *6*, 177–187 (1981).
120   Arnsten, A.F.T., Cai, J.X., Steere, J.C. and Goldman-Rakic, P.S.: J. Neurosci. *15*, 3429–3439 (1995).
121   Davis, K.L., Kahn, R.S., Ko, G. and Davidson, M.: Am. J. Psychiatr. *148* (1991).
122   Wang, S., et al.: Nature Genetics *10*, 41–46 (1995).
123   Straub, R.E., et al.: Nature Genetics *11*, 287–293 (1995).
124   Schwab, S.G., et al.: Nature Genetics *11*, 325–327 (1995).
125   Moises, H.W., et al.: Nature Genetics *11*, 321–324 (1995).
126   Giros, B., Jaber, M., Jones, S.R., Wightman, R.M. and Caron, M.G.: Nature *379*, 606–21 (1996).

Progress in Drug Research, Vol. 48 (E. Jucker, Ed.)
© 1997 Birkhäuser Verlag, Basel (Switzerland)

Novel and unusual nucleosides as drugs

Vera M. Kolb

Department of Chemistry, University of Wisconsin-Parkside, Kenosha, WI 53141-2000, USA

1   Introduction

The most important function of nucleosides is that they are components of the nucleic acids. The latter represent the blue print of organisms and determine the biochemical processes and the ability to reproduce [1, 2]. Nucleosides are composed of a heterocyclic nitrogenous base linked typically to a pentose via a beta-N-glycosidic bond. The nucleoside bases are derivatives of purine, commonly adenine and guanine, and pyrimidine, commonly cytosine, thymine, and uracil. The pentose moiety is ribose in ribonucleosides, and deoxyribose in deoxyribonucleosides. Nucleotides are nucleoside derivatives in which pentose is phosphorylated, usually at the 5'-hydroxyl group [1, 2]. Figure 1 shows structures of common nucleosides which are the components of nucleic acids and thus are the basis of the genetic system.

Nucleosides and the corresponding nucleotides, either by themselves or in combination with other molecules, serve many functions in the organisms other than that of the nucleic acid constituents. Examples include catalysis, transfer of energy, mediation of hormone signals, regulatory function, blood pressure control, and coenzyme function, to name a few [1]. A number of nucleosides which have been isolated from microorganisms differ from those occurring as part of nucleic acids or nucleotide coenzymes [3, 4]. Many of these nucleosides have antibiotic properties [3, 4]. The structures of both their nucleobases and sugar moieties may vary. For example, the ribose or 2'-deoxyribose moieties may be replaced by 3'-deoxyribose, ketohexoses, D-arabinose, or 4- or 5-aminohexuronic sugars. The oxygen of the furanosyl ring may be replaced by a methylene group. The nucleobases may be modified to an S-triazine, a pyrrolopyrimidine, a pyrazolopyrimidine, a maleimide, or an isoguanine.

One cannot help but marvel at the structural complexity and diversity of these naturally occurring nucleosides. Several representative structures are shown in Figure 2.

The antibiotic activity of the naturally occurring nucleosides may be directed against bacteria, viruses, fungi, yeast, or neoplastic tissues, depending on their biochemical mode of action [3–5]. In search of new drugs, especially antivirals, chemists synthesized a large number of nucleoside analogs. Much of the early drug design [6] followed the usual path, that is the structures of the natural lead compounds were partially modified with intent to improve the activity. It is fascinating that several of these early designer drugs were subsequently found in nature [6]. Examples include arabinoadenosine (Ara-A), 2'-amino-2'-deoxyadenosine (2'-

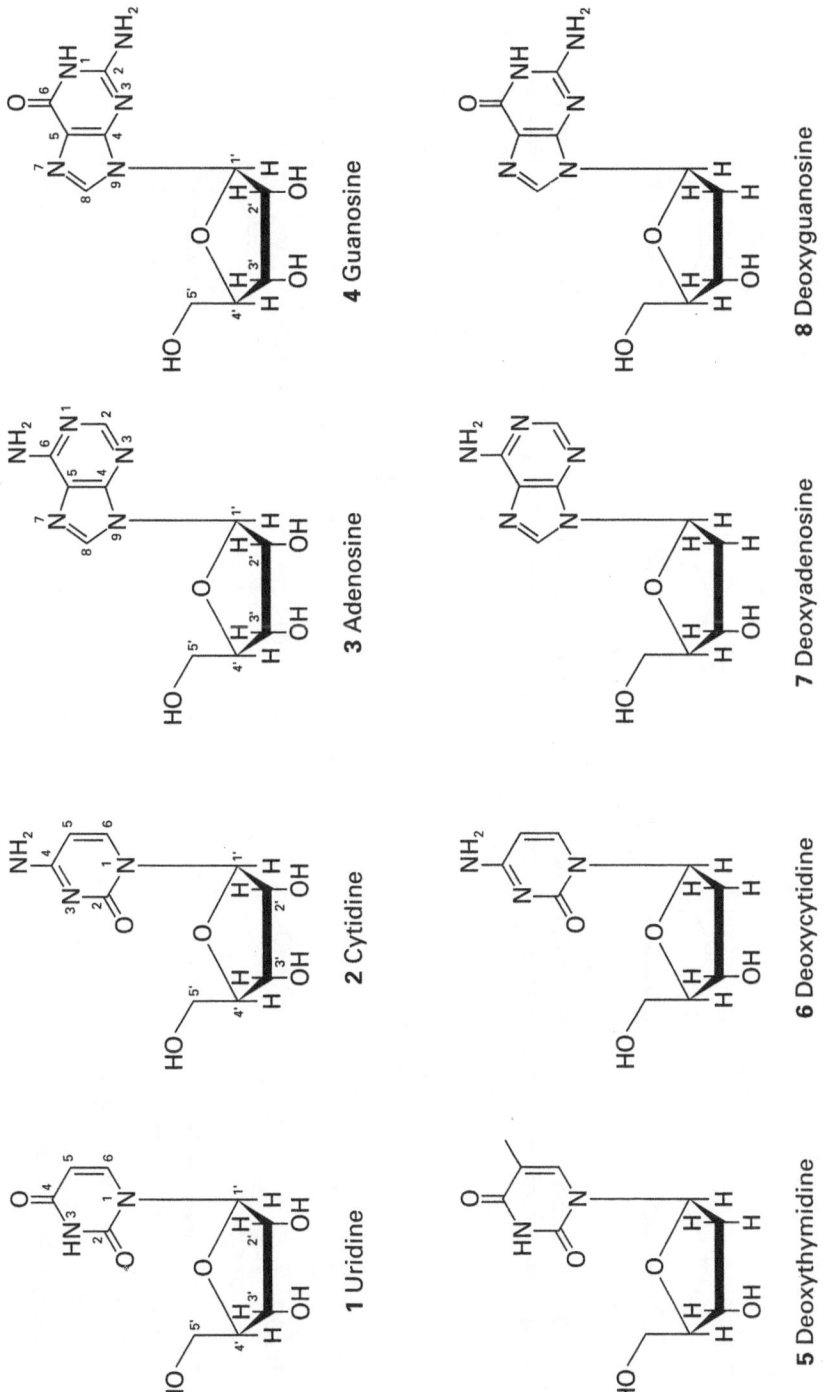

Fig. 1
Structures of common nucleosides which are the basis of the genetic system.

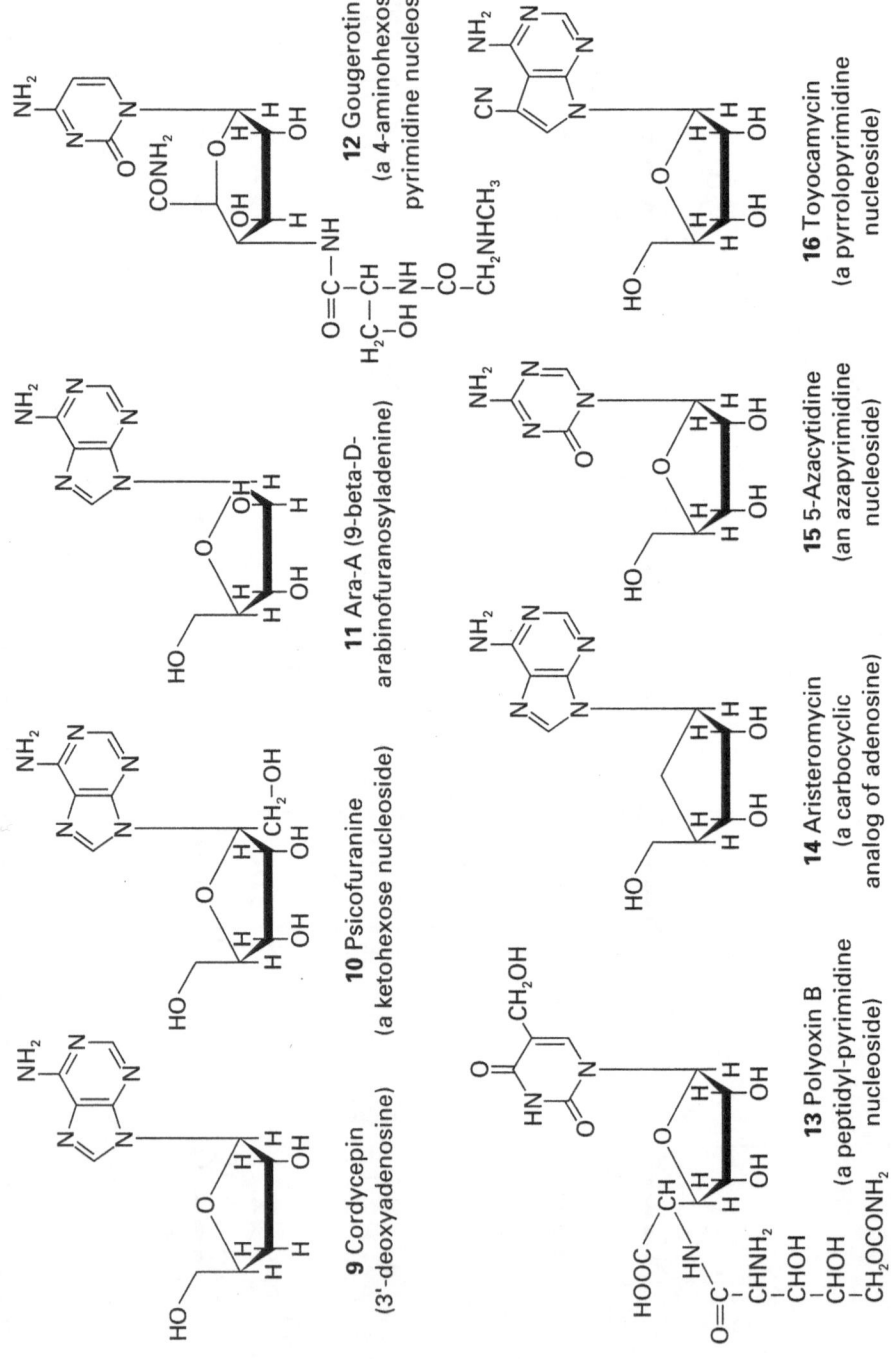

9 Cordycepin
(3'-deoxyadenosine)

10 Psicofuranine
(a ketohexose nucleoside)

11 Ara-A (9-beta-D-
arabinofuranosyladenine)

12 Gougerotin
(a **4**-aminohexose
pyrimidine nucleoside)

13 Polyoxin B
(a peptidyl-pyrimidine
nucleoside)

14 Aristeromycin
(a carbocyclic
analog of adenosine)

15 5-Azacytidine
(an azapyrimidine
nucleoside)

16 Toyocamycin
(a pyrrolopyrimidine
nucleoside)

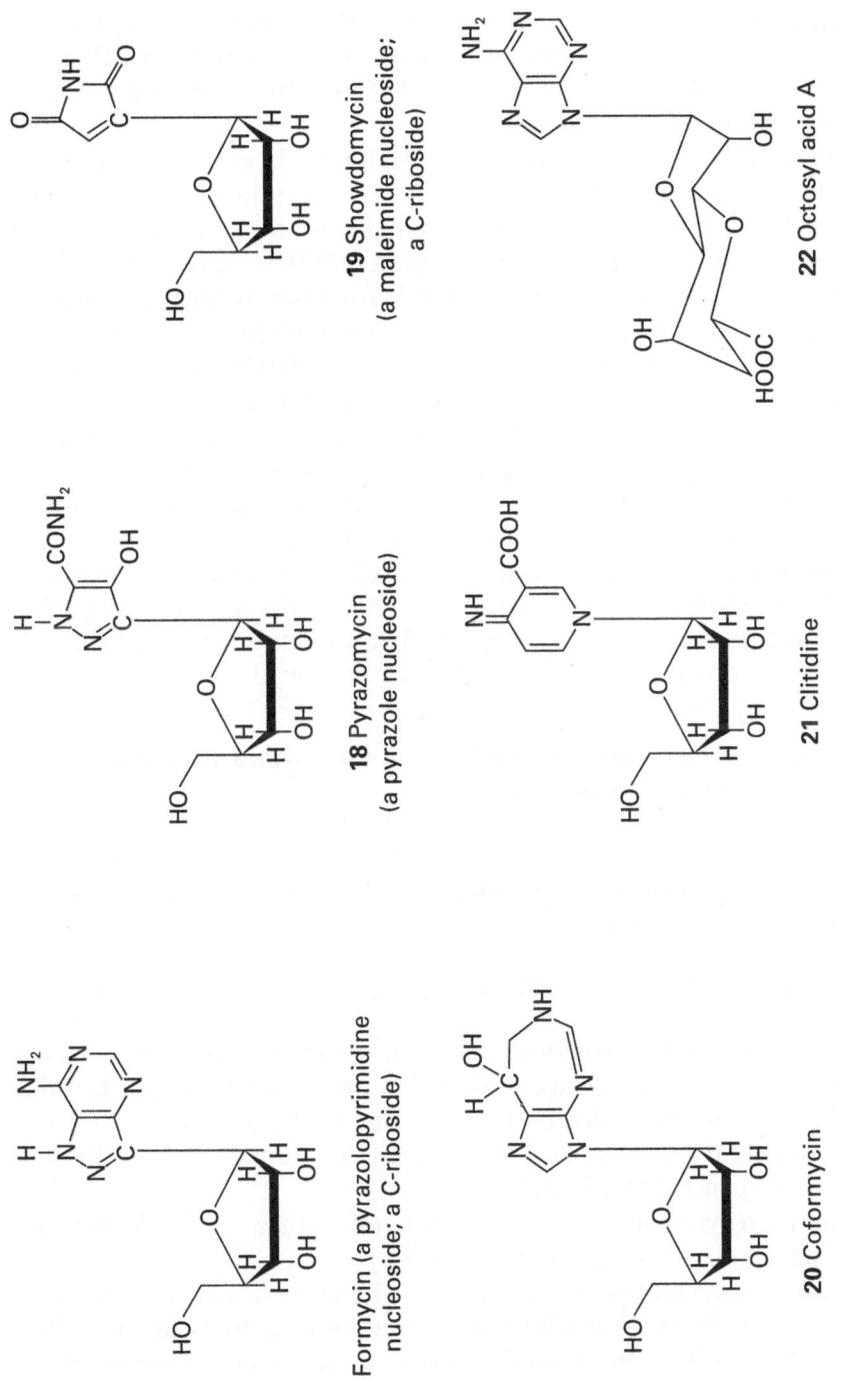

17 Formycin (a pyrazolopyrimidine nucleoside; a C-riboside)

18 Pyrazomycin (a pyrazole nucleoside)

19 Showdomycin (a maleimide nucleoside; a C-riboside)

20 Coformycin

21 Clitidine

22 Octosyl acid A

Fig. 2
Structures of some naturally occurring nucleoside antibiotics.

ADA), aristeromycin, and 5-azacytidine [6]. The cleverness of nature can be appreciated on the example of aristeromycin (compound 14), a carbocyclic analog of adenosine which was designed by chemists as a hydrolytically resistant adenosine analog.

Most of the efforts in nucleoside drug design have been directed towards antivirals. Thus, our review concentrates mostly on these drugs. The pre- and early-1980's era focused on the design of nucleosides to combat DNA viruses, such as herpes simplex virus type 1 (HSV-1) or type 2 (HSV-2), and RNA viruses, such as those responsible for major respiratory diseases in humans [7]. In the early- to mid-1980's an epidemic of a devastating disease, acquired immunodeficiency syndrome (AIDS), and the discovery of human immunodeficiency virus (HIV) as its cause, posed new challenges in the design of antivirals. The HIV belongs to the class of retroviruses, whose mode of action required new strategies for drug design [8]. These discoveries further stimulated research on nucleosides as antivirals, which continues strongly to the present time.

In this review we focus on recent nucleosides reported as antivirals or potential antivirals, whose structures we consider novel and unusual as compared to the structures of established natural or synthetic nucleoside antivirals. The established drugs are briefly reviewed in the next section.

2   Selected examples of established natural and synthetic antiviral nucleoside drugs

The structures of several established antiviral nucleoside drugs are shown in Figure 3. These drugs are grouped according to their activity against DNA, RNA, or retroviruses.

2.1   Drugs active against DNA viruses

IDU, iododeoxyuridine (structure 23, Fig. 3), was the first clinically effective antiviral [9]. It was used to treat corneal infection of humans, herpes keratitis. BVDU, a bromovinyl analog of deoxyuridine (structure 24, Fig. 3), is recognized mainly for its activity against HSV-1 in animals and against varicella-zoster virus (VZV) in children [7, 10, 11].

FIAC, an iodo cytosine fluoroarabinoside (structure 25, Fig. 3), is active against VZV and cytomegalovirus (CMV) [7, 10, 11].

Ara-A, an adenine arabinoside (structure 11, Fig. 2), was licensed for therapy of systemic herpes virus infections. It exhibits activity against HSV-1, HSV-2, VZV, CMV, and Epstein-Barr virus (EBV) [7]. Poor solubility of Ara-A in aqueous solution limits its use [7, 11].

Acyclovir, an acyclic guanosine analog (structure 26, Fig. 3), is a highly potent drug active specifically against HSV-1 and HSV-2 in humans [7, 10, 11]. Its common use is for genital herpes infections [7, 10]. This drug is proven to be prophilactically effective against HSV infection [12]. DHPG, or gancyclovir, is an analog of acyclovir (structure 27, Fig. 3). It is more soluble than acyclovir and has greater bioavailability and also enhanced *in vivo* activity [7, 10, 11]. DHPG is used for treatment of patients with CMV [12]. DHPG cyclic phosphate is water soluble and has a broad spectrum of activity against DNA viruses.

2.2   Drugs active against RNA viruses

Ribavirin, a ribofuranosyltriazolecarboxamide (Structure 28, Fig. 3), is a broad spectrum antiviral active against both RNA and DNA viruses [7, 10–12]. Naturally occurring carbocyclic nucleosides aristeromycin (structure 14, Fig. 2) and neplanocin A (structure 29, Fig. 3) are described as potent antivirals [10–12]. 3-Deaza analogs of compounds 14 and 29, as well as of adenosine (structure 3, Fig. 1), are also useful antivirals [10, 11].

2.3   Drugs active against retroviruses

A number of nucleosides having a 2', 3'-dideoxyribose moiety are effective antivirals against HIV [8, 13, 14]. Examples are AZT, an azidodideoxythymidine (structure 30, Fig. 3), which was the first drug effective against AIDS [15], ddC, a dideoxycytidine (structure 31, Fig. 3), ddI, a dideoxyinosine (structure 32, Fig. 3)[8, 13, 14, 16], and 3TC, a dideoxythiacytidine (structure 33, Fig. 3)[14, 16].

3   Selected strategies for design of nucleoside drugs

3.1   Prodrugs, combination drugs, and hybrid drugs

In this section we give selected examples of both antiviral and antitumor drugs based on recognized nucleosides or nucleobases as their key active components. The latter are creatively modified, combined and/or packaged for enhanced performance.

Let us start with an interesting design of a double prodrug from Menger's laboratory [17]. The drug is composed of two cytotoxic drugs, Ara-C and 5-fluorouracil (5-FU), which are joined by a short hydrolyzable linker, by an amide bond at NH2 of Ara-C, and an acyloxymethylene at N-1 of 5-FU (structure 34, Fig. 4). The amine acylation at Ara-C usually decreases

25 FIAC (2'-fluoro-5-iodo-1-beta-D-arabinofuranosylcytosine)

28 Ribavirin (1-beta-furanosyl-1,2,4-triazole-3-carboxamide)

24 BVDU (E-5(2-bromovinyl)-2'-deoxyuridine)

27 DHPG (9-(1,3-dihydroxy-2-propoxymethyl)guanine)

23 IDU (Idoxuridine, 2'-deoxy-5-iodouridine)

26 Acyclovir (9-(2-hydroxyethoxymethyl)guanine)

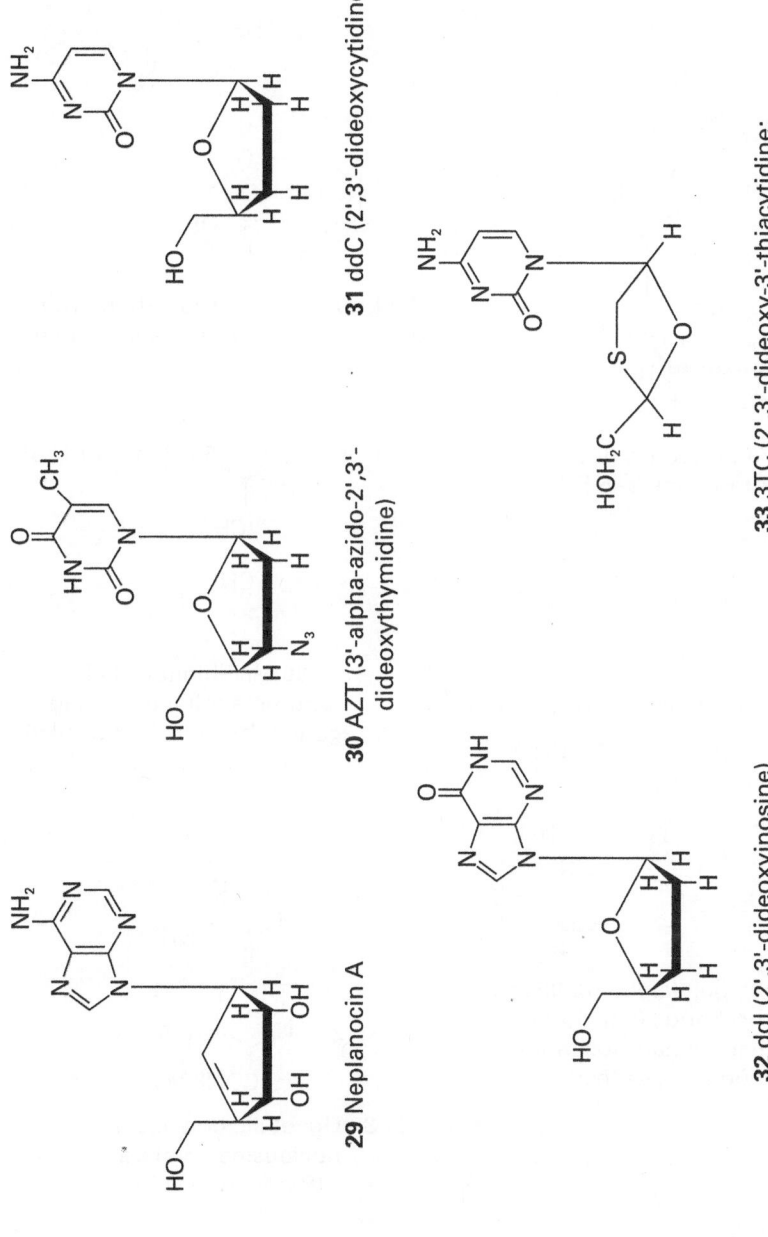

Fig. 3
Structures of some established antiviral nucleoside drugs.

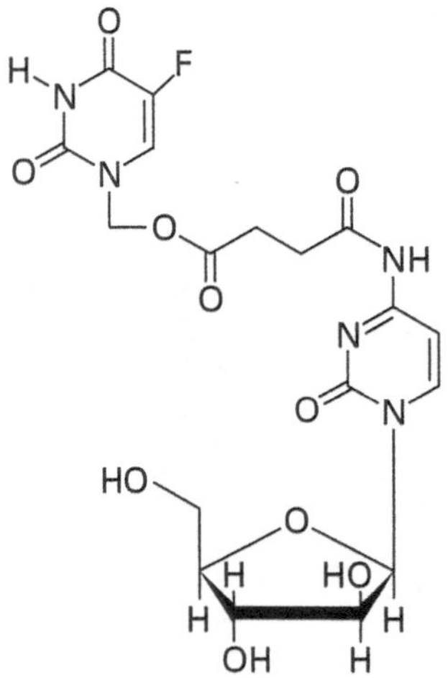

34 Menger and Rourk's double prodrug (Ara-C -linker- 5-FU)

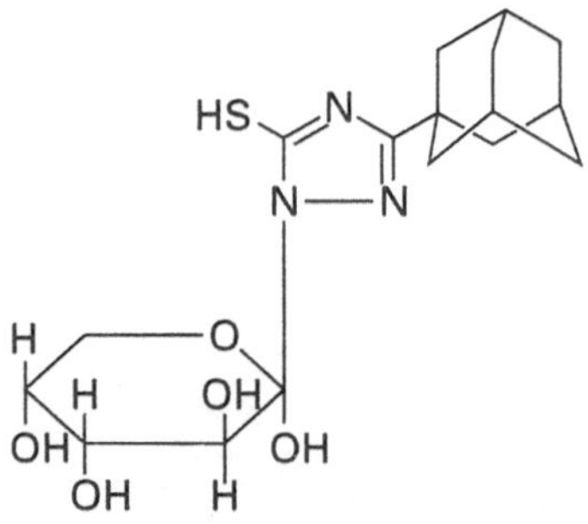

35 Ertan et al., combination drug (Ara-mercaptotriazole – Adamantane)

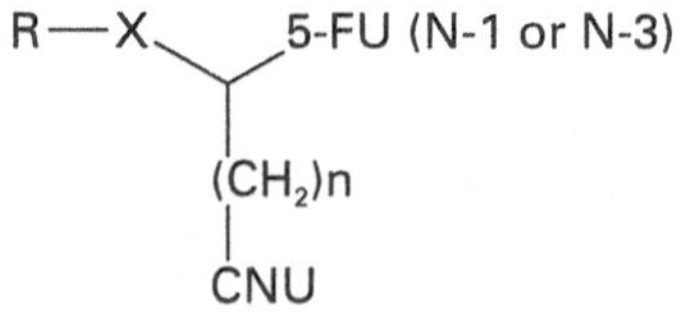

R—X   5-FU (N-1 or N-3)

$(CH_2)n$

CNU

36 McElhinney et al., antimetabolite-alkylating agent hybrids (R= small alkyl group; X= O,S; n=1,2)

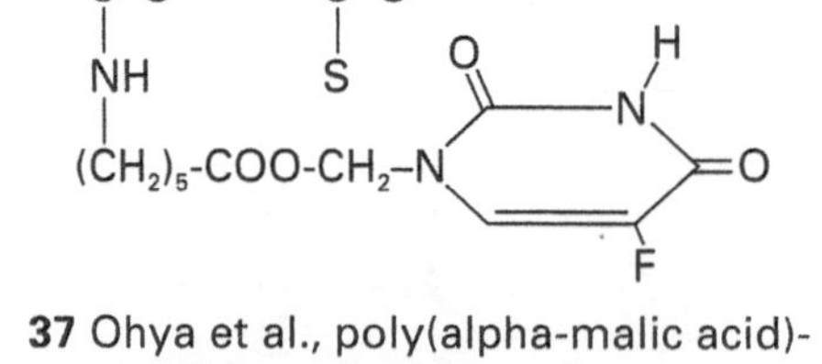

$-(OCHCO)x-(OCHCO)y-(OCHCO)1-x-y$

CH_2 CH_2 CH_2COOH

C=O   C=O

NH   S

$(CH_2)_5$-COO-CH_2-N

37 Ohya et al., poly(alpha-malic acid)-5-FU-saccharide conjugate (S=saccharide: galactosamine and others, see text)

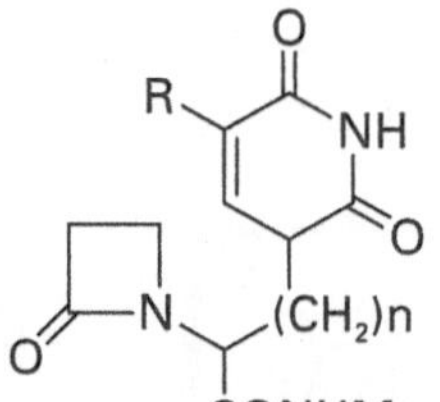

38 Ugi et al., beta-lactam-nucleoside chimera (R=Me, H; n=1,2)

CONHMe

$(CH_2)n$

Fig. 4
Structures of some prodrugs, combination drugs, and hybrid drugs, discussed in the text.

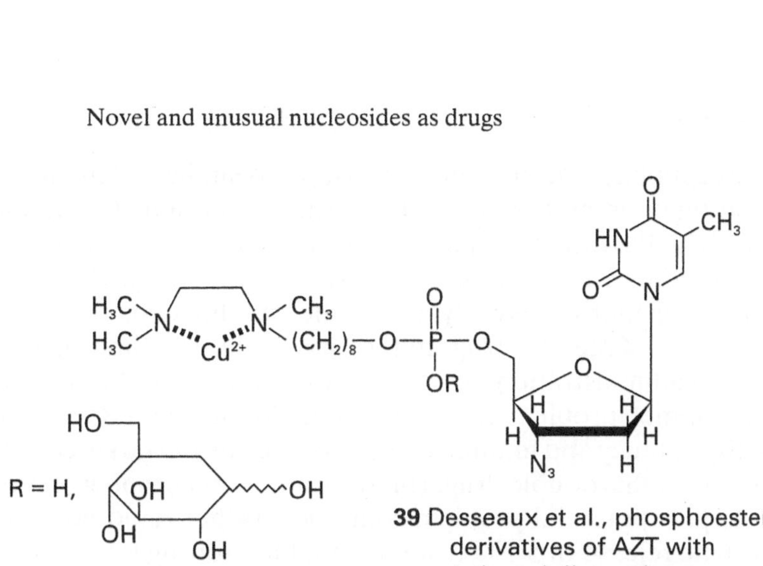

39 Desseaux et al., phosphoester derivatives of AZT with tethered ribonucleases

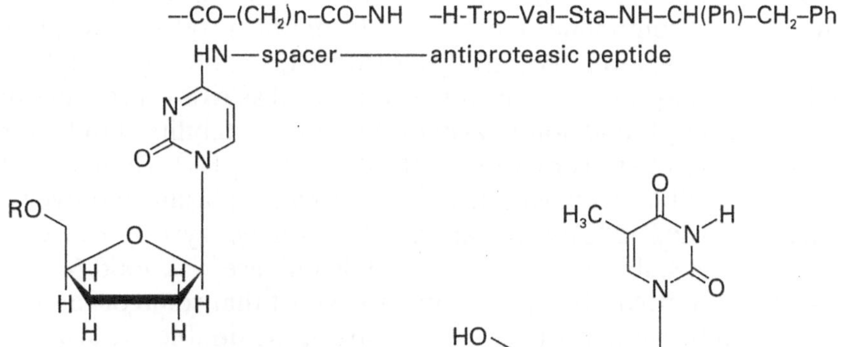

$-CO-(CH_2)n-CO-NH$ $-H-Trp-Val-Sta-NH-CH(Ph)-CH_2-Ph$

HN—spacer————antiproteasic peptide

40 Kraus et al., peptide-nucleoside conjugate (n=2-6; R=H, TBDPS)

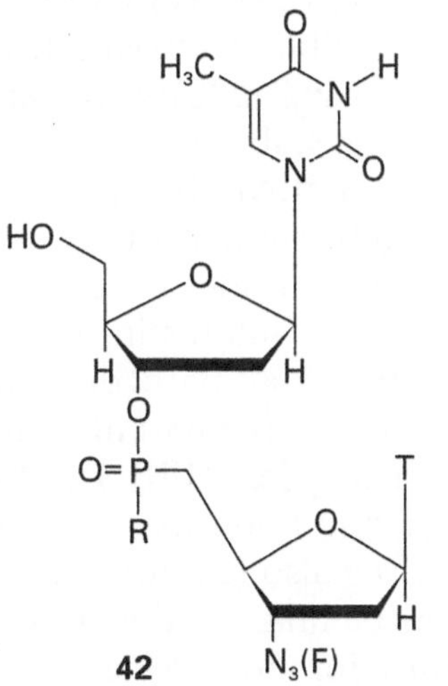

42 $N_3(F)$

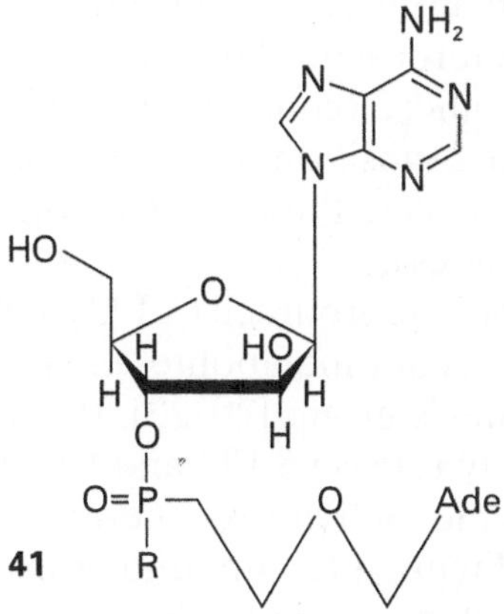

41 R

41,42 Hakimelahi et al., dinucleotide phosphonoamidates;
41 : R=OH, MeO$_2$CMeCHNH–, L;
42: R=OH, MeO$_2$CMeCHNH– L and D
T=thymine

Fig. 4 continued

the drug's susceptibility to deactivation by cytidine deaminase. This imparts an additional function on the linker. This drug was designed as an anti-cancer agent, with the rationale that it will be more effective than the two separate drugs administered simultaneously or sequentially. The former administering does not necessarily assure the simultaneous delivery of the equal amounts of the two drugs to the target cells. The time lag in the sequential drug administration may lead to the development of the drug resistance, a common problem in cancer therapy. Menger and Rourk hope to improve the potency and minimize the resistance by the targeted delivery of their more lethal double drug. This drug is now undergoing pharmaceutical testing. A potential problem could be a rather rapid non-enzymatic hydrolytic release of 5-FU from the double prodrug ($t1/2 = 9$ min, at pH 7, at 25 deg.). However, the amide bond to Ara-C is very stable to non-enzymatic degradation at pH 7. The latter result was also confirmed on a series of compounds identical to the double prodrug, except that the 5-FU unit is substituted by groups R (Me, Et, n-propyl, n-pentyl, n-octyl) or benzyl. These compounds were synthesized as Ara-C prodrugs by Fadl et al.[18]. They found non-enzymatic hydrolytic stability at pH 7, but high susceptibility towards hydrolysis (to Ara-C) at pH 2. Their compounds were susceptible to enzymatic hydrolysis by rat plasma and liver homogenate showing half lives from 0.14 hrs (for benzyl) to 4.19 days (for methyl). The stability against cytidine deaminase was good (e.g. t 1/2 of 9.45 days for ethyl). It is reasonable to expect that some of these kinetic values will be similar for the Ara-C part of the double prodrug of Menger and Rourk (vide supra).

A conceptually interesting design of a combination drug was reported by Ertan [19]. This antiviral drug, effective against poliovirus, is a composite of adamantane, the parent compound of adamantine, a recognized anti-influenza drug (e.g. [14]), 1, 2, 4-triazole, the heterocyclic core of the antiviral ribavirin (vide supra), and the sugar arabinose (compound 35, Fig. 4). The drug also features a thio moiety on the 5-position of the triazole ring, which enhances the activity. The arabinose is in the pyranose form (vide infra for more designs of pyranonucleosides).

A series of papers on hybrid drugs composed of 5-fluorouracil (5-FU) and N-(2-chloroethyl)-N-nitrosourea (CNU), namely antimetabolite-alkylating agent hybrids, was reported by McElhinney's group [20–22]. It was hoped that these hybrid drugs would gradually release 5-FU and CNU, both of which would contribute towards antitumor activity. A general formula of one series of such drugs is shown in Figure 4 (compound 36). 5-FU was linked either via N-1 as in natural nucleosides or via N-3. Seco-nucleoside moiety was an open-chain sugar rather than a normal cyclic.

At the carbon which would correspond to C-1' in normal nucleosides an alkyl chain of varying lengths was attached which terminated with CNU. Numerous other variations of this general structure were introduced, some having 5-FU (N-1), 5-FU (N-3) and CNU, and some having 5-FU in the position which would correspond to C-5' of the normal nucleosides. Many of the compounds from this series were potent antitumor agents, much more than what one would expect from the CNU and 5-FU moieties alone. Interestingly, studies showed that in most of these compounds, the 5-FU moiety is not likely to be released at physiological pH at a rate sufficient to contribute significantly to the antitumor activity. (Note that this problem is opposite to that of Menger and Rourk's compound 34 discussed above, in which 5-FU was released almost too fast). This would suggest that these drugs act primarily as alkylating agents, which, however, have particularly effective carriers. Additional role(s) of 5-FU unit are not fully elucidated.

A conceptually similar design was reported by Zhou et al. [23] in which polyphosphate polymers were prepared containing both 5-FU and nitrogen mustard. These polymers were water soluble and exhibited low toxicity and high anti-tumor activity. Other nucleic acid bases were also used, again in conjunction with nitrogen mustard.

An interesting polymer design for delivery of 5-FU was reported by Ohya et al. [24]. They designed poly (alpha-malic acid)-5-FU saccharide conjugate as a biodegradable and bioresorbable prodrug of 5-FU (Figure 4, structure 37). Poly(malic acid) was chosen since it is bioresorbable and can be chemically modified. 5-FU and different saccharides were attached to this poly-acid as shown in structure 37. The saccharides used were galactosamine, glucosamine, N-acetyl-D-glucosamine, mannose, and mannosamine. The idea behind the saccharide choice was to establish if the drug can target specifically the hepatoma cells (malignant liver cells), which are known to possess galactose receptors. The conjugate drug was a success. Indeed, the galactosamine conjugate had specific affinity for hepatoma cells. In addition, the chemical linkages of 5-FU to the polymer carrier were well chosen since the release of 5-FU had favorable kinetics (ca. 30% within 24 hrs) and produced only 5-FU and no other derivatives. Moreover, both acute toxicity and side effects of 5-FU were diminished when 5-FU was delivered as the polymer conjugate.

Ugi et al. reported a hybrid drug composed of a beta-lactam antibiotic and a nucleoside (compound 38, Fig. 4)[25]. This beta-lactam-nucleoside chimera, as the authors call it, is now being screened for antiviral and antibacterial activity. The hope is that this dual action drug will yield a new drug.

Hybrids between AZT (compound 30) and steroids were prepared as pro-drugs [26]. They were steroidal carboxylic esters, prepared from steroidal 17-beta-carboxylic acids and AZT, or alkyl steroidal phosphotriesters of AZT. The former showed anti -HIV activity comparable to AZT, while the latter were less active. Hybrids between cordycepin (compound 9) and lipids or vitamins E, D2, and A, were prepared via succinate or carbonate linkages [27]. These hybrids inhibited HIV-1 reverse transcriptase (RT) activity in 28–49% as compared to a 13% inhibition by cordycepin. There are several very recent reports of nucleoside-lipid hybrids which are promising. Coupling of hexadecylphosphonic acid and ara-cytidine monophosphate morpholide (morpholine-N, N'-dicyclohexylcarbox-amidine) salt gave a nucleoside-lipid adduct with cytostatic activity against human mammary cells [28]. Antitumor phospholipids with 5-FU as a cyto-toxic polar head were prepared [29]. These compounds have the same backbone structure as that of natural phospholipids, but the polar head group of usual phospholipids is replaced by 5-FU. These compounds had antitumor activity against both P388 leukemia and Meth A fibrosarcoma in mice.

Ether lipid-nucleoside hybrids were prepared as anti HIV -1 agents [30]. An example of such structure is 3'-azido-3'deoxythymidine-5'-monophos-phatoxypropane. Lipophilic nucleosides were prepared from uridine via either a 2'-O-hexylamino linker or the corresponding 3'-group [31]. These compounds were used for site-specific lipophilization of antisense oligo-nucleotides.

Lipophilic anti-HIV drugs were designed especially for the treatment of HIV in the central nervous system (CNS) [32, 33]. The drug design involved synthesis of molecules with increased lipophilicities which would enable them to pass the blood-brain barrier. These compounds were analogs of ddI (compound 32), or ddA, which had groups such as 6-halo, -alkoxy-, alkylamino, and -methoxyamino, as well as 2'-beta-F as substituent. The latter imparted stability towards acid-catalyzed cleavage of the glycosidic bond. Among the compounds with anti-HIV activity many were more lip-ophilic than ddI or F-ddI, e.g. 6- and 60-fold for 6-Cl and 6-OEt groups, respectively, and 100-fold for the ethylamino and dimethylamino groups. These new drugs were prodrugs of F-ddI or F-ddA which were activated by adenosine deaminase.

Prodrugs of AZT with potential RNase activity were reported [34]. These prodrugs were phosphate ester derivatives of AZT with tethered N,N,N'-trimethylethylenediamine (TMED), N-methylpiperazine, and 2,6-diacetyl pyridine (structure 39, Fig. 4). The metal complexes of these compounds were expected to combine a RT inhibition and the ability to hydrolyze the RNA of HIV. The antiviral activity of these drugs is caused by the AZT moiety, and the Cu(II) has RNase activity. The preliminary anti-HIV *in vitro* assays on Cu(II)-TMED drugs did not show enhancement of the RNA hydrolytic activity in comparison with CuCl2 alone. However, the planned *in vivo* testing could provide more encouraging results, since these Cu(II) drugs are expected to introduce Cu(II) ion inside the cells, where it can effect hydrolysis of RNA of HIV. This would not be possible with the plain CuCl2, since it cannot cross lipophilic membranes.

A series of papers appeared very recently also on hybrids between nucleosides and amino acids or peptides. Peptide-nucleoside hybrids were designed which consisted of an anti-RT nucleoside and an anti-protease peptide [35] (compound 40, Fig. 4). The authors first briefly review synergistic effects that have been reported previously for a combination of nucleoside drugs and antiprotease peptides, and then they offer their own new design. The nucleoside component of the new hybrid drug was ddC (compound 31). The peptide moiety featured various residues which mimic the transition state during HIV-protease hydrolysis. This peptide was found in a separate study to be a potent inhibitor of HIV-protease *in vitro*, and was also active against HIV-replication in cell cultures. The peptide moiety was hooked to ddC as shown in Fig. 4, compound 40. The 5'-OH group of ddC component was either free or substituted with tert-butyldiphenyl silyl group (TBDPS). The antiviral activity of these ddC-peptide hybrids was found to be lower than the component pieces, which was a disappointment. However, an interesting observation was made, that the silylated hybrids (5'-TBDPS) had activity very similar to that of the 5'-OH compounds. These results were surprising, since previous studies showed that the substitution at 5' (by ester or silylated groups) is detrimental for the anti-HIV activity. The reason is that the RT inhibition requires enzymatic phosphorylation of the 5'-OH group. While the mode of action of these hybrid drugs is not known, it was suggested that a possible interaction of these compounds at a non-substrate binding site of the RT could occur, based on an analogy with the action of the drug TSAO (vide infra), which also has the 5'-OH silylated.

Amino acid derivatives of nucleoside drugs have been prepared to improve their water solubility. Some examples include amino acid derivatizations of 5-fluoro-2'-deoxyuridine [36] to yield potent antitumor drugs, and 3'-amino-2',3'-dideoxycytidine [37] to give its chymotrypsin-activated pro-drugs which were potent antileukemic agents *in vivo*.

We chose to highlight here an interesting design in which esters of D- or L-amino acids were incorporated into dinucleotide phophonates [38]. The dimer of two different nucleotides was constructed first, by using a phosphonate linkage (structures 41, 42, Fig. 4). The expectation was that a lower dosage of two drugs in a dimeric form would be required to improve their efficacy in comparison with an individual drug applied alone. When dinucleotide phosphonates showed moderate antiviral activity, the latter was ascribed to their inefficient transport through cell membranes. To improve lipophilicity, phosphonoamidate derivatives were prepared possessing methyl L- or D-alanine moieties. These derivatives showed excellent antiviral activities. Interestingly, the dinucleotide phosphonamidates bearing a D-amino ester group showed less cellular toxicity than those carrying an L-amino ester moiety (structure 42, Fig. 4).

3.2   Nucleosides containing unusual elements

In this section we briefly review the newest work on nucleosides which incorporate B, Se, As, and Si.

Schinazi et al. reported preparation of carboranyl-containing nucleosides and their use in treatment of urogenital cancer [39, 40]. The design is to make boron-containing drugs which are sufficiently lipophilic to pass through the appropriate urogenital membrane and achieve concentrations high enough for successful boron neutron capture therapy (BNCT). The latter is based on the property of non-radioactive boron-10 nuclei to absorb low energy neutrons, and then release alpha particles and lithium-7 nuclei via a nuclear reaction which produces about 100 million times more energy than what was initially used.

If concentration of boron inside the tumor cells is high enough the BNCT will destroy such cells. For successful therapy a sufficient number of alpha-particles must be generated inside the cell to overwhelm the cellular DNA repair capacity. Quantitative studies have been done to estimate the concentration of carboranyl units, each of which being a cluster of 10 boron atoms, required to produce a lethal BNC reaction. A plateau is reached when there are two carboranyls per carrier molecule [40]. Examples of successful carboranyl nucleoside drugs are 5-carboranyl-2'-deoxyuridine (CDU) (compound 43, Fig. 5), and 5-O-carboranyl-1-(2'-deoxy-2'-fluoro-beta-D-arabinofuranosyl) uracil (CFAU). CDU was localized in the prostate tumor in 11 times higher concentrations than in the brain and in 2-3 fold higher levels than in serum [39]. Carboranyl oligonucleotides have also been prepared for antisense/antigene oligonucleotide therapy (AOT) of cancer and viral infections, and as molecular probes for diagnosis of genetic diseases [39].

Cyanoboryl nucleosides, such as compound 44, Fig. 5, were reported [41, 42]. Boronation was also performed on the phosphate group of nucleo-

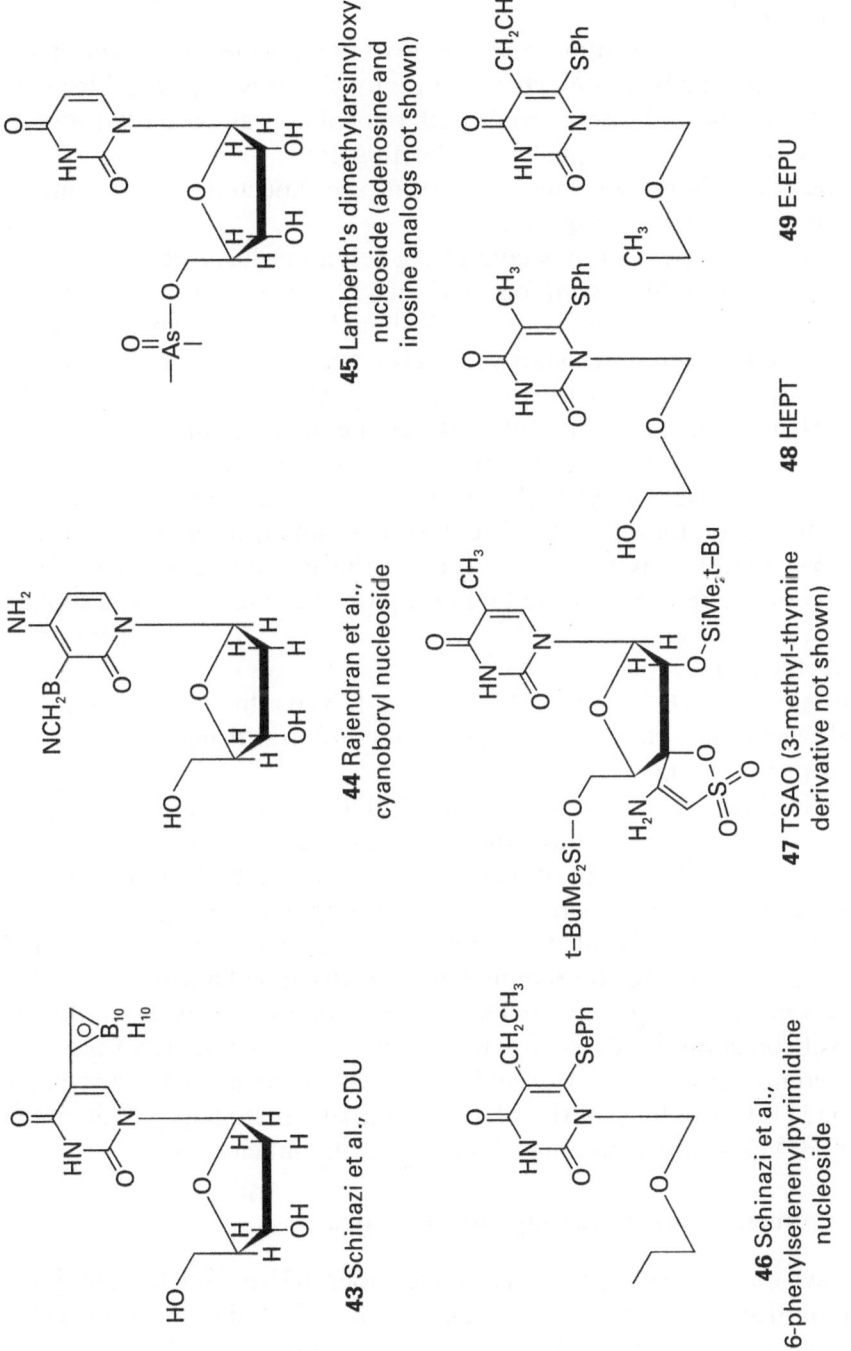

Fig. 5
Structures of some nucleosides containing unusual elements.

tides. Such compounds possess anti-inflammatory, anti-osteoporotic, and analgesic activities.

The first synthesis of 5'-dimethylarsinyloxy nucleosides (compound 45, Fig. 5) was reported by Lamberth [43]. Previously known nucleoside arsenates are isosteric and isoelectronic with phosphates and are tolerated in enzymatic reactions in its place. Lamberth's new 5'-dimethylarsinyloxy derivatives of uridine, adenosine, and inosine are expected to possess interesting pharmacological properties.

Anti-HIV acyclic pyrimidines containing selenium have been reported by Schinazi's group [44] (compound 46, Fig. 5). The design was to have a 6-phenylselenenyl group, which, like a 6-phenylthio group, when incorporated in acyclic pyrimidines, shows anti HIV activity. The new addition to the design was to substitute the primary hydroxyl group in the acyclic side chain with hydrogen. The rationale was that the presence of the OH group is not necessary for antiviral activity, since the previously made 6-phenylthio and 6-phenylselenenyl nucleosides did not require phosphorylation in order to exhibit their anti-HIV activity. The substitution of OH with H may impart better antiviral activity. Indeed, the activity was improved (or retained) by the removal of the OH group on the side chain. The 6-phenylselenenyl drugs have their spectrum of activity different from drug HEPT (vide infra).

Synthesis of novel D-1, 3-dioxolane and L-1, 3-oxathiolane 5-phenylselenenylpyrimidine nucleosides as potential antiviral drugs has been recently reported [45].

Drugs TSAO (compound 47, Fig. 5) and HEPT (compound 48, Fig. 5) [14] represent classes of compounds which contain structural elements in common with nucleosides, but they exert their anti-HIV activity as non-nucleoside RT inhibitors. HEPT analog E-EPU (compound 49, Fig. 5), in which the primary hydroxyl is substituted by H, is especially promising (compare a similar design for 6-selenenyl analogs discussed above).

The presence of silyl groups in TSAO is just one of many examples of organosilicon compounds as antiviral drugs. Recently the use of organosilicon compounds in the rational design of antiviral drugs has been described [46], including a series of nucleoside sila-analogs as potent inhibitors of HIV RT, and as mimics of antisense oligonucleotides.

3.3   ·   Nucleosides containing different sugars

Furanosyl arabino-, xylo-, and lyxo- nucleosides [47] and nucleotides [48], both natural and synthetic, have been known for a long time. Marine nucleosides and their analogs possessing 2'-deoxyribo-, arabino-, xylo-, and rhamno-moieties have been reviewed very recently [49]. Mashida and Sakata reviewed 5-substituted ara-uracil nucleosides as anti herpes virus agents [50]. Fucosylated nucleoside derivatives have been patented as excitatory amino acid antagonists [51]. A very recent patent on lyxofuranosyl analogs of adenosine which selectively inhibit adenosine kinase appeared [52].

A systematic study of beta vs. alpha xylofuranosyl nucleosides including their biological evaluation was published [53]. Mikhailov et al. studied disaccharide nucleosides [54]. Interest in such compounds exists because several nucleoside antibiotics, such as amicetin and tunicamycins, have disaccharide units, as do some modified nucleosides in t-RNA. Ribosylated pyrimidine 2'-deoxynucleosides reported in ref. 54 (structures 50, 51, Fig. 6), were found, however, to be inactive against a number of viruses.

3.4 Pyranosyl nucleosides

3.4.1 Introduction, statement of the problem and the early studies

A number of nucleosides which possess a pyranosyl carbohydrate moiety have been known for a long time [3–6]. Examples include antibiotics gougerotin, blasticidin, amicetin, hikizimycin, mildiomycin, and neosidomycin. In addition to antimicrobial activities, antifungal, anthelmintic, antitumor, and antiviral activities have also been observed for some of such compounds.

It was not until the mid 1980's that the first systematic study of pyranosyl nucleosides was reported (Nord, 1985 [55]; Nord et al., 1987 [56]). A series of 2'-deoxy-D-ribo-hexopyranosyl nucleoside and nucleotide analogs of adenosine, inosine, guanosine, cytidine, and uridine were prepared, and used as probes for the structural requirements of selected nucleic acid metabolizing enzymes. In addition, the compounds were evaluated for antiviral and antitumor activities. The rationale behind choosing 2'-deoxy-D-ribo-hexopyranosides (structure 52, Fig. 6) was as follows. This type of nucleoside has the capability of mimicking either the 2'-deoxyribonucleosides found in DNA via their 2'-deoxy moiety, or the ribonucleotides found in RNA by virtue of their 3', 4'-alpha-dihydroxy grouping, which could assume the role of cis-2', 3'-ribo-hydroxyls. In addition, the corresponding 6'-triphosphate analogs would have 6',4'- or 6',3'- centers available for incorporation into nucleic acids.

These compounds indeed served as useful probes for the objectives as they have been set. For example, two 2'-deoxyribohexopyranosyl purines, 6-amino and 2, 6-diamino, were substrates for adenosine deaminase, thus dispelling the previously held belief that this enzyme has little bulk tolerance for a carbohydrate larger than the ribofuranose ring. However,

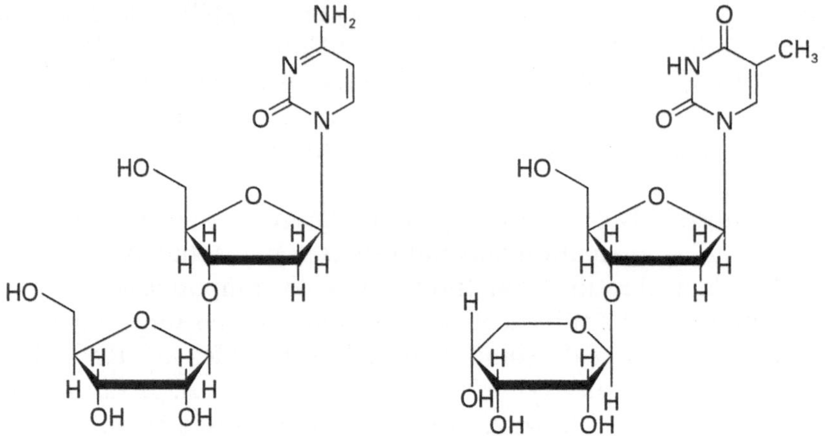

50,51 Mikhailov et al., ribosylated pyrimidine
2'-deoxynucleosides

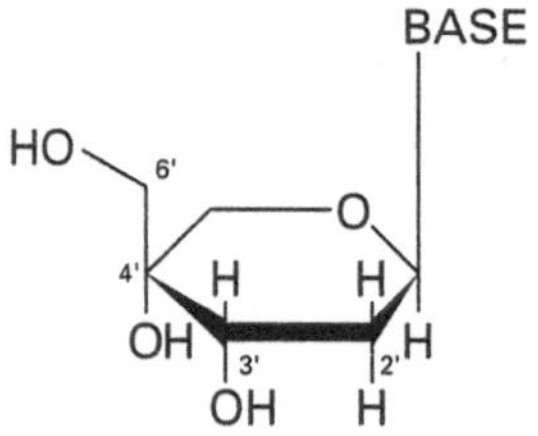

52 Nord et al.,
2'-ribohexopyranosides
(Base = adenine, hypoxanthine,
guanine, cytosine, uracil)

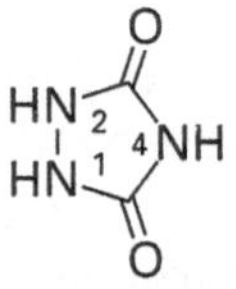

53 Urazole, an
alternative nucleobase

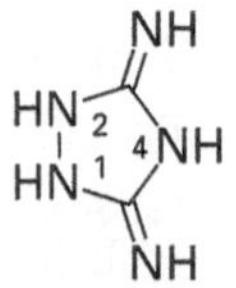

54 Guanazole, an
alternative nucleobase
(other tautomers are possible)

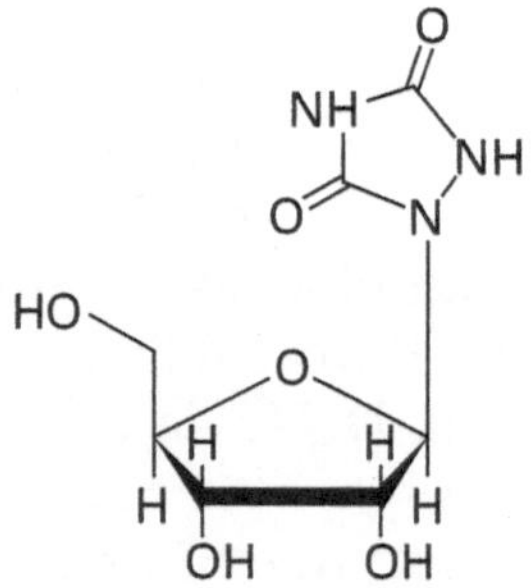

55 Kolb et al., urazole D-riboside
(only beta-f isomer is shown)

Fig. 6
Nucleosides containing different sugars or sugars in the pyranose form.

56 Pseudouridine

57 Robinson et al.,
urazole alpha-p-deoxyriboside

58 Kolb et al., pyrazolidine-dione
alpha-p-deoxyriboside

59 Herdewijn et al.,
hexopyranosyl-like nucleoside,
which is the constituent
of a potential antisense drug

Fig. 6 continued

only two pyranosides in this study demonstrated antiviral activity – the guanosine analog and the UMP uridine analog. The latter also exhibited antileukemic activity. These activities were moderate.

In terms of the search for the magic bullet antiviral nucleosides, the above described moderate antiviral activities of pyranosyl nucleosides were disappointing. This was not entirely unexpected, since the nucleosides which are part of the genetic system are exclusively furanosyl nucleosides (e.g. [2, 3]). Also, the inspection of the biosynthetic paths to nucleosides, both de novo and salvage pathways, reveals that all the intermediates contain furanosyl carbohydrate moieties (e.g. [2, 3, 57, 58]). One needs more insight into the pyranosyl nucleoside structures/behavior to be able to design them to act as substitutes for the furanosyl structures.

3.4.2   Some recent studies including those inspired by the primordial chemistry

Very recent basic chemical research addressed issues of pyranosyl nucleosides [59–61] and pyranosyl nucleic acids [62–68] from a prebiotic point of view. These findings shed light on the properties of pyranosyl systems, which subsequently stimulated further drug research based on such structures. We summarize the main findings below.

There are two different approaches to the chemical evolution of pyranosides. One is bottom-to-top, bases to nucleosides (Kolb's research group), and the other one is top-to-bottom, starting from nucleic acids (Eschenmoser and co-workers). The first approach is to question how were the nucleosides made prebiotically. The second approach is to question why are pentose nucleic acids represented in present-day genetic systems, and not, for example, hexose ones.

Since prebiotic nucleoside synthesis by direct coupling of nucleobases with sugars has been found to be poor [69, 70], Kolb et al. proposed that alternative bases, which could couple with sugars readily, were constituents of prebiotic nucleosides. Kolb stumbled upon urazole (compound 53, Fig. 6) during her unrelated research on carbazones' spectroscopic properties. She was intrigued by the urazole molecule since it had hydrogen-bonding moiety similar to that of uracil. She found that urazole reacts readily with ribose in the aqueous solution. The work was completed with Miller's research group, which added guanazole (compound 54, Fig. 6) to the menu of alternative nucleo-bases [59]. Urazole gives a mixture of four isomeric nucleosides when reacted with ribose in the aqueous solution, alpha and beta furanosides (f) and alpha and beta pyranosides (p) (structure 55, Fig. 6) [59]. The beta-p is the major form. The four isomers are isomerizable, and equilibrate in solution at room temperature to give a mixture of 78%

beta-p, 8% alpha-p, 9% beta-f, and 5% alpha-f. It is interesting that Witkowski and Robins made urazole beta-furanoriboside (via a standard coupling of protected activated sugar with a protected urazole) as a potential drug [71]. Their reasoning was that this compound would mimic natural nucleoside showdomycin, which specifically inhibits uridine MP-kinase and phosphorylase (compound 19, Fig. 2) and pseudouridine, a minor component of various t-RNA's (compound 56, Fig. 6). They have not reported the isomerization of beta-f-urazole riboside. Biological activity of this coupound was not reported, which suggests that it was inactive. A possible explanation for this presumed inactivity is that during the testing the urazole beta-f-riboside equilibrated with the more stable p-form. The latter would not be expected to be active based on a showdomycin resemblance model. It is interesting that urazole nucleosides are isomerizable similar to pseudouridine [72, 73]. (More about isomerizable nucleosides on examples of "homo-urazole" and "homo-iso-urazole" systems will be presented in Section 3.7).

We have found that urazole reacts also with 2-deoxyribose, again to give all four isomers, but this time the main product was alpha-pyranoside [60]. The alpha structure was proven by the X-ray method both for the product of the reaction with urazole [74] and its 4-carbon analog (4, 4-dimethylpyrazolidine-3, 5-dione) [75]. Interestingly, both urazole and its 4-carbon analog's moieties within the crystalline alpha 2-deoxyribonucleosides were optically active, having 1R, 2R stereochemistry on the hydrazide nitrogens, despite the fact that the starting urazoles are racemic (compounds 57, 58, Fig. 6). Further studies are needed to determine if this stereochemical feature will translate itself into a distinctive biological activity. Guanazole's reactions with ribose [59] and 2-deoxyribose [61] in the aqueous solution have many similarities with those of urazole, but with a difference that a double sugar substitution may occur under certain reaction conditions, and that additional positional isomers are possible [61]. Guanazole itself exhibits antitumor activity [76, 77]. Its nucleosides are promising also as components of potential antigene drugs [61]. Such drugs are oligonucleotides which are capable of making specific triplexes (triple-stranded structures) with double-stranded DNA, thus controlling the gene expression [78]. Guanazole nucleosides resemble pseudocytidine (C*) which allows formation of the triplex when part of a C*GC triad [78].

In the first part of a series of seven papers entitled "Why Pentose- and not Hexose- Nucleic Acids" [67] Eschenmoser and Dobler give the philosophical set of principles for this study. They state that there are two criteria for rationalizing the structure of a biomolecule. The first is the well-known structure-activity relationship (SAR). The second one is the structure's potential for self-assembly, which includes chemical potential for its preformation and selection to become a biomolecule. To rationalize the structure of DNA, the authors set a goal to design, synthesize and study some structural alternatives to DNA which might have become biomolecules on the basis of the above two criteria, but which are not present in nature. One way of looking at this goal is that a study of the unnatural has been undertaken to learn about the natural. Before we discuss the actual findings of Eschenmoser et al. on hexose-DNA (homo-DNA) [64–67] and a related system, pyranosyl-RNA (p-RNA) [62, 63, 68], let us discuss the philosophical principles first, and see how they can be related to drug design.

From the chemical evolution point of view, another chemical world might have preceded our current one, which was populated with chemically feasible structures such as our urazole nucleosides (vide supra) or Eschenmoser's p-RNA (vide infra). Such structures probably existed, but were replaced in the evolution process by more fit structures in a genetic takeover process, similar to the one described in [79]. However, there may be sufficient similarities between the unnatural potential primordial nucleosides and pre-RNA's and DNA's, that some of such compounds may become useful drugs. They could be similar enough to the present day genetic system to interact with it at various levels of its assembly and/or function, and yet sufficiently different to interfere with or abort various of its crucial functions. Along the lines "unnatural as a potential drug" we recommend a wonderful chapter by Roald Hoffmann titled "Natural/Unnatural, Just a Little Bit Unnatural" in a new and conceptually different book "Organic Reactions, Simplicity and Logic", by Pierre Laszlo [80].

A complete analysis of work by Eschenmoser et al. on pyranosyl DNA's and RNA's is beyond the scope of this review. We just show some salient points which emerged from their studies. Qualitative conformational analysis of 2', 3'-dideoxyglucopyranosyl oligonucleotides ("homo-DNA's") shows that their strands are linear [67]. In addition, a comparative analysis reveals that the backbones of normal DNA single strands are predisposed to give helical DNA duplexes because of the 5-membered ring structure of the sugar [67]. The actual homo-DNA's were synthesized [66], and their pairing properties examined [65]. Among numerous interesting findings we select again the formation of linear structures which have been found to give linear duplexes. Such duplexes were thermodynamically more stable than the helical DNA duplexes [65]. The formation of linear duplexes of homo-DNA was also confirmed and further studied via NMR [64]. To come closer to the natural systems, Eschenmoser and co-workers synthesized and studied hydroxylated pyranosyl systems (rather than the 2', 3'-deoxy ones, discussed above). These systems are now well known as pyranosyl-RNA, or p-RNA's [62, 63]. (These structures should not be confused with PNA's, which stand for peptide nucleic acids, which are RNA analogs which have an amide linkage in their backbone; these structures will be mentioned later). The p-RNA's also form very strong linear duplexes, and show Watson-Crick pairing between the bases.

Sanghvi and Cook evaluate Eschenmoser et al.'s work from the point of view of use of hexose-modified oligonucleotides as potential antisense drugs [81]. Oligonucleotides that interact with single-stranded RNA have been given the name antisense oligonucleotides. They are designed to bind the mRNA sequence, and thus disrupt the mRNA function or expression. Chemically, they should be stable toward nuclease degradation [78]. Herdewijn et al. commented that since Eschenmoser's homo-DNA and p-RNA do not show base pairing with natural DNA, their predicted therapeutic value would be low [82–84]. However, the principle demonstrated by Eschenmoser that the Watson-Crick rules are not only a consequence of the chemical properites of the four bases but also of the furanose structure of the DNA backbone, was used by Herdewijn et al. to design novel hexopyranosyl-like nucleosides as potential antisense drugs [82–84]. These authors also stressed the importance of the principle that pyranosyl oligonucleotides should have a free energy advantage over the flexible furanosyl oligomers during hybridization. A series of pyranose nucleosides having all four native heterocyclic bases have been prepared. Preliminary results are encouraging. For example, oligonucleotides constructed from the hexopyranosyl nucleosides such as 1, 5-anhydro-2, 3-dideoxy-2(thymin-1-yl)-D-arabinohexitol (structure 59, Fig. 6) are able to hybridize with natural DNA [82]. Also, oligonucleotides built from another hexopyranosyl nucleoside, 2'3'-dideoxy-3'-C-hydroxymethyl-alpha-threo-pentopyranosyl adenine, form duplexes with oligothymidylate [83].

Several of the designs in this subsection, as well as some in the next ones, have been motivated by the search for novel antisense drugs. The subject of general design of such drugs has been reviewed extensively (e.g. [81, 85], and, for most part, is beyond the scope of this review. Since our topic is nucleosides, we limit ourselves to novel designs in regard to the nucleoside constructs as components of antisense drugs. Since we exclude a major set of designs, let us give some information on those for the sake of completeness. In these designs the novelty is in the modification of phosphodiester groups in nucleotides, as phosphorothioates, or their substitution by e.g. methyleneimino, guanidine, or peptide linkages (the latter give PNA's, or peptide nucleic acids) and others [81, 85–87]. We refer the interested reader to the recent review by Sanghvi and Cook who list 58 different linkages, which include amides, carbamates, sulfides, sulfones, silyl, and other constructs [81]. New results are being published literally as this chapter is written. For example, fully nonionic oligomers of RNA, which are based on the sulfone backbone, are reported by Benner's group [88]. (The nonionic antisense designs, including sulfone backbones, have been previously described by Maddry et al. [87].) Prebiotic implications of 2',5'-linked DNA (iso-DNA) [89], in addition to its antisense potential [89, 90] have been reported. Iso-DNA does not bind normal DNA, but recognizes RNA. The 2', 5'-antisense oligonucleotides have been described also by Torrence et al. [91].

3.5   Alpha nucleosides and nucleosides possessing L vs. D sugars, and related systems

Surprisingly, many unnatural, L, nucleosides possess antiviral (or other) activity in their alpha and/or beta, furano-and/or pyrano forms. We list below some recent examples.

There are several recent patents in this area. Some dideoxyribofuranosyl nucleosides having L-configuration showed activity against Hepatitis-B virus (HBV) [92]. A compound from this class, 2'3'-dideoxy-beta-L-ribofuranosyl-5-fluorocytosine was shown to be a potent anti-HIV agent with low toxicity to host cell [92]. Beta-L-pyrimidine and beta-L-purine nucleosides as agents against AIDS [93] and HBV viruses are described [93, 94]. Examples include dideoxy systems with 3'-fluoro and 5-chloro- or 5-methyl cytidine moieties. L-Ribofuranosyl nucleosides, alpha and beta, have been described as antitumor and antiviral agents [95]. L-Ribopyranosyl, alpha and beta, nucleosides were described as useful against viral and other agents, as well as against tumors [96]. L-Nucleosides have been reported as active also against Epstein-Barr virus [97].

In addition to patents, numerous papers also appeared on this subject. Rather than singling out particular structure(s) as novel and unusual, we feel that this whole class of nucleosides is novel and unusual. We are giving here some useful and interesting references as a guide to the reader. These include works by Young et al. on both enantiomeric series of 2',3'-dideoxy and other 4'-thionucleosides [98], by Gosselin et al. on 2',3'-dideoxy-beta-L-pentofuranosyl nucleosides [99], and by Lin et al. on purine [100] and pyrimidine [101] 2'3'-dideoxy-L-nucleoside analogs. All of these compounds were active as antivirals against a variety of viruses. Nair and Jahnke reviewed the topic of isomeric dideoxynucleosides having D- and L-stereochemistry and concluded that some structure-activity relationships are emerging from this new work [102]. They pointed out that the compounds which exhibited potent antiviral activities may belong to either D or L families. They felt that a new chapter has been opened in the field of antiviral nucleosides. Spadari et al. reviewed the molecular basis for the antiviral activity of unnatural L-beta-nucleosides [103]. They pointed out exceptions to the universal rule that enzymes act only on one enantiomer of a chiral substrate, and that only one enantiomer may effectively bind to the catalytic site and display biological activity. Among exceptions listed are cellular enzymes deoxycytidine kinase, deoxynucleoside mono- and diphosphate kinase, some DNA polymerases, and viral enzymes herpes virus thymidine kinases, some viral DNA polymerases, and HIV-1 reverse transcriptase. These enzymes have the ability to utilize unnatural L-beta-nucleosides or nucleotides as substrates. These properties obviously may be exploited in drug design.

Another review appeared by Furman et al. [104], on the effect of absolute configuration on the anti-HIV and anti-HBV activity of nucleoside analogs. Again, it was pointed out that the activity is associated primarily with one of the two enantiomers, 1-beta-D or 1-beta-L. The more potent activity is not necessarily displayed by the natural 1-beta-D-configuration. The differences in activity were analyzed in terms of the differential metabolism of the isomers and their differential inhibition of the target enzymes.

An interesting therapeutical application of L-nucleosides is their use in combination with clinically approved anti-HIV nucleoside drugs [105]. For example, L-(2', 3'-dideoxy) drugs having 3'-thiacytidine, 5-fluorocytidine, or 5-fluoro-3'-thiacytidine moieties, when given in combination with AZT synergistically inhibited replication of HIV (*in vitro*).

Structure-activity relationship (SAR) has been reported for 150 analogs of uridine, in which both uracil and sugar moieties have been modified, in respect to their binding to uridine phosphorylase from Toxoplasma gondii [106]. The latter parasite is responsible for congenital toxoplasmosis and for toxoplasmic encephalitis in immunocompromised individuals. The parasite replicates rapidly and requires large amounts of pyrimidines. The salvage pathways for the latter synthesis differ from those in the mammalian host, and depend on a single nonspecific uridine phosphorylase. This enzyme is a target for inhibition by drugs or by blockage with inadequate substrates. For this reason, the knowledge of SAR is of the utmost importance. The effect of the alpha and beta anomers, the L- and D-enantiomers, the restricted syn- and anti-rotamers, ribosyl, arabinosyl, xylosyl, lyxosyl, deoxy, or anhydro moieties in various positions, and other were examined. The results of the SAR are beyond the scope of this subsection, other than for the alpha and beta anomers and D- and L-enantiomers. In terms of the anomers, the general conclusion is that this parasite's enzyme is more tolerant to anomeric modifications than the host (mammalian) enzyme, since the latter does not bind some alpha anomers. For D- and L-series, it was found that the best binding is not necessarily associated with the natural isomer.

The L- structure and L/D chimeric constructs have been exploited for the antisense drug design. This has been reviewed by Sanghvi and Cook [81]. The alpha anomeric oligodeoxyribonucleotides ("alpha-DNA") and their alpha phosphorothioate analogs are anti-HIV agents [107]. The alpha anomeric oligoribonucleotides ("alpha-RNA") have also been synthesized and were found to have promising biological properties [108].

3.6   Carbocyclic nucleosides

The original idea behind the synthesis of carbocyclic nucleosides was to replace hydrolytically and enzymatically unstable aminal (acetal-like) bond between the base and the sugar with a more stable C–C bond. This was accomplished initially by substituting the furanose oxygen with carbon. Interestingly, some such synthetic analogs were later discovered in nature (e.g. aristeromycin, compound 14, Fig. 2).

A review or carbocyclic nucleosides by Marquez with 329 references [109] just appeared. This author states that "creativity, be it from nature or from the minds of synthetic organic chemists, has no limits", and illustrates this by giving examples of carbocyclic nucleosides with excellent activities. They include compounds 60–65 in Fig. 7. The synthetic cytosine analog of neplanocin A (compound 29, Fig. 3), cyclopentenyl cytosine or CPE-C (compound 60), is in phase I clinical trials as an antitumor and antiviral agent. Carbovir (compound 61), a potent and specific antiretroviral agent, has the double bond in the cyclopentyl ring shifted to a different position, relative to the neplanocins. Carbocyclic oxetanocins, such as the guanine analog carba-oxetanocin C (compound 62) show superb antiherpetic activity. Compounds 63 and 64, (+) and (–) iso-ddA, respectively, are novel retroviral agents. The new transposed isonucleoside BMS-181, 164 (compound 65), is an antiherpetic agent. The review by Marquez contains sections of purine and pyrimidine carba-nucleosides, fluorinated-, 5'-nor-, cyclopentene-containing carba-nucleosides, carba- oxetanocins and their ring-contracted or expanded versions, carba-nucleosides modified with a heteroatom, conformationally constrained, and phosphate-mimics. The structure-activity aspect is emphasized throughout the review.

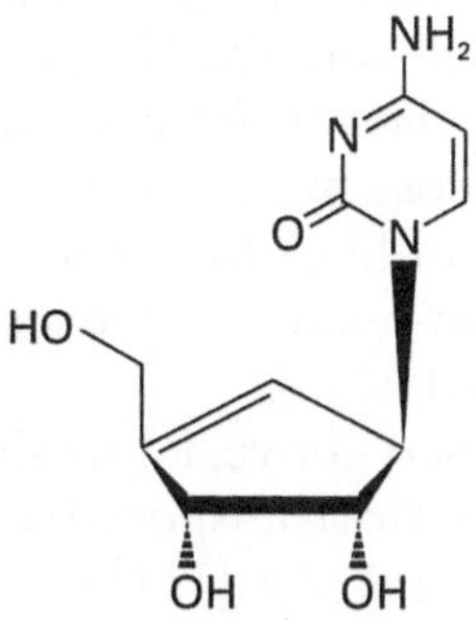

60 CPE-C

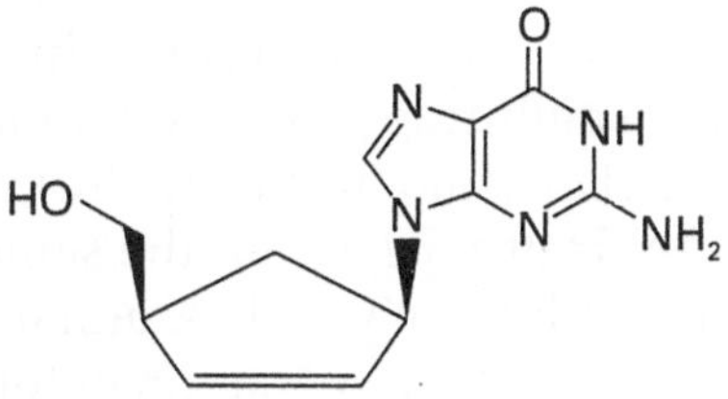

61 Carbovir

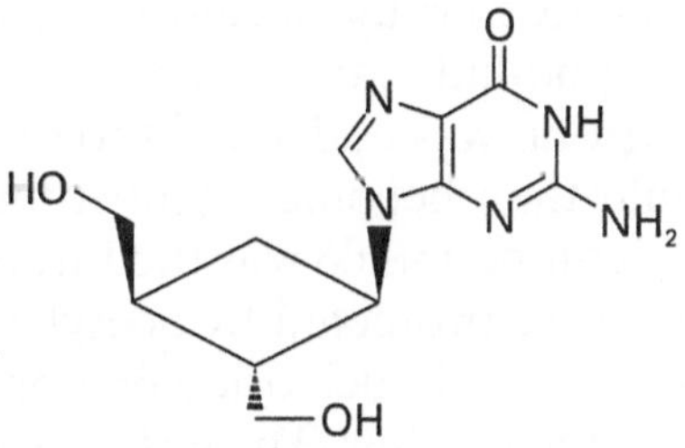

62 Carba-oxetanocin G

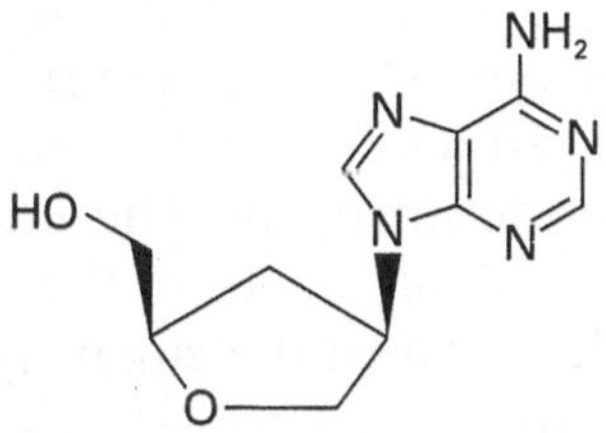

63 (+)-iso-ddA

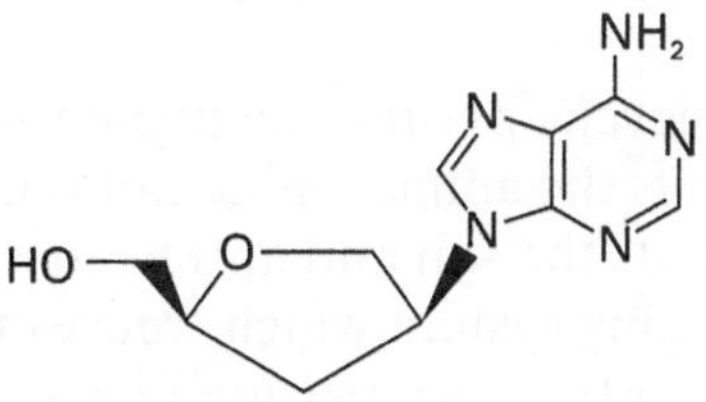

64 (−)-iso-ddA

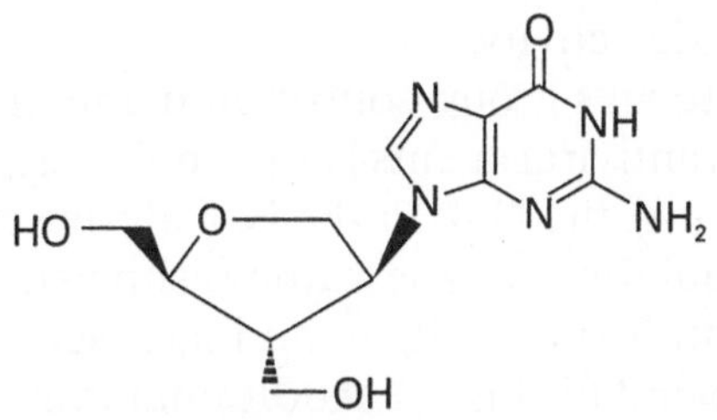

65 BMS-181,164

Fig. 7
Structures of some active carbocyclic nucleosides.

One cannot help but marvel at nature's synthetic ability when one inspects the biosynthetic pathways to carbocyclic nucleosides, published in a recent review by Jenkins and Turner [110]. For example, the carbocyclic ring of neplanocin A and aristeromycin is made from glucose by joining C-2 and C-6, in a multistep process (shikimate-like or inositol-like), to give a cyclopentenyl intermediate (1-hydroxymethyl-cyclopent-1-ene-3,4,5-triol; the 3,4,5-OH groups are on the same face of the ring).

In line with the natural vs. unnatural topic discussed above, let us single out creative work by Nair on natural and regioisomeric (transposed) dideoxynucleosides, which yielded numerous active drugs (e.g. [111]).

3.7   Miscellaneous examples of nucleosides having an unusual base, nucleosides as probes, and nucleosides as overall unusual constructs

Krausz's group investigated new non-aromatic triazinic nucleosides (compounds 66 and 67, Fig. 8) [112]. These compounds can be considered as "homo" urazoles, in which a methylene group was added next to one of the hydrazide nitrogens. The latter would then become a (substituted) hydrazine. The precursor of the furanose compound 66 was the furanose nucleoside in which the sugar hydroxyls were protected by acetylation. Upon deprotection with NH3/MeOH the desired nucleoside 66 was not obtained; instead, its pyranoside form was the product. The latter proved stable in solution. Here we see another example of furanoside to pyranoside isomerization, similar to the one discussed previously for urazole beta-furanoside. Very interestingly, the isomer of 66, compound 67, in which the sugar is attached to the hydrazide rather than the hydrazine nitrogen, did not undergo isomerization. Even more interestingly, the only active compounds in the series were actually pyranosides. They showed cytotoxic activity.

Brown's group contributed a number of bicyclic pyrimidine nucleosides as antiviral agents [113]. Their design exploits the amino-imino tautomerism at the N-4. In the N-4 alkoxy compounds the syn and anti forms are equilibrated. The authors showed that the ring system which freezes the anti form results in an increased stability in the base pairing (e.g. compound 68, Fig. 8). Additional cyclic designs were described as well as 3'-azido derivatization. Many compounds exhibited good antiviral activity against a number of viruses (except for HIV).

The first nucleoside derivative in which two ethynyl groups are present in the same molecule has been reported by Gossauer's group (structure 69, Fig. 8) [114]. The two ethynyls are at the positions 3' and 5' and replace

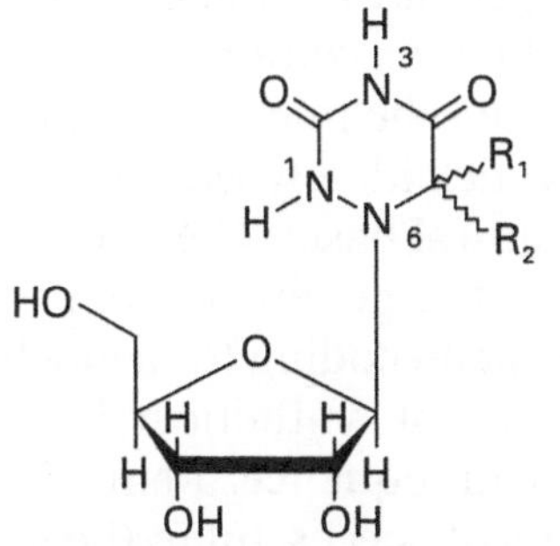

66 Isomerizable triazinic
nucleoside from Krausz's group
(R1=propyl,methyl,H; R2=H,methyl,H)

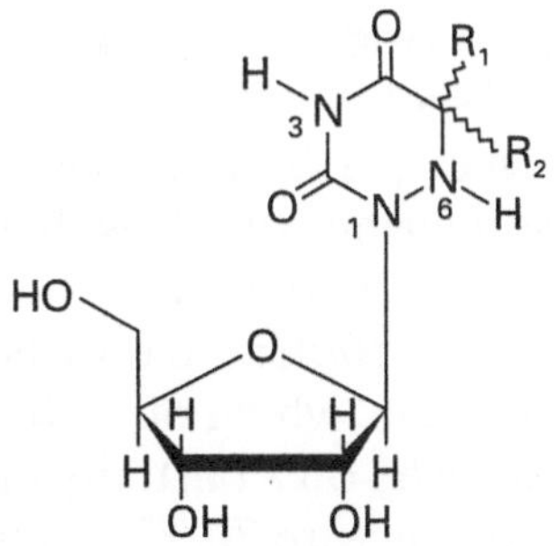

67 Non-isomerizable triazinic
isomeric nucleoside from
Krausz's group

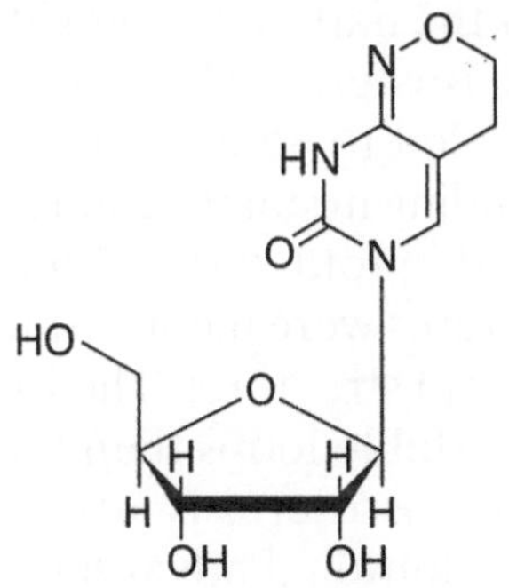

68 Bicyclic pyrimidine nucleoside
from Brown's group

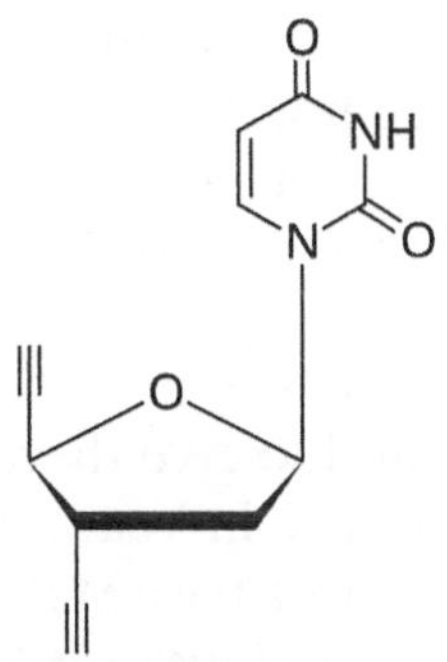

69 Gossauer et al.,
self-polymerizable nucleoside

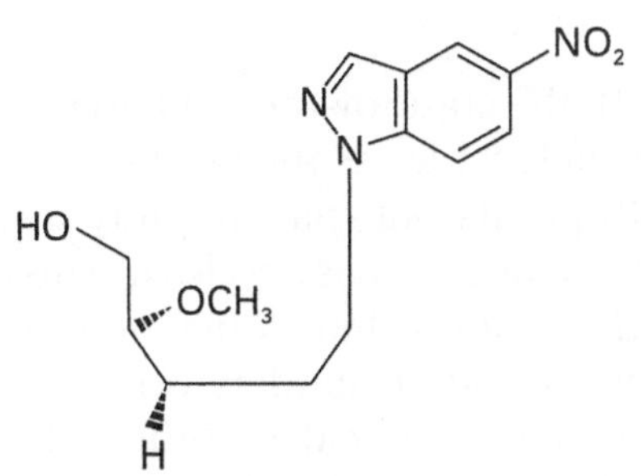

70 Van Aerschot et al.,
5-nitroindazole
as universal nucleoside

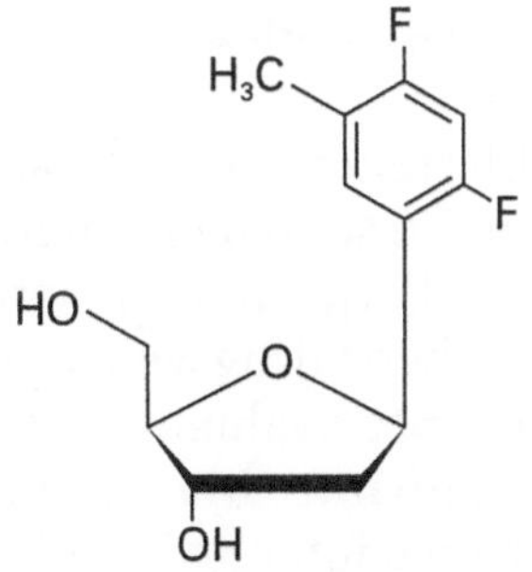

71 Non-hydrogen-bonding
nucleoside isostere
from Kool's group

Fig. 8
Examples of miscellaneous unusual nucleosides.

the substituents which are involved in the polymerization process of natural nucleosides. Preliminary results on oligomerization are promising. Van Aerschot et al. [115, 116] reported on acyclic nucleoside analogs as "universal", or "ambiguous" nucleosides, which ideally would be capable of base-pairing equally well with all four natural bases. The need for such nucleosides is related to the redundancy of the genetic code. The latter becomes a problem in efforts to isolate the gene coding for a newly identified protein, which often depends on the use of synthetic hybridization probes based on a partially known amino acid sequence. 5-Nitroindazole analog (structure 70, Fig. 8) has been the most successful in the series of compounds prepared.

Kool's research group contributed a series of non-hydrogen bonding nucleoside isosteres (e.g. structure 71, Fig. 8) [117]. These compounds were designed to act as nearly perfect isosteres for the natural nucleosides thymidine and deoxyadenosine. However, these isosteres exhibit little or no hydrogen bonding capability. They were needed to address the relative importance of base stacking and hydrogen bonding in stabilization of DNA loops. Such loops are hairpin structures found in folded RNA and DNA sequences in nature. The non-H-bonding isosteres were incorporated into DNA sequences and compared with the natural structures. The isosteres were found to give thermodynamically more stable loops than the natural loops. The increase in stabilization by these isosteres is attributed to their superior base stacking propensity. An additional advantage of the isostere-based loops is their resistance to degradation by nucleases.

4   Perspectives

Many different views exist about both the state-of-the-art and the future of antiviral research in general, and nucleosides as the antiviral agents in particular. For example, Darby [118] points out that the only truly successful antiviral drug which can be given long term is acyclovir. This author offers a sober evaluation of side-effects and other deficiencies of most present antivirals. Marquez [109], on the other hand, is very optimistic. Our personal interest in this field, which is chemical evolution of nucleosides, influences our own perspective. Our belief is that the overall progress in antiviral drug design is tied in part to the new knowledge about the biochemistry of the present and past, advanced and primitive, enzymatic pathways in both viruses and their hosts, and to the detailed understanding of the structural requirements of the substrates for these enzymes. However, a quick win in drug design may be achieved by following the route of the unusual. Surprise Mother Nature! (but expect Mother Nature to surprise you too.)

To conclude this review, let us state that there may be many differing opinions among scientists as to which nucleosides are novel and unusual. In this review we made a personal choice, and selected just a few examples of each novel design of a particular interest to us. In no way does this imply that these are the only novel and unusual nucleosides. It just reflects our choice among literally hundreds of recent references on nucleoside drugs. We regret that we could not cite works of all the fine scientists in the field. However, we sincerely hope that the readers of this review will find our examples interesting, intriguing, and inspiring.

References

1 L. A. Moran, K. G. Scrimgeour, H. R. Horton, R. S. Ochs and J. D. Rawn: Biochemistry, Second Ed., Neil Patterson Publ., Prentice Hall, Englewood Cliffs, NJ 1994; pp. 10.1–10.19, and the references cited therein.

2 A. Kornberg and T. A. Baker: DNA Replication, Second Ed., W. H. Freeman and Co., New York, 1992; a) pp. 53–97; b) pp. 439–470, and the references cited therein.

3 R. J. Suhadolnik: Nucleoside Antibiotics, Wiley-Interscience, J. Wiley and Sons, Inc., New York 1970; a review of 35 naturally occurring nucleosides.

4 R. J. Suhadolnik: Nucleosides as Biological Probes, Wiley-Interscience, J. Wiley and Sons, New York 1979; a review of 70 naturally occurring nucleosides and their nucleotide analogs; the author reviewed over 4,000 publications.

5 J. Goodchild: The Biochemistry of Nucleoside Antibiotics, in Topics in Antibiotic Chemistry, Vol. 6, P. G. Sammes, Ed., J. Wiley and Sons, New York 1982, pp. 101–227; a review of 620 references.

6 J. G. Buchanan and R. H. Wightman: The Chemistry of Nucleoside Antibiotics, in: Topics in Antibiotic Chemistry, Vol. 6, P. G. Sammes, Ed., J. Wiley and Sons, New York 1982, pp. 231–339; a review of 384 references.

7 R. Dolin: Science 227, 1296–1303 (1985), and the reference cited therein.

8 H. Mitsuya, R. Yarchoan and S. Broder: Science 249, 1533–1544 (1990), and the references cited therein.

9 H. E. Kaufman: The First Effective Antiviral, in: The Search for Antiviral Drugs, Case Histories from Concept to Clinic, J. Adams and V. J. Merluzzi, Eds., Birkhäuser Publ., Boston, Massachusetts 1993, pp 1–21.

10 M. M. Mansuri and J. C. Martin: Annual Reports in Medicinal Chemistry 22, 147–157 (1987), and the references cited therein.

11 R. K. Robins and G. R. Revankar: Design of Nucleoside Analogs as Potential Antiviral Agents, in: Antiviral Drug Development, A Multidisciplinary Approach, E. De Clercq and R.T. Walker, Eds., Plenum Press, New York 1988, pp. 11–36.

12 M. M. Mansuri and J. C. Martin: Annual Reports in Medicinal Chemistry 23, 161–170 (1988), and the references cited therein.

13 M. M. Mansuri and J. C. Martin: Annual Reports in Medicinal Chemistry 26, 133–140 (1991), and the references cited therein.

14 J. C. Barrish and R. Zahler: Annual Reports in Medicinal Chemistry *28*, 131–140 (1993), and the references cited therein.

15 K. H. Pattishall: Discovery and Development of Zidovudine as the Cornerstone of Therapy to Control Human Immunodeficiency Virus Infection, in: The Search for Antiviral Drugs, Case Histories from Concept to Clinic, J. Adams and V. J. Merluzzi, Eds., Birkhäuser Publ., Boston, Massachusetts 1993, pp. 23–43.

16 D. D. Richman: Science *272*, 1886–1888 (1996).

17 F. M. Menger and M. J. Rourk: Simultaneous Delivery of two Drugs: The Double Prodrug. Presented at the Fourth European Symposium on Controlled Drug Delivery (held in Noordwijk aan Zee, The Netherlands, April 3–5, 1996), manuscript in preparation.

18 T. A. Fadl, T. Hasegawa, A. F. Youssef, H. H. Farag, F. A. Omar and T. Kawaguchi: Die Pharmazie *50*, 382–387 (1995).

19 M. Ertan, S. Ersan, R. Ertan and C. Artuk: Acta Pharm. Turcica *30*, 185–195 (1988).

20 R. S. McElhinney, J. E. McCormick, M.C. Bibby, J. A. Double, M. Radacic and P. Dumont: J. Med. Chem. *39*, 1403–1412 (1996).

21 M. C. Bibby, J. A. Double, J.E. McCormick, R. S. McElhinney, M. Radacic, G. Pratesi and P. Dumont: Anti-Cancer Drug Design *8*, 115–128 (1993).

22 R. S. McElhinney, J. E. McCormick, M. C. Bibby, J. A. Double, G. Atassi, P. Dumont, G. Pratesi and M. Radacic: Anti-Cancer Drug Design *4*, 191–207 (1989).

23 N. Zhou, Q. Chen and R. Zhuo: Gaofenzi Xuebao *6*, 417–422 (1987); CA 109: 122075.

24 Y. Ohya, H. Kobayashi and T. Ouchi: Reactive Polymers *15*, 153–163 (1991).

25 A. Domling, M. Starnecker and I. Ugi: Angew. Chem. Int. Ed. English *34*, 2238–2239 (1995).

26 M. I. Balagopala, A. P. Ollapally and H. J. Lee: Cell. Mol. Biol. *41* (Suppl. 1), S1–S7 (1995).

27 M. Wasner, R. J. Suhadolnik, S. E. Horvath, M. E. Adelson, N. Kon, M-X, Guan, E. E. Henderson and W. Pfleiderer: Helv. Chim. Acta *79*, 609–618 (1996).

28 H. Brachwitz, P. Langen, I. Fichtner, W. E. Berdel , M. Baeseler, U. Lachmann, K. Dressler and Y. Thomas: German Patent, No. 4,400,310, July 13, 1995.

29 S. Shuto, H. Itoh, A. Sakai, K. Nakagami, S. Imamura and A. Matsuda: Bioorg. Med. Chem. *3*, 235–243 (1995).

30 C. Piantadosi, C. J. Marasco, Jr. and L. S. Kucera: US Patent 5,512,671, April 30, 1996.

31 M. Manoharan, K. L. Tivel and P. D. Cook: Tetrahedron Lett. *36*, 3651–3654 (1995).

32 H. Ford, Jr., M. Siddiqui, J. S. Driscoll, V. E. Marquez, J. A. Kelley, H. Mitsuya and T. Shirasaka: J. Med. Chem. *38*, 1189–1195 (1995).

33 J. S. Driscoll, M. A. Siddiqui, H. Ford, Jr., J. A. Kelley, J. S. Roth, H. Mitsuya, M. Tanaka and V. E. Marquez: J. Med. Chem. *39*, 1619–1625 (1996).

34 C. Desseaux, C. Gouyette, Y. Henin and T. Huynh-Dinh: Tetrahedron *51*, 6739–6756 (1995).

35 N. Mourier, C. Trabaud, J. C. Graciet, V. Simon, V. Niddam, P. Faury, A. S. Charvet, M. Camplo, J.-C. Chermann and J. L. Kraus: Nucleosides Nucleotides *14*, 1393–1402 (1995), and the references cited therein.

36 N. Harada, M. Hongu, T. Kawaguchi, M. Ohohashi, K. Oda, T. Hashiyama and K. Tsujihara: Chem. Pharm. Bull. *44*, 1196–1201 (1996).

37 T. Kawaguchi, H. Sakairi, S. Kimura, T. Yamaguchi and M. Saneyoshi: Chem. Pharm. Bull. *43*, 501–504 (1995).

38 G. H. Hakimelahi, A. A. Moosavi-Mohavedi, M. M. Sadeghi, S.-C. Tsay and J. R. Hwu: J. Med. Chem. *38*, 4648–4659 (1995).

39   R. F. Schinazi, T. E. Keane and D. C. Liotta: Patent 9,614,073 (wo), May 17, 1996.
40   R. F. Schinazi, Z. J. Lesnikowski, G. Fulcrand-El Kattan and D. W. Wilson: Carbor-
      anyl Oligonucleotides for Antisense Technology and Boron Neutron Capture
      Therapy of Cancers, in: Carbohydrate Modifications in Antisense Research, Y. S.
      Sanghvi and P. D. Cook, Eds., American Chemical Society (ACS) Symposium Series
      No.580, ACS, Washington DC 1994, pp. 169–182.
41   B. F. Spielvogel, A. Sood, I. H. Hall, B. R. Shaw and J. Tomasz: US patent 5,362,732,
      Nov. 8, 1994.
42   K. J. Rajendran, B. S. Burnham, S. Y. Chen, A. Sood, B. F. Spielvogel, B. R. Shaw and
      I. H. Hall: J. Pharm. Sci. 83, 1391–1395 (1994).
43   C. Lamberth: Pharmazie 50, 768 (1995).
44   N. M. Goudgaon, A. McMillan and R. F. Schinazi: Antiviral Chem. Chemother. 3,
      263–266 (1992), and the references cited therein.
45   J. M. Yoo, H. J. Moon, B. H. Chung, B. G. Choi, J. H. Hong and M. W. Chun: Yakhak
      Hoechi 40, 46–51 (1996); CA 124: 343952.
46   G. Deleris: Met. Based Drugs 2, 143–151 (1995).
47   G. A. LePage: Purine Arabinosides, Xylosides and Lyxosides, Ch. 49 in: Handbook
      of Experimental Pharmacology (New Series), Vol. 38, Pt. 2, Springer-Verlag, New
      York 1975, pp. 426–433.
48   K. H. Scheit: Nucleotide Analogs, Synthesis and Biological Function, Wiley-Inters-
      cience, J. Wiley and Sons, New York 1980, pp. 143–153.
49   D. S. Bhakuni: Proc. Natl. Acad. Sci., India, Section B 65, 97–112 (1995).
50   H. Mashida and S. Sakata: 5-Substituted Arabinofuranosyluracil Nucleosides as Anti-
      herpesvirus Agents: From araT to BV-araU, in: Nucleosides and Nucleotides as Anti-
      tumor and Antiviral Agents, C. K. Chu and D. C. Baker, Eds., Plenum Press, New
      York 1993, pp. 245–264.
51   S. Goldin, J. Fisher, K. Kobayashi, L. Reddy, A. Knapp, L. Margolin and K. D. McCor-
      mick: Patent 9,415,622 (wo), July 21, 1994.
52   M. D. Erion, B. G. Ugarkar and A. J. Castellino: US Patent 5,506,347, April 9, 1996.
53   G. Gosselin, M-C. Bergogne, J. de Rudder, E. DeClercq and J-L. Imbach: J. Med.
      Chem. 29, 203–213 (1986).
54   S. N. Mikhailov, E. DeClercq and P. Herdewijn: Nucleosides Nucleotides 15, 1323–
      1334 (1996), and the references cited therein.
55   L. D. Nord: The Synthesis, Structure and Biochemistry of 2-Deoxy-D-ribo Hexo-
      pyranosyl Nucleosides and Nucleotides, PhD Dissertation, Brigham Young Uni-
      versity, 1985, 97 pages.
56   L. D. Nord, N. K. Dalley, P. A. McKernan and R. K. Robins: J. Med. Chem. 30, 1044–
      1054 (1987).
57   R. T. Walker and M. J. Gait: Biosynthesis of Nucleotides, in Nucleic Acids in Che-
      mistry and Biology, G. M. Blackburn and M. J. Gait, Eds., IRL Press, Oxford Uni-
      versity Press, New York 1990, pp. 135–163.
58   D. Voet and J. G. Voet: Biochemistry, J. Wiley and Sons, New York 1990, pp. 740–768.
59   V. M. Kolb, J. P. Dworkin and S. L. Miller: J. Molecular Evolution 38, 549–557 (1994).
60   V. M. Kolb and P. A. Colloton: On the Mechanism of Formation of Urazole Nucleo-
      sides: Reaction of Open-Chain and Cyclic Analogs of Urazole with D-Ribose and
      2-Deoxy-D-Ribose, in: Mission to Planet Earth, Proceedings of the Sixth Annual
      Wisconsin Space Conference, G.T. Moore and S.D. Brandt, Eds., Wisconsin Space
      Grant Consortium, Univ. of Wisconsin-Milwaukee, Milwaukee, WI 1997.
61   V. M. Kolb and P. A. Colloton: Chemical Evaluation of Guanazole Ribosides and

2-Deoxyribosides as Primordial Nucleosides and Potential Drugs, manuscript in prep.

62 A. Eschenmoser: Toward a Chemical Etiology of the Natural Nucleic Acids' Structure, Ch. 14 in: Proceedings of the Robert A. Welch Foundation, 37th Conference on Chemical Research, 40 Years of the DNA Double Helix, Houston, Texas, 1994, pp. 201–235.

63 S. Pitsch, S. Wendeborn, B. Jaun and A. Eschenmoser: Helv. Chim. Acta 76, 2161–2183 (1993).

64 G. Otting, M. Billeter, K. Wüthrich, H-J. Roth, C. Leumann and A. Eschenmoser: Helv. Chim. Acta 76, 2701–2756 (1993).

65 J. Hunziker, H-J. Roth, M. Böhringer, A. Giger, U. Diederichsen, M. Göbel, R. Krishnan, B. Jaun, C. Leumann and A. Eschenmoser: Helv. Chim. Acta 76, 259–352 (1993).

66 M. Böhringer, H-J. Roth, J. Hunziker, M. Göbel, R. Krishnan, A. Giger, B. Schweizer, J. Schreiber, C. Leumann and A. Eschenmoser: Helv. Chim. Acta 75, 1416–1477 (1992).

67 A. Eschenmoser and M. Dobler: Helv. Chim. Acta 75, 218–259 (1992).

68 A. Eschenmoser: Pyranosyl-RNA, Natl. Meeting of Amer. Chem. Soc., Orlando, Florida, August 25–29, 1996, Abstract BIOL-095.

69 W. D. Fuller, R. A. Sanchez and L. E. Orgel: J. Mol. Biol. 67, 25–33 (1972).

70 W. D. Fuller, R. A. Sanchez and L. E. Orgel: J. Molecular Evolution 1, 249–257 (1972).

71 J. T. Witkowski and R. K. Robins: J. Org. Chem. 35, 2635–2641 (1970).

72 W. E. Cohn: J. Biol. Chem. 235, 1488–1498 (1960).

73 R. W. Chambers: The Chemistry of Pseudouridine, Progr. Nucleic Acid Res. Mol. Biol. 5, 349–398 (1966).

74 P. D. Robinson, C. Y. Meyers, V. M. Kolb and P. A. Colloton: Acta Cryst. C52, 1215–1218 (1996).

75 V. M. Kolb, P. A. Colloton, P. D. Robinson, H. G. Lutfi and C. Y. Meyers: Acta Cryst., C52, 1781–1784 (1996).

76 R. W. Brockman, S. Shaddix, W. R. Laster, Jr. and F. M. Schabel, Jr.: Cancer Res. 30, 2358–2368 (1970).

77 M-A. Hahn and R. H. Adamson: J. Natl. Cancer Inst. 48, 783–790 (1972).

78 P. S. Miller: Antisense/Antigene Oligonucleotides, in: Bioorganic Chemistry: Nucleic Acids, S. M. Hecht, Ed., Oxford Univ. Press, New York 1996, pp. 347–374, and the references cited therein.

79 C. Böhler, P. E. Nielsen and L. E. Orgel: Nature 376, 578–581 (1995), and the reference cited therein.

80 R. Hoffmann: Natural/Unnatural, Just a Little Bit Unnatural, in: P. Laszlo: Organic Reactions, Simplicity and Logic, J. Wiley and Sons, New York 1995, pp. 226–232.

81 Y. S. Sanghvi and P. D. Cook: Carbohydrates: Synthetic Methods and Applications in Antisense Therapeutics, An Overview, in: Carbohydrate Modifications in Antisense Research, Y. S. Sanghvi and P. D. Cook, Eds., American Chemical Society (ACS) Symposium Series No. 580, ACS, Washington, DC 1994, pp. 1–12.

82 P. Herdewijn, H. De Winter, B. Doboszewski, I. Verheggen, K. Augustyns, C. Hendrix, T. Saison-Behmoaras, C. de Ranter and A. Van Aerschot: Hexopyranosyl-Like Nucleotides, in: Carbohydrate Modifications in Antisense Research, Y. S. Sanghvi and P. D. Cook, Eds., American Chemical Society (ACS) Symposium Series No. 580, ACS, Washington, DC 1994, pp. 80–99.

83 B. Doboszewski, H. De Winter, A. Van Aerschot and P. Herdewijn: Tetrahedron 51, 12319–12336 (1995).

84   A. Van Aerschot, I. Verheggen, C. Hendrix and P. Herdewijn: Angew. Chem. Int. Edn. Engl. *34*, 1338–1339 (1995).

85   M. D. Matteucci and R. W. Wagner: In Pursuit of Antisense, Nature, Suppl. to Vol 384, Issue No. 6604, Nov. 7, 1996, pp. 20–22.

86   A. De Mesmaeker, A. Waldner, J. Lebreton, V. Frisch and R. M. Wolf: Novel Backbone Replacements for Oligonucleotides, in: Carbohydrate Modifications in Antisense Research, Y. S. Sanghvi and P. D. Cook, Eds., American Chemical Society (ACS) Symposium Series No. 580, ACS, Washington, DC 1994, pp. 24–39.

87   J. A. Maddry, R. Reynolds, J. A. Montgomery and J. A. Secrist III: Synthesis of Nonionic Oligonucleotide Analogues, in: Carbohydrate Modifications in Antisense Research, Y. S. Sanghvi and P. D. Cook, Eds., American Chemical Society (ACS) Symposium Series No. 580, ACS, Washington, DC 1994, pp. 40–51.

88   C. Richert, A. L. Roughtor and S. A. Benner: J. Amer. Chem. Soc. *118*, 4518–4531 (1996).

89   A. M. Rouhi: Natural Product's Scope Expanding, Chemical And Engineering News, Oct. 21, 1996, pp. 34–44.

90   T. L. Sheppard and R. C. Breslow: J. Amer. Chem. Soc. *118*, 9810–9811 (1996).

91   P. F. Torrence, W. Xiao, G. Li, K. Lesiak, S. Khamnei, A. Maran, R. Maitra, B. Dong and R. H. Silverman: 2',5'-Olygoadenylate Antisense Chimeras for Targeted Ablation of RNA, in: Carbohydrate Modifications in Antisense Research, Y. S. Sanghvi and P. D. Cook, Eds., American Chemical Society Symposium Series No. 580, ACS, Washington, DC 1994, pp. 118–132.

92   T-S. Lin and Y-C. Cheng: Patent 9,427,616 (wo), December 8, 1994.

93   E. Matthes, M. Von Janta-Lipinski: Patent 9,611,204 (wo), April 18, 1996.

94   E. Matthes, M. Von Janta-Lipinski: German Patent 19,518,216, April 11, 1996.

95   A. L. Weiss, C. T. Goodhue and K. Shanmuganathan: Patent 9,613,512 (wo), May 9, 1996.

96   A. L. Weiss and C. T. Goodhue: Patent 9,612,728 (wo), May 2, 1996.

97   C. K. Chu, Y-C. Cheng, B. S. Pai and G-Q. Yao: Patent 9,520,595 (wo), August 3, 1995.

98   R. J. Young, S. Shaw-Ponter, J. B. Thomson, A. J. Miller, J. G. Cumming, A. W. Pugh and P. Rider: Bioorg. Med. Chem. Lett. *5*, 2599–2604 (1995).

99   G. Gosselin, C. Mathe, M-C. Bergogne, A-M. Aubertin, A. Kirn, J-P. Sommadossi, R. Schinazi and J-L. Imbach: Nucleosides Nucleotides *14*, 611–617 (1995).

100   T-S. Lin, M-Z. Luo, J-L. Zhu, M-C. Liu, Y-L. Zhu, G. E. Dutschman and Y-C. Cheng: Nucleosides Nucleotides *14*, 1759–1783 (1995).

101   T-S. Lin, M-Z. Luo and M-C. Liu: Tetrahedron *51*, 1055–1068 (1995).

102   V. Nair and T. S. Jahnke: Antimicrob. Agents Chemother. *39*, 1017–1029 (1995).

103   S. Spadari, G. Maga, A. Verri, A. Bendiscioli, L. Tondelli, M. Capobianco, F. Colonna, A. Garbesi and F. Focher: Biochimie *77*, 861–867 (1995).

104   P. A. Furman, J. E. Wilson, J. E. Reardon and G. R. Painter: Antiviral Chem. Chemother. *6*, 345–355 (1995).

105   E. G. Bridges, G. E. Dutschman and E. A. Gullen: Biochem. Pharmacol. *51*, 731–736 (1996).

106   M. H. el Kouni, F. N. M. Naguib, R. P. Panzica, B. A. Otter, S-H. Chu, G. Gosselin, C. K. Chu, R. F. Schinazi, Y. F. Shealy, N. Goudgaon, A. A. Ozerov, T. Ueda and M. H. Ilitzsch: Biochem. Pharmacol. *51*, 1687–1700 (1996).

107   F. Morvan, B. Rayner and J-L. Imbach: Anti-Cancer Drug Design *6*, 521–529 (1991).

108   F. Debart, C. Chaix, B. Rayner and J-L. Imbach: Modified Oligoribonucleotides: Synthesis and Preliminary Evaluation of alpha-RNA, in: Nucleosides and Nucleotides

as Antitumor and Antiviral Agents, C. K. Chu and D. C. Baker, Eds., Plenum Press, New York 1993, pp. 303–310.

109   V. E. Marquez: Carbocyclic Nucleosides, Advances in Antiviral Drug Design 2, 89–146 (1996).

110   G. N. Jenkins and N. J. Turner: Chem. Soc. Rev. 24, 169–176 (1995).

111   V. Nair: Approaches to Novel Isomeric Nucleosides as Antiviral Agents, in: Nucleosides and Nucleotides as Antitumor and Antiviral Agents, C. K. Chu and D. C. Baker, Eds., Plenum Press, New York 1993, pp. 127–140, and the references cited therein.

112   J. Depelley, R. Granet, M. Kaouadji, P. Krausz, S. Piekarski, S. Delebassee and C. Bosgiraud: Nucleosides Nucleotides 15, 995–1008 (1996).

113   D. Loakes, D. M. Brown, N. Mahmood, J. Balzarini and E. De Clercq: Antiviral Chem. Chemother. 6, 371–378 (1995).

114   M. A. Amin, H. Stoeckli-Evans and A. Gossauer: Helv. Chim. Acta 78, 1879–1886 (1995).

115   A. Van Aerschot, J. Rozenski, D. Loakes, N. Pillet, G. Schepers and P. Herdewijn: Nucleic Acid Res. 23, 4363–4370 (1995).

116   A. Van Aerschot, C. Hendrix, G. Schepers, N. Pillet and P. Herdewijn: Nucleosides Nucleotides 14, 1053–1056 (1995).

117   X-F. Ren, B. A. Schweitzer, C. J. Sheils and E. T. Kool: Angew. Chem. Int. Ed. Engl. 35, 743–745 (1996).

118   G. Darby: Only 35 Years of Antiviral Nucleoside Analogues!, in: Symposia of the Society for General Microbiology, Cambridge Univ. Press, Cambridge 1995, pp. 279–297.

Index Vol. 48

The references of the Subject Index are given in the language of the respective contribution.
Die Stichworte des Sachregisters sind in der jeweiligen Sprache der einzelnen Beiträge aufgeführt.
Les termes repris dans la Table des Matières sont donnés selon la langue dans laquelle l'ouvrage est écrit.

Index of titles
Verzeichnis der Titel
Index des titres
Vol. 1–48 (1959–1997)

Author and paper index
Autoren- und Artikelindex
Index des auteurs et des articles
Vol. 1–48 (1959–1997)

Some neuropathologic and cellular aspects of leprosy 18, 53 (1974)	D. K. Dastur Y. Ramamohan A. S. Dabholkar
Autonomic dysfunction as a problem in the treatment of tetanus 19, 245 (1975)	F. D. Dastur G. J. Bhat K. G. Nair
Studies on *Vibrio parahaemolyticus* infection in Calcutta as compared to cholera infection 19, 490 (1975)	B. C. Deb
Biochemical effects of drugs acting on the central nervous system 8, 53 (1965)	L. Decsi
Some reflections on the chemotherapy of tropical diseases: Past, present and future 26, 343 (1982)	E. W. J. de Maar
Drug research – whence and whither 10, 11 (1966)	R. G. Denkewalter M. Tishler
Immunization of a village, a new approach to herd immunity 19, 252 (1975)	N. S. Deodhar
Profiles of tuberculosis in rural areas of Maharashtra 18, 91 (1974)	M. D. Deshmukh K. G. Kulkarni S. S. Virdi B. B. Yodh
The interface between drug research, marketing, management, and social political and regulatory forces 20, 181 (1976) Medicinal research: Retrospectives and perspectives 29, 97 (1985) Serendipity and structured research in drug discovery 30, 189 (1986) Medicinal chemistry: A support or a driving force in drug research? 34, 343 (1990) Heterocyclic diversity: The road to biological activity 44, 9 (1995)	G. deStevens
Hypolipidemic agents 13, 217 (1969)	G. deStevens W. L. Bencze R. Hess

Drug receptors and control of the cardiovascular system: Recent advances *36*, 117 (1991)	Robert R. Ruffolo Jr J. Paul Hieble David P. Brooks Giora Z. Feuerstein Andrew J. Nichols
Behavioral correlates of presynaptic events in the cholinergic neurotransmitter system *32*, 43 (1988)	Roger W. Russell
Epidemiology of pertussis *19*, 257 (1975)	J. A. Sa
Surgical amoebiasis *18*, 77 (1974)	A. E. de Sa
Role of beta-adrenergic blocking drug propranolol in severe tetanus *19*, 361 (1975)	G. S. Sainani K. L. Jain V. R. D. Deshpande A. B. Balsara S. A. Iyer
Studies on *Vibrio parahaemolyticus* in Bombay *19*, 586 (1975)	F. L. Saldanha A. K. Patil M. V. Sant
Leukotriene antagonists and inhibitors of leukotriene biosynthesis as potential therapeutic agents *37*, 9 (1991)	John A. Salmon Lawrence G. Garland
Pharmacology and toxicology of axoplasmic transport *28*, 53 (1984)	Fred Samson Ralph L. Smith J. Alejandro Donoso
Clinical experience with bitoscanate *19*, 96 (1975)	M. R. Samuel
Tetanus: Situational clinical trials and therapeutics *19*, 367 (1975)	R. K. M. Sanders M. L. Peacock B. Martyn B. D. Shende
Epidemiological studies on cholera in non-endemic regions with special reference to the problem of carrier state during epidemic and non-epidemic period *19*, 594 (1975)	M. V. Sant W. N. Gatlewar S. K. Bhindey
Epidemiological and biochemical studies in filariasis in four villages near Bombay *18*, 269 (1974)	M. V. Sant W. N. Gatlewar T. U. K. Menon

Hookworm anaemia and intestinal mal-absorption associated with hookworm infestation *19*, 108 (1975)	A. K. Saraya B. N. Tandon
The effects of structural alteration on the anti-inflammatory properties of hydrocortisone *5*, 11 (1963)	L. H. Sarett A. A. Patchett S. Steelman
The impact of natural product research on drug discovery *23*, 51 (1979)	L. H. Sarett
Aldose reductase inhibitors: Recent developments *40*, 99 (1993)	Reinhard Sarges Peter J. Oates
Anti-filariasis campaign: Its history and future prospects *18*, 259 (1974)	M. Sasa
Barbiturates and the $GABA_A$ receptor complex *34*, 261 (1990)	Paul A. Saunders I. K. Ho
Platelets and atherosclerosis *29*, 49 (1985)	Robert N. Saunders
Immuno-diagnosis of helminthic infections *19*, 119 (1975)	T. Sawada K. Sato K. Takei
Immuno-diagnosis in filarial infection *19*, 128 (1975)	T. Sawada K. Sato K. Takei M. M. Goil
Quantitative structure-activity relationships *23*, 199 (1979)	Anil K. Saxena S. Ram
Advances in chemotherapy of malaria *30*, 221 (1986) Developments in antihistamines (H_1) *39*, 35 (1992) Developments in anticonvulsants *44*, 185 (1995)	Anil K. Saxena Mridula Saxena
Pyrimidinones as biodynamic agents *31*, 127 (1987)	Anil K. Saxena Shradha Sinha
Phenothiazine und Azaphenothiazine als Arzneimittel *5*, 269 (1963)	E. Schenker H. Herbst

Advances in the treatment and control of tissue-dwelling helminth parasites *30*, 473 (1986) The benzimidazole anthelmitics chemistry and biological activity *27*, 85 (1983) Treatment of helminth diseases, challenges and achievements *31*, 9 (1987) Vector-borne diseases *35*, 365 (1990)	Satyavan Sharma
Chemotherapy of cestode infections *24*, 217 (1980)	Satyavan Sharma S. K. Dubey R. N. Iyer
Chemotherapy of hookworm infections *26*, 9 (1982)	Satyavan Sharma Elizabeth S. Charles
Ayurvedic medicine – past and present *15*, 11 (1971)	Shiv Sharma
Mechanisms of anthelmintic action *19*, 147 (1975)	U. K. Sheth
Aspirin as an antithrombotic agent *33*, 43 (1989)	Melvin J. Silver Giovanni Di Minno
Immunopharmacological approach to the study of chronic brain disorders *30*, 345 (1986) Implications of immunomodulant therapy in Alzheimer's disease *32*, 21 (1988)	Vijendra K. Singh H. Hugh Fudenberg
Neuroimmune axis as a basis of therapy in Alzheimer's disease *34*, 383 (1990) Immunoregulatory role of neuro-peptides *38*, 149 (1992) Neuropeptides as native immune modul-ators *45*, 9 (1995) Immunotherapy for brain diseases and mental illnesses *48*, 129 (1997)	Vijendra K. Singh
Natural products as anticancer agents *42*, 53 (1994)	Shradha Sinha Sudha Jain
Biologically active quinazolones *43*, 143 (1994)	Shradha Sinha Mukta Srivastava

Age profile of diphtheria in Bombay *19*, 412 (1975)	N. S. Tibrewala R. D. Potdar S. B. Talathi M. A. Ramnathkar A. D. Katdare
On conformation analysis, molecular graphics, fentanyl and its derivatives *30*, 91 (1986)	J. P. Tollenaere H. Moereels M. van Loon
Antibakterielle Chemotherapie der Tuberkulose *7*, 193 (1964)	F. Trendelenburg
Alternative approaches to the discovery of novel antipsychotic agents *38*, 299 (1992)	M. D. Tricklebank L. J. Bristow P. H. Hutson
Diphtheria *19*, 423 (1975)	P. M. Udani M. M. Kumbhat U. S. Bhat M. S. Nadkarni S. K. Bhave S. G. Ezuthachan B. Kamath
Biologische Oxydation und Reduktion am Stickstoff aromatischer Amino- und Nitroderivate und ihre Folgen für den Organismus *8*, 195 (1965) Stoffwechsel von Arzneimitteln als Ursache von Wirkungen, Nebenwirkungen und Toxizität *15*, 147 (1971)	H. Uehleke
Mode of death in tetanus *19*, 439 (1975)	H. Vaishnava C. Bhawal Y. P. Munjal
Comparative evaluation of amoebicidal drugs *18*, 353 (1974) Comparative efficacy of newer anthelmintics *19*, 166 (1975)	B. J. Vakil N. J. Dalal
Cephalic tetanus 19, 443 (1975)	B. J. Vakil B. S. Singhal S. S. Pandya P. F. Irami

The effect and usefulness of early intravenous beta blockade in acute myocardial infarction *30*, 71 (1986)	Anders Vedin Claes Wilhelmsson
Methods of monitoring adverse reactions to drugs *21*, 231 (1977) Aspects of social pharmacology *22*, 9 (1978)	J. Venulet
The current status of cholera toxoid research in the United States *19*, 602 (1975)	W. F. Verwey J. C. Guckian J. Craig N. Pierce J. Peterson H. Williams Jr
Systemic cancer therapy: Four decades of progress and some personal perspectives *34*, 76 (1990)	Charles L. Vogel
Cell-kinetic and pharmacokinetic aspects in the use and further development of cancerostatic drugs *20*, 521 (1976)	M. von Ardenne
The problem of diphtheria as seen in Bombay *19*, 452 (1975)	M. M. Wagle R. R. Sanzgiri Y. K. Amdekar
Drug nephrotoxicity – The significance of cellular mechanisms *41*, 51 (1993)	Robert J. Walker J. Paul Fawcett
Nicotine: An addictive substance or a therapeutic agent? *33*, 9 (1989)	David M. Warburton
Cell-wall antigens of *Vibrio cholerae* and their implication in cholera immunity *19*, 612 (1975)	Y. Watanabe R. Ganguly
Steroidogenic capacity in the adrenal cortex and its regulation *34*, 359 (1990)	Michael R. Watermann Evan R. Simpson
Antigen-specific T-cell factors and drug research *32*, 9 (1988)	David R. Webb
Where is immunology taking us? *20*, 573 (1976) Immunology in drug research *28*, 233 (1984)	W. J. Wechter Barbara E. Loughman